AORTIC VALVE SURGERY

Edited by **Noboru Motomura**

Aortic Valve Surgery
Edited by Noboru Motomura

Published by InTech
Janeza Trdine 9, 51000 Rijeka, Croatia

Publishing Process Manager Alenka Urbancic

Technical Editor Teodora Smiljanic

Cover Designer InTech Design Team

Additional hard copies can be obtained from orders@intechopen.com

Aortic Valve Surgery, Edited by Noboru Motomura
p. cm.
ISBN 978-953-307-600-3

For EU product safety concerns:
IN TECH d.o.o., Prolaz Marije Krucifikse Kozulić 3, 51000 Rijeka, Croatia,
info@intechopen.com or visit our website at intechopen.com.

Meet the editor

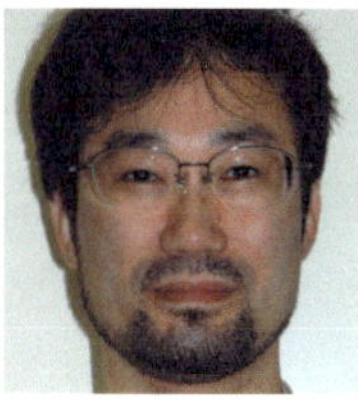

Professor Motomura is an Associate Professor at the Department of Cardiac Surgery, University of Tokyo, who graduated from Kyoto Prefectural University of Medicine in 1985. Following the training in National Cardiovascular and Research Center in Osaka, Georgetown University in Washington DC, and St. George Hospital in Sydney, he was appointed staff surgeon at the University of Tokyo.

Contents

Preface

The aortic valve is located at the center of the heart and is the core of the cardiac anatomy. In the history of cardiac surgery, the aortic valve prosthesis was the first target of the cardiac surgery, which was performed by Dr. Hufnagel at Georgetown University, Washington DC, in 1952. Since then, aortic valve surgery has led the field of cardiac surgery. Many prosthetic heart valves have been developed to replace defective valves, and numerous surgical procedures have been created to deal with the complexities of aortic valve surgery.

Aortic valve surgery has developed from a single valve replacement to more complex procedures, such as the Ross procedure or valve sparing surgery. Recently, a trans-catheter aortic valve replacement has evolved as well. All aspects regarding of the aortic valve are addressed in this book, including anatomy, physiology, preoperative examination by techniques such as echocardiography, as well as various surgical procedures, operative risk analysis especially in the senile population, and newly emerging technologies. The authors are among the most active cardiac surgeons chosen from all over the world. I believe this book will help clarify daily questions regarding the clinical practice in aortic valve surgery, as well as induce inspiration and new insights into this field.

I would like to thank all the chapter authors who sent us splendid manuscripts albeit their tight schedules. I could not have accomplished editing this book without the help and tremendous support of the staff at INTECH. Finally, I thank my family for encouraging me to proceed with this project.

Noboru Motomura, M.D., Ph.D.
Associate Professor
Department of Cardiothoracic Surgery
Director, University of Tokyo Tissue Bank (UTTB)
Department of Healthcare Quality Assessment
University of Tokyo, Faculty of Medicine
Tokyo,
Japan

Part 1

Anatomy and Preoperative Estimation

1

Intraoperative Imaging in Aortic Valve Surgery as a Safety Net

Kazumasa Orihashi
Kochi Medical School
Japan

1. Introduction

In the modern era, the morbidity and mortality of aortic valve surgeries has been markedly reduced. These improvement have been seen in: 1) aortic valve replacement or repair; 2) aortic root replacement or valve-sparing operations; 3) surgery on aortic dissections complicated by aortic regurgitation; and 4) recently introduced transcatheter aortic valve implantations. However, the goal of consistent success without complication is hampered by a number of pitfalls listed in Table 1.

While some of these complications are preventable if essential and timely information is obtained, others are rare and unpredictable. For the latter, early diagnosis and the institution of appropriate measures without delay is important in minimizing serious sequelae. For this purpose, intraoperative imaging plays an important role in recognizing the events behind the scenes. This author has exclusively applied transesophageal echocardiography (TEE) and direct echo to aortic valve surgery. The aim of this chapter is to describe the details of echo imaging in aortic valve surgery with a number of tips and case presentations.

Difficulty in implanting prosthetic valve
inadequate annular size
small sino-tubular junction
Myocardial damage
inadequate cardioplegia (antegrade and retrograde)
obstruction of coronary artery by prosthetic valve
air embolism of coronary artery
dissection in coronary artery
Aorta
calcified aorta: aortic route, clamp, aortotomy
new dissection
Dysfunction of prosthetic valve
malfunction of prosthesis
perivalvular or transvalvular leakage
Systolic anterior motion of mitral leaflet

Table 1. Pitfalls and complications in aortic valve surgery

2. Visualization of aortic valve

The aortic valve is most clearly visualized in midesophageal aortic valve long- and short-axis view through the left atrium as an acoustic window (Fig. 1a,b). Aortic regurgitation is readily assessed in the former, and every cusp and the sinus of Valsalva are visualized in the latter. Because the direction of blood flow is nearly perpendicular to the ultrasound beam in both views, Doppler measurements as an assessment of the pressure gradient in aortic stenosis cases are done in transgastric long-axis view (Fig. 1c) with minimal incident angle.

Due to the bulbar shape of the cusps and the sinus of Valsalva, visualization is limited in two-dimensional imaging of the aortic valve. 3D TEE is useful for visualizing all three cusps in a single view as well as surrounding structures such as the coronary artery and the sinus of Valsalva (Fig. 1d).

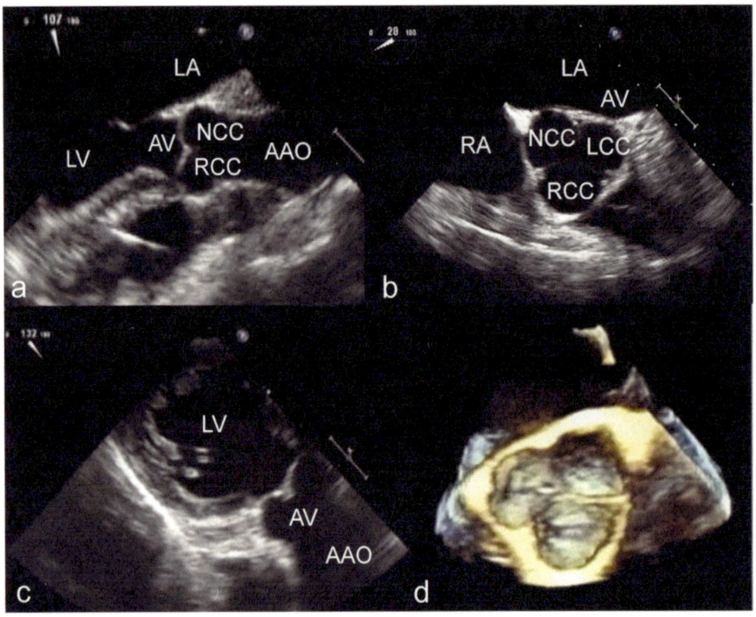

Fig. 1. Basic imaging of aortic valve. a: midesophageal aortic valve (AV) long-axis view; b: midesophageal aortic valve short-axis view; c: transgastritic long-axis view, d: 3D TEE view from the aortic side. AAO: ascending aorta, LA: left atrium, LCC: left coronary cusp, LV: left ventricle, NCC: noncoronary cusp, RCC: right coronary cusp

3. Sizing of annulus and sinotubular junction

In aortic valve replacement, the bioprosthetic valve has gained in popularity because of its long-term durability as well as its lack of dependence on anticoagulation. However, the annular size limits the use of bioprostheses in patients with small stature. Calcifications in the annulus also limit the size of the implanted valve.

In addition to preoperative transthoracic echocardiography, the annular size is measured with TEE following induction of anesthesia. In midesophageal aortic valve long-axis view, the aortic annulus is best visualized with the hinge points of the right coronary and non-coronary cusps identified as the intersection of the cusp and the sinus of Valsalva. The internal dimension of these points can then be measured (Fig. 2). In those patients with a calcified annulus, the external margin of calcium is calipered in order to assess the largest implantable valve size that would accommodate a single interrupted or non-everting mattress suture after the calcium is meticulously removed. When intraannular placement with everting mattress sutures is considered, a prosthesis one size smaller is chosen.

The internal diameter at the sinotubular junction level is important. When it is equal to or smaller than the annular dimension as in Fig. 2b, it is difficult to insert the prosthetic valve down to the annular level and a very narrow space for ligation is anticipated.

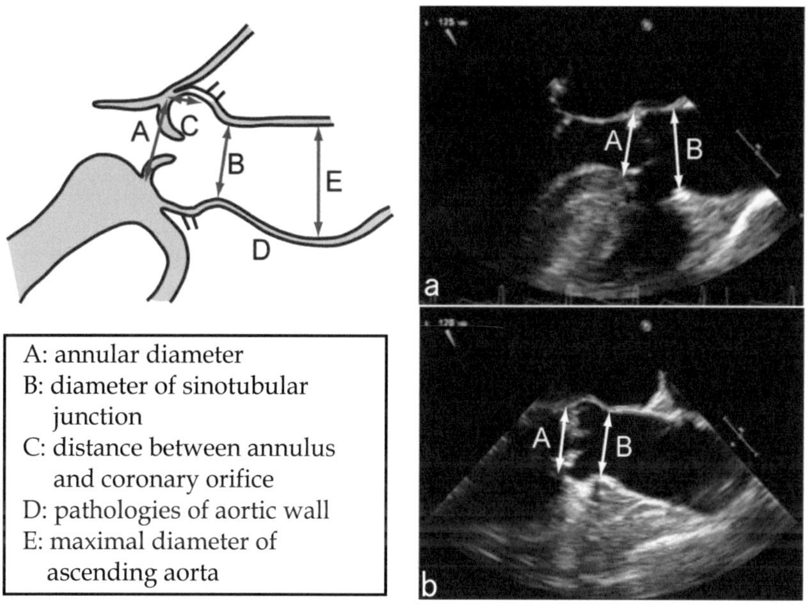

Fig. 2. Assessment of aortic valve and ascending aorta. Left: check points. a: measurement of annular dimension and sinotubular junction; b: small sinotubular junction

4. Assessment of aorta

The ascending aorta is exposed to various surgical procedures such as arterial cannulation, cross clamping, root cannula insertion and aortotomy, which is potentially responsible for intraoperative stroke and dissection. While the aorta is assessed for calcification or atheromatous changes in preoperative CT in most cases, TEE or direct echo facilitates a surgeon's ability to exactly locate these pathologies intraoperatively.

TEE assessment is beneficial in minimizing interruptions in the surgical procedure. The aorta is visualized with TEE in midesophageal ascending aorta long- or short-axis view. Although the distal portion of ascending aorta used for cannulation has been deemed to be a blind zone, this can be minimized by two tips. One is the *look-up method* (Fig. 3a,b). Instead of withdrawing the probe to visualize the distal portion, the probe is rather advanced and anteflexion is applied. Improved visualization is obtained through the left atrium and right pulmonary artery as an acoustic window. Another is the *xPlane mode* (Fig. 3c,d). In the midesophageal ascending aorta long-axis view with the probe tip anteflexed, the orthogonal scanning plane is tilted upward. Not only is the distal portion of ascending aorta seen, but the aortic arch is often visualized through the left atrium and left pulmonary artery as an acoustic window. From the upper esophageal arch long- and short-axis views, the ascending aorta can be visualized by tilting the orthogonal scanning plane downward.

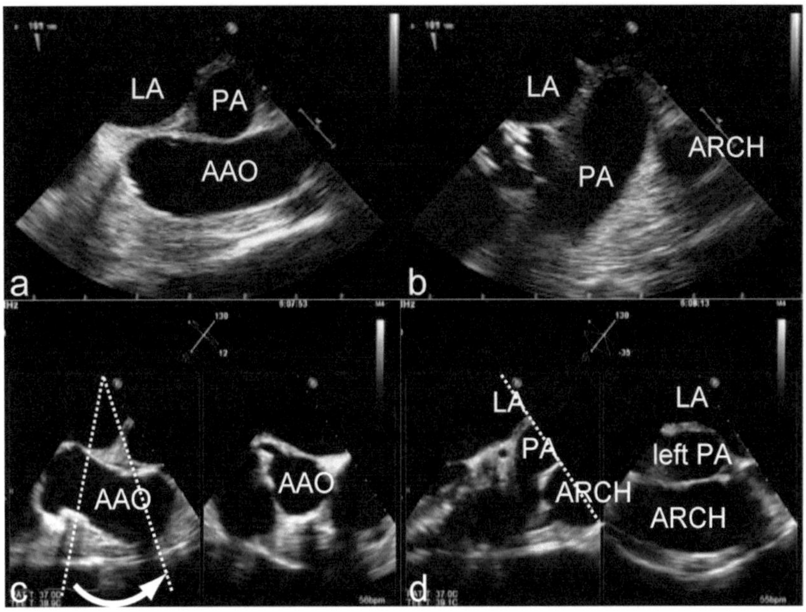

Fig. 3. Tips for visualizing the distal portion of ascending aorta (AAO). In the look-up method, the probe is rather advanced from the midesophageal ascending aorta long-axis view (a), and anteflexed. b: The arch is visualized via the left atrium (LA) and pulmonary artery (PA). In xPlane mode, the scanning plane is tilted upward (c). d: The arch is visualized through the LA and left PA

The ascending aorta is assessed for calcification and atheromatous plaque. The former is depicted as a strong echo accompanied by an acoustic shadow. When the aorta is severely calcified, it may be necessary to change the perfusion routes to the axillary artery or femoral artery. In the former, pathologies in the arch branches are checked (Orihashi, 2000). When femoral arterial perfusion is chosen, the atheromatous lesion in the descending aorta should be assessed. If the calcified aorta is clamped, it is checked for a new dissection immediately following declamping to minimize a delay in recognition and treatment.

5. Myocardial damage

Myocardial damage following aortic valve surgery can be permanent and is caused by several mechanisms. Even if the left ventricular function is transiently depressed by these mechanisms, it considerably prolongs the pump time and leads to sustained heart failure in the postoperative period. Prevention is important in avoiding these complications and can be done so through efficient and timely use of intraoperative imaging.

5.1 Visualization of the coronary arteries

Unfavorable events related to aortic valve surgeries mainly take place in the ostium and/or the proximal portion of the coronary arteries, which can be visualized with TEE.

The ostium of the right coronary artery is found in the right coronary sinus (Fig. 4a,b). Although only a few centimeters of right coronary artery can be visualized due to the large distance from the transducer, the posterior descending artery can be visualized in the posterior interventricular groove in the transgastric mid-short-axis view.

The left coronary ostium is visualized in the left sinus of Valsalva by rotating the TEE probe counterclockwise from the midesophageal aortic valve short- or long-axis view (Fig. 4c,d).

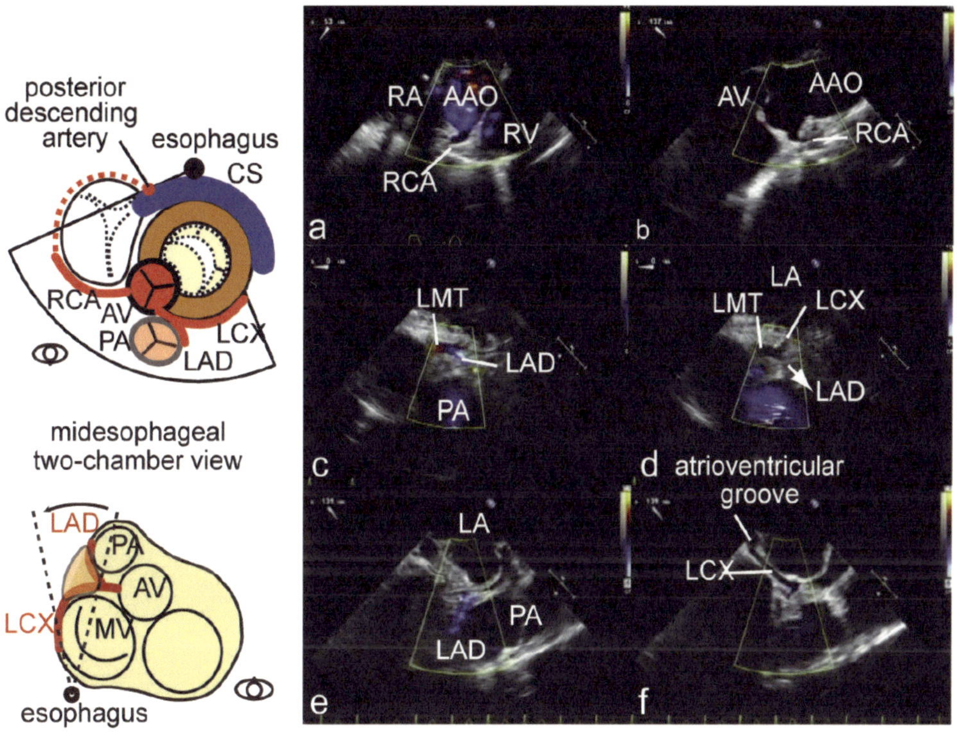

Fig. 4. Visualization of coronary arteries. Left top: diagram showing visualization of coronary arteries. The right coronary artery (RCA) is depicted in midesophageal ascending aorta (AAO) short- and long-axis view (a,b). c,d: The left main truncus (LMT) to the division to left anterior descending (LAD) and left circumflex arteries (LCX) is shown. Left bottom: method of visualizing the distal portion of LCX. e: LAD flow, f: LCX in the atrioventricular groove. AV: aortic valve, CS: coronary sinus, PA: pulmonary artery, RA: right atrium, RV: right ventricle

Further rotation visualizes the division of the left main truncus to left anterior descending artery and left circumflex artery. A few centimeters of left anterior descending artery is often visualized. The distal portion of the left circumflex artery is visualized in the left posterior atrioventricular groove in the 90° to 120° scanning plane (Fig. 4e,f) (Ender et al., 2010; Karthik et al., 2007).

3D TEE provides unique information of the coronary ostium (Fig. 5). This perspective view is helpful for recognizing the distance of the coronary orifice from the annulus.

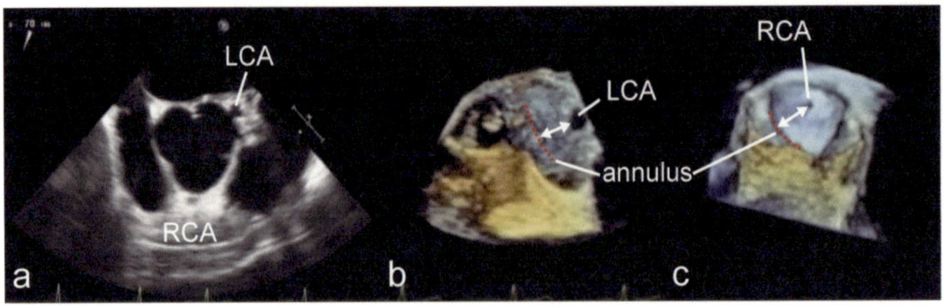

Fig. 5. 3D images of coronary ostia. a: Right and left coronary arteries (RCA, LCA) in midesophageal aortic valve short-axis view, b: 3D image of left coronary ostium, c: 3D image of right coronary ostium

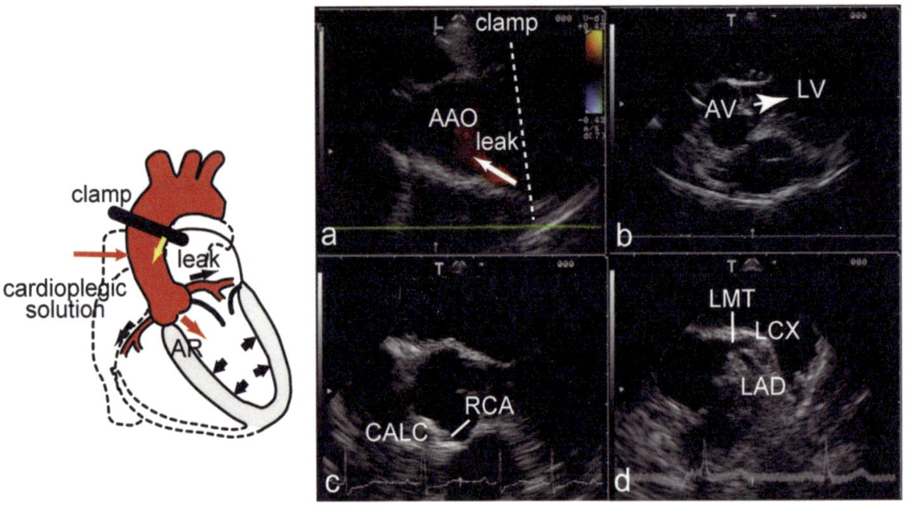

Fig. 6. Pitfalls in antegrade cardioplegia. a: incomplete aortic cross-clamp, b: Aortic regurgitation (AR) shown in B mode, c: calcification at the right coronary ostium, d: short left main truncus (LMT). AAO: ascending aorta, AV: aortic valve, LAD: left anterior descending artery, LCX: left circumflex artery, LV: left ventricle

5.2 Troubles in antegrade cardioplegia

There are two pitfalls in antegrade cardioplegia via a root cannula. In cases with a calcified aorta, the aorta may be incompletely clamped (Fig. 6a). As a result, cardioplegic solution can be washed out by leaking blood. When a patient goes into ventricular fibrillation soon after cardiac arrest, this pitfall needs to be checked. Furthermore, mild aortic reguritation may be responsible for regurgitation of cardioplegic solution, leading to distension of the left ventricle. Regurgitation is noted in the B mode as echo contrast below the aortic valve (Fig. 6b) as well as in color flow imaging.

Calcification at the coronary ostium is not uncommon in cases of aortic stenosis. This is seen as a highly echogenic area accompanied by an acoustic shadow (Fig. 6c). In such cases, the selective cannula occasionally fails to fit the ostium. Thus, infusion of cardioplegic solution is unintendedly delayed and myocardial protection becomes inadequate. Although the myocardium in the left coronary artery regions can be protected by retrograde cardioplegia, that in the right coronary artery region cannot be protected unless the right atrium is opened and coronary perfusion cannula is inserted with coronary sinus ostium tourniqueted. Otherwise, antegrade cardioplegia is essential in this region. Having TEE information on hand during these situations can help guide the surgeon in the choice of cannulas and prevent delays in the case.

In the case of a short left main truncus, the tip of the infusion cannula can be inserted into either the left anterior descending or left circumflex artery and cause inadequate myocardial protection (Fig. 6d). Therefore, a larger cannula is recommended. Adequate perfusion into both arteries is confirmed by either color flow imaging or checking blood flow in the myocardium (anterior wall for the left anterior descending artery, posterior wall for the left circumflex artery) by pulsed-wave Doppler mode with the sample volume placed on the myocardium.

5.3 Difficult cannulation of the coronary sinus

Retrograde cardioplegia is used as an adjunct method of cardioplegia in aortic valve or aortic surgery, especially in cases of coronary artery stenosis or difficult cannulation of the left coronary artery. While a coronary sinus cannula is placed with digital guidance in many institutions, it is difficult in minimally invasive cardiac surgery or in cases with an aneurysmal or angulated ascending aorta or in redo cardiac cases with marked adhesions around the heart. The author routinely uses TEE guidance in such instances.

The coronary sinus is visualized in the 0° and 90° scanning plane (Fig. 7 left). Since this image orientation is rather difficult for guidance, the view is rotated by 180° (flipped upside-down then right-left: Fig. 7 center). The upper image is oriented as viewed from the atrial side. The cannula enters the right atrium from the 1 o'clock position and is directed to the coronary sinus which is depicted in the 6 o'clock position. The cannula is often found to press the posterior wall of the right atrium near the orifice of the coronary sinus. As the

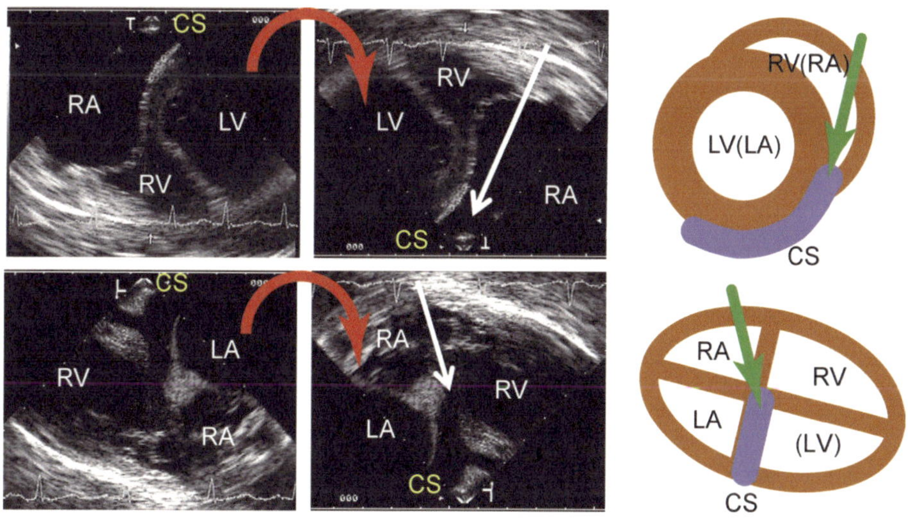

Fig. 7. TEE guided placement of coronary sinus cannula. The 0° and 90° images of coronary sinus (CS) are rotated by 180°. These images are oriented as shown in the right column, which is surgeon-friendly. LA: left atrium, LV: left ventricle, RA: right atrium, RV: right ventricle

cannula tip is tilted toward the left or the two-stage venous cannula is pulled forward to tighten the right atrial wall, cannulation is facilitated. The bottom view is oriented as viewed from the lateral side: the right atrium is depicted on the left and the right ventricle is on the right.

Once the cannula enters the coronary sinus, the location of the cannula tip is assessed with TEE. When it reaches the vicinity of the left atrial appendage, balloon inflation may interfere with the infusion of cardioplegic solution into the posterior branch of the great coronary vein. TEE assessment is helpful when palpation is not feasible in minimally invasive cardiac surgery or redo surgeries.

When the perfusion pressure of retrograde cardioplegia is low, there are two possible causes: 1) migration of the cannula to the right atrium and 2) an unusually large coronary sinus compared to the balloon. If the flow is undetectable in the coronary sinus and a flow signal is found in the right atrium, the former is probable. The coronary sinus should be checked beforehand to rule out the presence of a persistent left superior vena cava. It is diagnosed by the findings of: 1) a large coronary sinus; 2) a lumen between the left atrial appendage and left upper pulmonary vein; and 3) caudal blood flow in the lumen. However, the coronary sinus can be unusually large without such an anomaly. In this case, a cannula with a larger balloon size is used instead.

5.4 Injury of coronary artery

The coronary artery may be injured during selective infusion of cardioplegic solution by the cannula tip or the jet stream. Fig. 8 shows the echo views in a case of coronary artery damage during aortic valve replacement.

Before cardiopulmonary bypass, the TEE showed that the left coronary artery was rather small and calcification was present adjacent to the ostium (Fig. 8a). The surgeon needed to press the cannula to the ostium during perfusion. As the patient was weaned from cardiopulmonary bypass, TEE showed akinesis in the anterior and lateral left ventricular wall in the territory of the left coronary artery. Blood flow in the left coronary artery was undetectable (Fig. 8b) and there was another unusual echo-free space adjacent to it (Fig. 8c). Diagnosis of coronary artery occlusion was made and coronary revascularization to the left anterior descending artery was immediately performed. After reperfusion, direct echo was applied to clarify the mechanism of occlusion. A flap was found in the left main truncus which interrupted the flow in the left main truncus (Fig. 8d). Retrograde blood flow from the left anterior descending artery and continuous flow into the left circumflex artery was seen (Fig. 8e,f). The echo-free space adjacent to the coronary artery was the false lumen which developed due to dissection of the coronary artery.

5.5 Occlusion of coronary ostium

Aortic valve replacement can be complicated by occlusion of the coronary ostium. Although one should be aware of the potential risk of this event in cases with a low take off of the coronary artery, it is rather difficult to predict in preoperative coronary arteriography or transthoracic echocardiography.

In midesophageal aortic valve long-axis view, the ostium is located and placement of prosthetic valve is simulated (Fig. 9a). During weaning from cardiopulmonary bypass, the coronary ostium is checked for obstruction. While there is no obstruction in Fig. 9b, acceleration of flow is noted in Fig. 9c. In the latter case, even a small pannus formation can occlude the left coronary artery ostium. This intraoperative TEE assessment would be the last chance for confirming the exact spatial relationship between the coronary ostium and valve prosthesis.

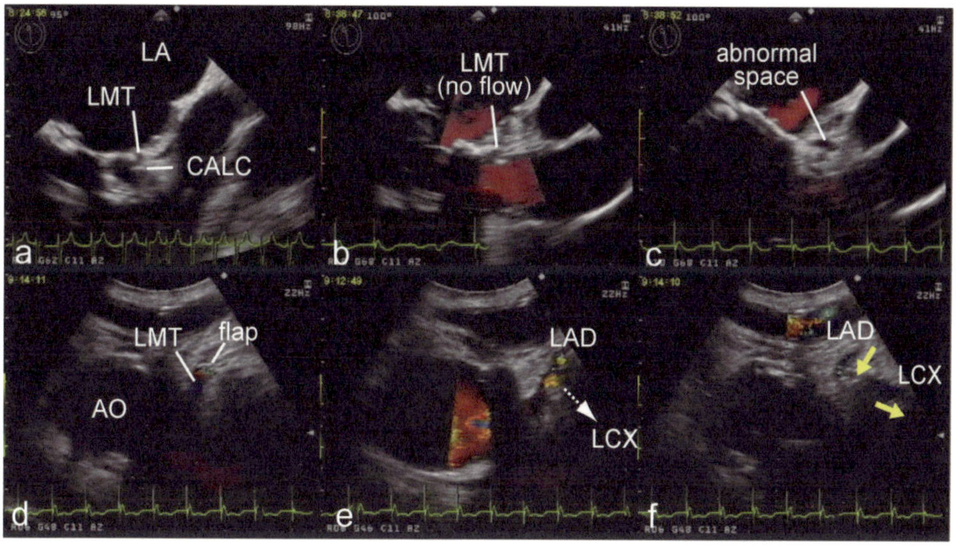

Fig. 8. A case of coronary artery damage. a: preoperative image showing small and calcified left coronary ostium, b: at weaning from bypass without flow in the left main truncus (LMT). c: abnormal space adjacent to the LMT. Direct echo following additional coronary revascularization, flap was noted in the LMT (c) with retrograde flow from the left anterior descending artery (LAD) (e) direct toward left circumflex artery (LCX) (f). AO: aorta, CALC: calcification, LA: left atrium

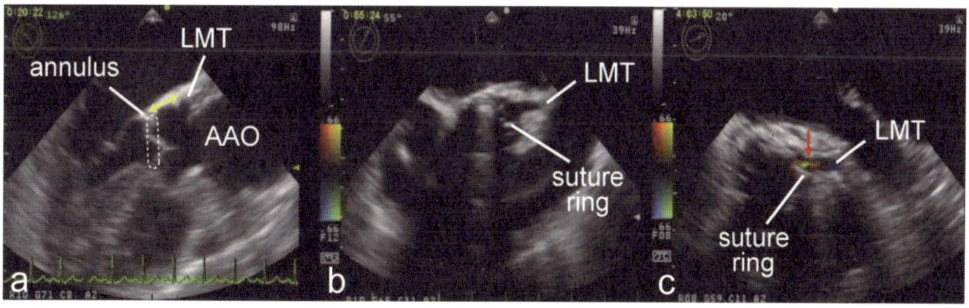

Fig. 9. Aortic valve replacement and coronary artery. a: Distance between the annulus and left coronary orifice is measured. b: no obstruction of left coronary orifice. c: accelerated flow in front of the left coronary orifice, suggesting the presence of narrowed space. AAO: ascending aorta, LMT: left main truncus

In aortic root repair procedures, the coronary anastomosis is routinely checked for stenosis immediately following declamping of the aorta. When there is significant stenosis, one should not proceed to weaning from bypass because it prolongs the duration of ischemic insults on the myocardium.

5.6 Air embolism of coronary artery

Air embolism in the coronary artery can occur in aortic valve surgery. Air not only enters the left ventricle during aortotomy, but also reaches the left atrium and even pulmonary veins. It moves to the left ventricular outflow tract during weaning from bypass and enters the coronary artery (predominantly the right coronary artery because of its buoyancy) (Orihashi et al, 1993, 1996).

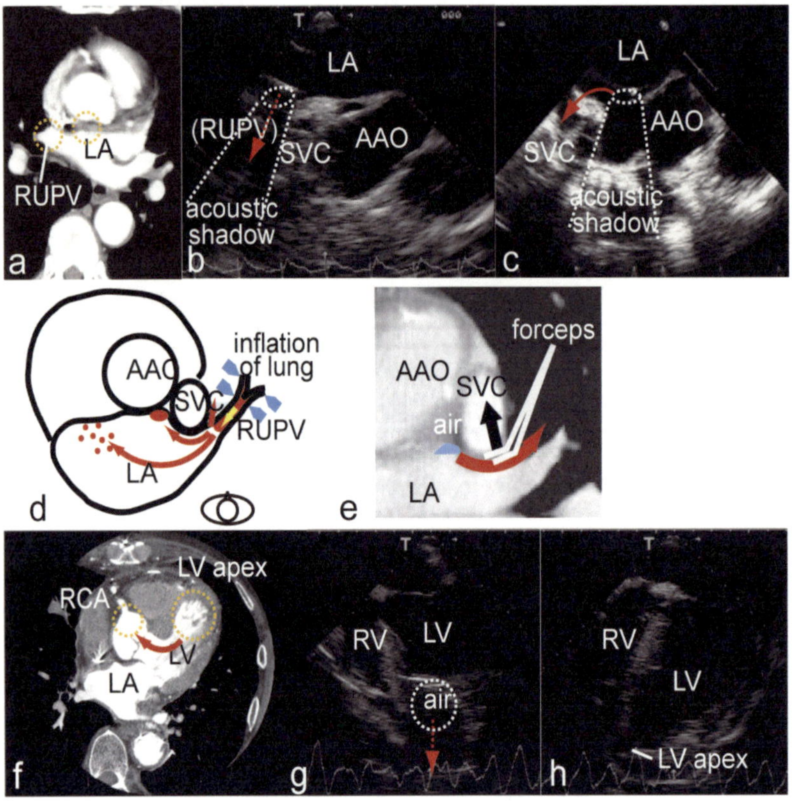

Fig. 10. Retained air visualized with TEE. a: Air retention in the right upper pulmonary vein (RUPV) and left atrium (LA), which is visualized with TEE (b: RUPV, c: LA). d: removal of air in the RUPV, e: removal of air in the LA. f: air in the left ventricular (LV) apex, which is depicted with TEE (g). h: after aspiration of air. AAO: ascending aorta, RCA: right coronary artery, RV: right ventricle, SVC: superior vena cava

Air embolism causes regional myocardial ischemia manifesting as a conduction disturbance and/or regional wall motion abnormality mainly in the inferior wall. Although the air is washed out within 10 to 30 minutes with gradual improvement of the ischemia, it prolongs the pump time and occasionally results in myocardial infarction. Despite the use of carbon dioxide gas inflation in the pericardial sac during cardiopulmonary bypass, wall suction easily removes the gas.

To prevent air embolism, it is important to detect air retention and remove it before it moves to the coronary artery. Common sites of air retention include the right upper pulmonary vein, left atrium, and left ventricle (Fig. 10a,f). TEE is useful for detecting and guiding aspiration of retained air.

Visualization of air in the right upper pulmonary vein is often tricky. The pooled air which fills it up to its ostium is hard to see, but a strong echo accompanied by side lobes and acoustic shadowing with a swinging motion indicates the presence of air at the orifice of the right upper pulmonary vein. As venous return resumes, the air pops up as bubbles in the left atrium or scrolls along the left atrial wall. The air in the left atrium often stays in a shallow pocket formed by the superior vena cava and ascending aorta (Fig. 10c). It can be aspirated directly with a needle or led to the vent port by lifting the superior vena cava with a forceps (Fig. 10d,e, c: red arrow). The adequacy of air removal can be immediately assessed by TEE.

The air in the left ventricle is visualized as a strong echo at the apex to the anteroseptal region. The air masks the image of the apex by acoustic shadowing (Fig. 10g). Aspiration by a needle often produces several milliliters of air. If the amount of air is small, it may be agitated to let the bubble out while the right coronary artery is pressed to avoid new air entry. Again, the outcome can be assessed by TEE (Fig. 10h).

When depressed ventricular contraction is associated with echogenic dots, especially in the inferior wall, air embolism is likely to be responsible and circulatory assist at a rather high perfusion pressure is advised. If such findings are not present, other causes are probable. Thus, TEE is helpful for differentiating the reasons for undesirable hemodynamics.

6. Assessment of prosthetic valve

The function of implanted prosthetic valves is assessed during weaning from cardiopulmonary bypass and is focused on transvalvular and perivalvular leakage. The former originates from inside of the suture ring and the leakage is usually directed inward. This type of leak is allowed to persist unless the regurgitant volume is high. The latter originates from the outside of the sewing ring and is directed outward. This is abnormal and should be addressed by the surgeon.

Unfortunately, the discs of the mechanical valve are hard to visualize by TEE. Instead, the ejected blood just above the valve prosthesis is checked. When the color signal fills the aortic lumen, an immobilized disc is unlikely.

A case of an everted leaflet of a bioprosthetic valve is demonstrated (Orihashi et al., 2010). This patient underwent aortic valve replacement with a Magna valve [TM] due to severe aortic regurgitation. Following aortic declamping, however, TEE showed an unusual transvalvular regurgitant flow in the left ventricular outflow tract. The noncoronary leaflet was fixed in an open position (Fig. 11). The 3D view from the aorta showed that the left ventricular outflow tract was visible in diastole on the noncoronary side. An attempt at weaning failed due to severe aortic regurgitation. Based on the TEE finding and the hemodynamic data, we decided to perform a second aortotomy.

There was no jammed thread or captured leaflet, but the noncoronary leaflet was everted. After it was manually corrected, the leaflet did not spontaneously evert. No needle hole or laceration on the leaflets was noted. Even if the bioprosthetic valve was replaced with another one, a similar event could have occurred. There was no reason for replacement with a mechanical valve. Reimplantation of the same valve would not have been beneficial as it would have prolonged the cardiac arrest time. Eversion of leaflet is unlikely to occur after it starts opening and closing. Thus, the aortotomy was just closed. After weaning from bypass, the leaflet was shown to close normally without significant leakage. Two years after discharge, this patient has had no recurrences of an everted leaflet.

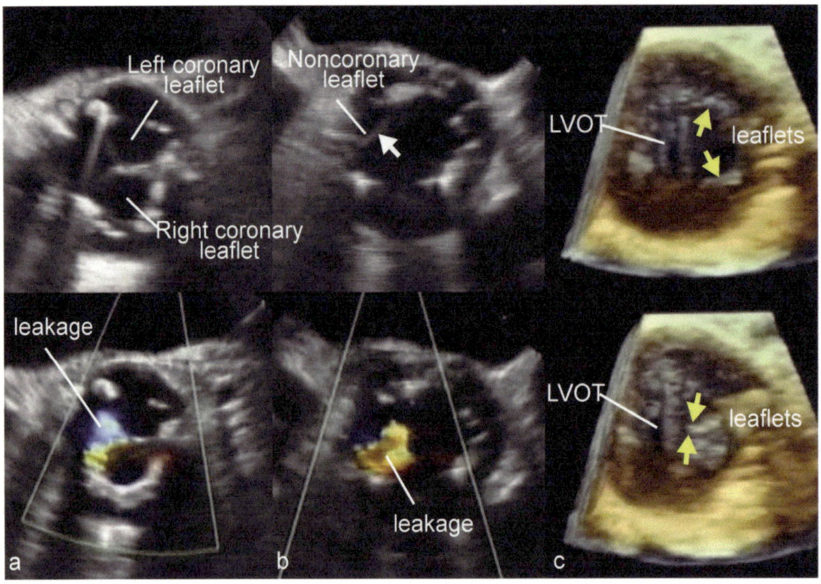

Fig. 11. A case of everted leaflet of Magna valve. a: severe aortic regurgitation in the noncoronary leaflet, b: immobilized leaflet visualized by lateral bending of the probe tip, c: 3D image of valve prosthesis. On the noncoronary side, the left ventricular outflow tract (LVOT) is seen from the aorta side

7. Echo-oriented aortic valve repair

In aortic valve repair or valve sparing surgery, aortic regurgitation is assessed by TEE. When significant regurgitation remains despite the best possible repair based on the preoperative assessment and acceptable coaptation by inspection, the mechanism of regurgitation under pressure loading needs to be identified in order to make additional repairs on the valve.

The origin and eccentricity of the regurgitant jet is an important key to assessing the problem. The former is assessed in midesophageal short-axis view which can examine which pair of cusps is responsible for incompetency. The latter is assessed in midesophageal aortic valve long-axis view to determine the mechanism of regurgitation. If the regurgitant jet is central and originates from the center of the three cusps, coaptation of the Arantius nodule is incompetent, either by deformity of the nodule or by tethering of the three commissures. When the regurgitant jet is deviated to the anterior mitral leaflet and originates from coaptation between the right coronary cusp and noncoronary cusp (Fig. 12b), prolapse of the right coronary cusp is most likely to be causative and plication of this cusp is indicated (Fig. 12c).

Aortic regurgitation can be caused by aortic dissection by three mechanisms: 1) prolapse of the leaflet due to detachment of the commissures from the aortic wall; 2) tethering of the commissures due to an enlarged sinotubular junction; and 3) invagination of an intimal flap into the aortic valve (Fig. 13 a,b,c). These scenarios can be repaired by reuniting the dissected layers and plicating the sinotubular junction to the size which is nearly equal to the aortic annulus diameter (Fig. 13 d,e). If significant regurgitation remains, the mechanism of regurgitation needs to be explored by TEE and additional interventions performed as necessary.

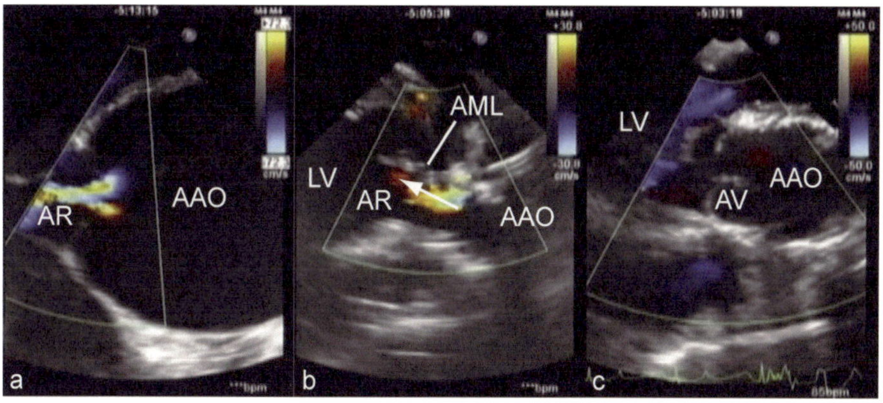

Fig. 12. Echo-oriented aortic valve repair. a: preoperative TEE image of aortic regurgitation (AR) by annuloaortic ectasia, b: residual regurgitation following initial repair with a Valsalva graft, which is directed to the anterior mitral leaflet (AML). c: no regurgitation after plication of right coronary cusp. AAO: ascending aorta, AV: aortic valve, LV: left ventricle

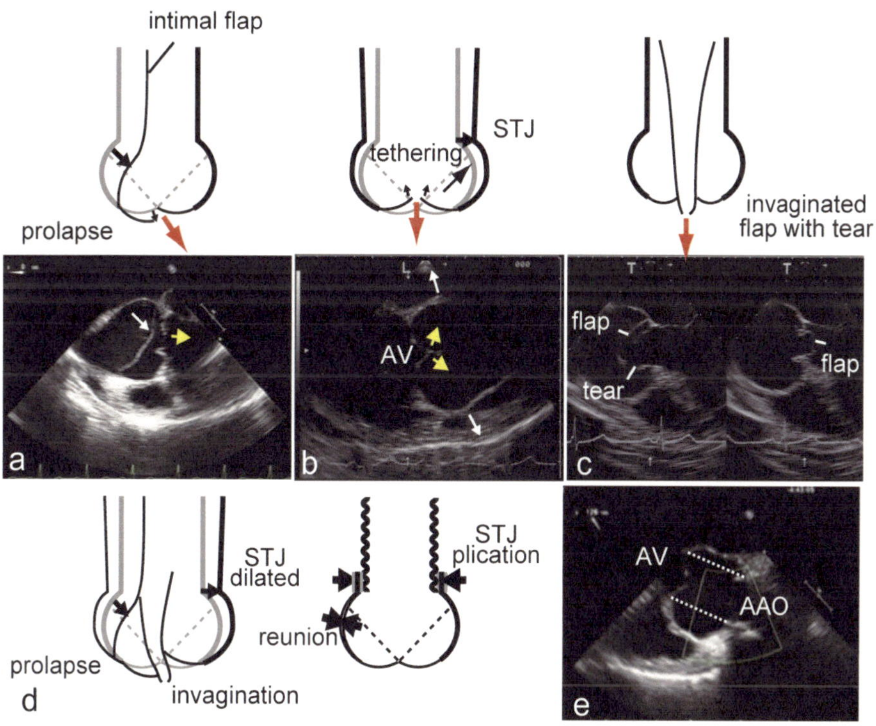

Fig. 13. Three mechanisms of aortic regurgitation in aortic dissection. a: prolapse of a leaflet due to a detached commisure, b: tethering of a leaflet due to an enlarged sinotubular junction (STJ), c: an invaginated flap with tear. d: repair of the sinus of Valsalva sinus based on these mechanisms. e: TEE view after repair. Note that the size of the aortic graft is nearly equal to the aortic valve (AV) annulus. AAO: ascending aorta

8. Systolic anterior motion of mitral leaflet

Systolic anterior motion (SAM) of the mitral leaflet occurs not only in cases with mitral valve repair but also in cases with aortic stenosis or hypertrophic cardiomyopathy. SAM may develop following aortic valve replacement and necessitates additional mitral valve replacement. The mechanism of SAM has been reported as being due to a Venturi effect or drag effect (Cape et al, 1989; Sherrid et al, 1993, 2003). There are several risk factors for developing SAM in mitral valve repair, including a short distance between the coaptation point and interventricular septum (C-Sept), a large angle between the mitral and aortic annular plane, an decreased length ratio of the anterior and posterior mitral leaflets, excess valvular tissue, and a hyperkinetic left ventricle (Maslow et al., 1999).

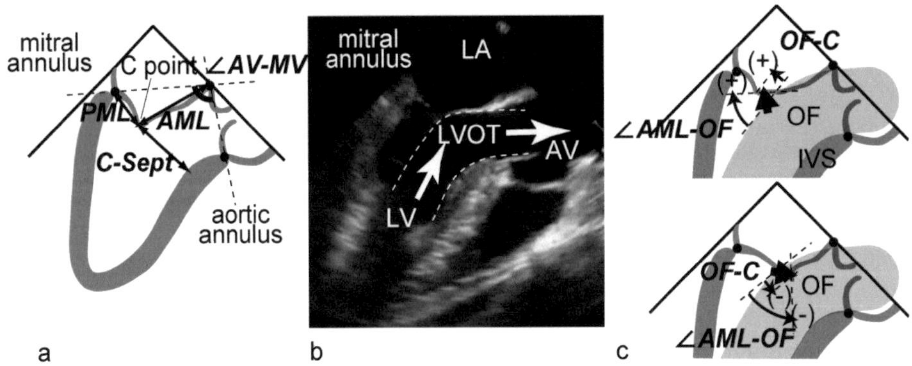

Fig. 14. Measurements for mechanisms of systolic anterior motion. a: conventional parameters, b: assumed outflow in the LV. c: newly introduced two parameters. AML: anterior mitral leaflet, ∠AML-OF: angle between AML and outflow (OF), AV: aortic valve, C-Sept: distance between coaptation and interventricular septum, LA: left atrium, LV: left ventricle, OF-C: distance between OF and coaptation, PML: posterior mitral leaflet

The author believes that there should be a common mechanism of SAM beyond the causative diseases and has analyzed the TEE images obtained in cases of mitral valve repair and septal hypertrophy. In the midesophageal long-axis view, several parameters related to SAM were examined (Fig. 14a): 1) C-Sept; 2) the ratio of lengths of anterior and posterior mitral leaflets (AL/PL ratio); and 3) the angle between the aortic and mitral annular planes (∠AV-MV). Since the LV to LVOT forms a curved but an isometric path (Fig. 14b), the virtual outflow (OF) was assumed as an isometric route along the interventricular septum with a width equal to the dimension of the aortic annulus. The angle and location of the AML tip relative to the OF (∠AML-OF, C-OF) was measured and defined as positive when the AML was away from the outflow and negative when it was within the outflow (Fig. 14c). Measurements were done in 27 cases of mitral valve repair (before and after repair: 54 measuring points including 6 measuring points with SAM and one point of missing data) and 7 cases with septal hypertrophy which underwent mitral valve replacement. The above parameters were compared among three groups: MVP-SAM Group (valve repair without SAM: n=47), MVP+SAM Group (valve repair with SAM: n=6), and SH+SAM Group (septal hypertrophy with SAM: n=7). Among these three groups, there was no significant difference in the ∠AV-MV and AL/PL ratios. However, C-Sept, ∠AML-OF, and C-OF was significantly smaller in the SAM positive groups than in the negative group (Fig. 15).

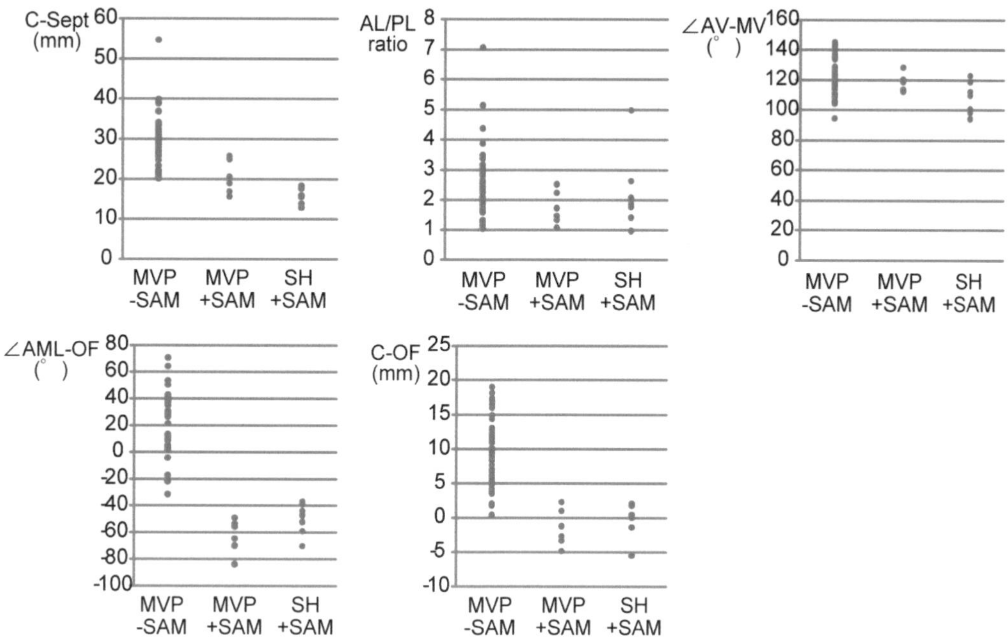

Fig. 15. Comparison between three groups. Among the three groups (mitral valve repair with or without SAM and septal hypertrophy with SAM), there was no significant difference in ∠AV-MV and AL/PL ratio, but C-Sept, ∠AML-OF, and C-OF was significantly smaller in the SAM positive groups than in the negative groups

These results indicate that a dragging effect is the common mechanism in mitral valve disease and septal hypertrophy. SAM occurs when the tip of the anterior mitral leaflet is located in the outflow with a tilted angle to be dragged toward the septum. To prevent SAM in aortic valve replacement, septal myectomy should be adequate so that the anterior mitral leaflet is located out of the new outflow after myectomy. To solve the tilting problem of anterior mitral leaflet, Alfieri's stitch, especially on the A1-P1 side, may be beneficial (Pareda et al, 2010).

In conclusion, intraoperative imaging by means of echocardiography provides a variety of data which can help guide the operation including: 1) avoiding unexpected complications; 2) enhancing the efficacy of surgical treatment; and 3) making immediate and appropriate decisions in cases of rare and unpredictable events. To take the best advantage of this capability, it is essential to efficiently and effectively utilize the modalities available with echocardiography.

9. References

Cape EG, Simons D, Jimoh A, Weyman AE, Yoganathan AP, & Levine RA. (1989) Chordal geometry determines the shape and extent of systolic anterior mitral motion: In vitro studies. *J Am Coll Cardiol* 13, 1438-48.

Ender J, Selbach M, Borger MA, Krohmer E, Falk V, Kaisers UX, Mohr FW, & Mukherjee C. (2010) Echocardiographic identification of iatrogenic injury of the circumflex artery during minimally invasive mitral valve repair. *Ann Thorac Surg* 89, 1866–72.

Karthik S, Mahmood F, Panzica PJ, Khabbaz KR, & Lerner AB. (2007) Intraoperative transesophageal echocardiographic visualization of a left anterior descending coronary artery aneurysm. *Anesth Analg* 104, 263-264.

Maslow AD, Regan MM, Haering JM, Johnson RG, & Levine RA. (1999) Echocardiographic predictors of left ventricular outflow tract obstruction and systolic anterior motion of the mitral valve after mitral valve reconstruction for myxomatous valve disease. *J Am Coll Cardiol* 34, 2096–2104.

Orihashi K, Matsuura Y, Hamanaka Y, Sueda T, Shikata H, Hayashi S, & Nomimura T. (1993) Retained intracardiac air in open heart operation examined by transesophageal echocardiography. *Ann Thorac Surg* 55, 1467-71.

Orihashi K, Matsuura Y, Sueda T, Shikata H, Mitsui N, & Sueshiro M. (1996) Pooled air in open heart operations examined by transesophageal echocardiography. *Ann Thorac Surg* 61, 1377-80.

Orihashi K, Matsuura Y, Sueda T, Watari M, Okada K, Sugawara Y, & Ishii O. (2000) Aortic arch branches are no longer blind zone for transesophageal echocardiography: a new eye for aortic surgeons. *J Thorac Cardiovasc Surg* 120, 466-472.

Orihashi K, Kurosaki T, & Sueda T. (2010) Everted leaflet of a bovine pericardial aortic valve. *Interact Cardiovasc Thorac Surg* 10, 1059-60.

Pereda D, Topilsky Y, Nishimura RA, & Park SJ. (2010) Asymmetric Alfieri's stitch to correct systolic anterior motion after mitral valve repair. *Eur J Cardio-thorac Surg* (ePub).

Sherrid MV, Chu Ck, DeLia E, Mogtader A, & Dwyer EM Jr. (1993) An echocardiographic study of the fluid mechanics of obstruction in hypertrophic cardiomyopathy. *J Am Coll Cardiol* 22, 816–25.

Sherrid MV, Chaudhry FA, & Swistel DG. (2003) Obstructive hypertrophic cardiomyopathy: Echocardiography, pathophysiology, and the continuing evolution of surgery for obstruction. *Ann Thorac Surg* 75, 620–32.

2

Revealing of Initial Factors Defining Results of Operation in Patients with Aortic Valve Replacement and Coronary Artery Disease

A. M. Karaskov[1], F. F. Turaev[2] and S. I. Jheleznev[1]
[1]*E.N. Meshalkin Novosibirsk State Research Institute of Circulation Pathology, Novosibirsk,*
[2]*V. Vakhidov Republican Specialized Center for Surgery, Tashkent,*
[1]*Russia*
[2]*Uzbekistan*

1. Introduction

Moderate aortic valve stenosis is a common condition in patients with coronary heart disease (Gullinov and Garsia, 2005). Recent studies have shown that progression of aortic valve stenosis depends on the degree of valvular leaflets calcification; that aortic valve replacement does not increase mortality after coronary artery bypass grafting (CABG); moreover,valve replacement performed after CABG leads to decreased mortality, it was especially confirmed in patients with severe aortic valve stenosis. However, review of the literature concerning integration of the mathematical approaches in medicine has demonstrated that, the simple prognosis is more significant than an evaluation based on organ and system modeling for choice of treatment method and options for patients with such combined pathology. Repeated intervention is one of the most significant prognostic factors. Thus, after analyzing of 13,346 CABG cases Yap et al (2007) have shown that mortality of repeated interventions is approximately 3 times higher than that of primary interventions (4.8% and 1.8%, respectively). Patient's age is another such a factor. Urso et al. (2007) have established that one-year survival after aortic valve replacement in patients aged over 80 years (86,1%) is significantly less than that in the younger group. Analyzing of 1567 patients after valve replacement combined with CABG, Doenst et al.(2006) have demonstrated patients' gender influence on surgery outcomes, postoperatively women had higher stroke possibility (risk index was 1.52). We believe that various influences of parameters characterizing patient's baseline status on surgery outcome require more complex multivariate statistical analysis to be used. It allows defining rational number of the most significant factors determining the surgery prognosis related both to baseline status of patients with heart defects and immediate postoperative complications caused by interventional injury and heart hemodynamic changes (1, 2, 3, 4, 5, 6). Moreover, one of the authors of the article (Wann and Balkhy, 2009) considers that application of the most modern diagnostics tests (i.e. computed tomography coronary angiography) allows predicting an outcome of the scheduled surgery more accurately.

The objective of this study was to investigate factors affecting the outcomes of combined interventions performed in patients with aortic valve defects and coronary artery lesions and to evaluate anatomical and hemodynamic parameters influencing the prognosis.

2. Material and methods of the study

One hundred twenty eight (128) patients who underwent one-step aortic valve replacement and CABG were enrolled in the study (104 men and 24 women aged from 40 to 73, mean age was 56.4±1.5 years). Aortic valve stenosis was predominant in 82.8% (106) cases; aortic insufficiency was predominant in 17.2% (22) cases. Aortic valve lesions were caused by rheumatic process (65.6%), atherosclerotic degeneration and calcification (15.6%), and infective endocarditis (18.8%). All patients underwent examination including chest X-ray, ECG, EchoCG. Increase in cardiothoracic index and change in pulmonary circulation were observed on X-ray scans. Enlargement of ascending aorta was revealed in all patients. Left ventricle hypertrophy and intraventricular conduction disturbance were observed on ECG. Aortic valve defect was complicated by valvular and extravalvular calcification in 87.1% patients: 3.2% - Grade I, 22.6% -Grade II, 32.3% - Grade III, 29% - Grade IV, absolutely, it was a complicating factor for surgery. Table 1 presents the distribution of patients by chronic heart failure (CHF) and New York Heart Association Functional Class (NYHA FC).

NYHA Functional Class	Number of patients	HF	Number of patients
II	21 (16.1%)	IIA	88 (68.7%)
III	78 (61.3%)	IIБ	40 (31.3%)
IV	29 (22.6%)		

Table 1. Distribution by chronic heath failure stage and functional class

All patients were operated using cardiopulmonary bypass and cardioplegia. Mean time of cardiopulmonary bypass was 178.5±7.8 min, time of aortic occlusion was 132.8±5.0 min. One hundred eight (108) mechanical (75 bicuspid, 33 unicuspid) and 20 biological prostheses were implanted. The most common aortic valve prostheses were MEDINZH, SorinBicarbon, EMIKS, KEM-AV-MONO, KEM-AV -COMPOZIT.

All patients who had significant coronary artery lesions (stenosis >50%) underwent coronary artery bypass grafting: one artery – in 56 (43.8%) patients, two arteries – in 42 (32.8%) patients, three arteries – in 30 (23.4%) patients. Concomitant mitral and tricuspid insufficiency was corrected in 25 and 23 patients, respectively. Atrioventricular valve insufficiency was in all cases caused by fibrous annulus dilatation, which was treated with support ring implantation. Patient status at baseline was a landmark to determine all totality of defect pathogenetic disorders, and evaluation of the factors affecting the separate components of complete clinical picture creation permitted to consider specially the causes, conditions and consequences of systemic positions. Calculations were performed using «STATISTICA for Windows», v.6.0 and original programs developed in "Excel - 2000" on "Visual Basic for Application" integrated computer language. Group data were divided into numeral and classification ones; additional tables for deviations (abs. and %) of variables from baseline levels were calculated. Difference significance was evaluated by $\chi 2$ criterion and 2x2 tables by adjusted Fisher test.

Distribution parameters were evaluated by formulas as follows:

$$M = \frac{1}{N}\sum_{i=1}^{n} Xi; \qquad S = \sqrt{\frac{1}{N-1}\sum_{i=1}^{n}} (Xi\text{-}M)2; \qquad m = M\frac{S}{\sqrt{N}}$$

Consistency of numerical data with normal distribution law was assessed with Kolmogorov test. If the numerical data did not correspond to normal distribution law, non-parametric statistical methods were used - Wilcoxon rank test. Power and direction of correlation between the signs were determined by Pearson correlation coefficient **(r)** and Spearman rank correlation, if distribution of the baseline data was not normal. The values of these tests range from -1 to +1. The extreme values are observed in signs associated with linear functional relation. The significance of selected correlation coefficient is assessed by statistics value r* $\sqrt{n-2}\,/\,\sqrt{1-r2}$ = ta,f (1). Expression (1) permits to determine a, i.e. possibility of correlation coefficient difference from zero depending on r and sample size n. This, in turn, allows comparing the correlation of the same signs in the different sample sizes by possibility. Correlation power was assessed by a value of the correlation coefficient: strong, if r ≥0.7, moderate, if r = 0.3-0.7, weak, if r<0.3. The differences between compared values were significant if p<0.5, it is consistent with criteria accepted in medical and biological researches. Prognosis model is based on the regression analysis.

Regression analysis was directed to the test of significance of one (dependent) variable Y from set of other ones, so called independent variables Xj = {X1, X2, ... Xp}. The values of the prognostic parameter are defined as a result of determination of the risk factors based on analysis of the clinical materials. The purpose of linear regression analysis in this study was to predict the values of the resulted variable Y using the known values of physical parameters, EchoCG parameters and various additional features related to surgery specificity. Parameter of favorable surgery outcome was calculated as an arithmetic mean of risk factors. As a result of these calculations, the model was developed. Based on this model the program was created in "Excel–2000»: «Program for outcome prognosis of aortic valve replacement combined with coronary heart disease» (CERTIFICATE SPD RUz № DGU 01380») allowing to calculate a percentage of favorable surgery outcome and dynamics of LV ejection fraction after a surgery with prognostic significance 75-90%.

3. Results and discussion

As a result of the performed analysis the variables pooled in factor groups **(F)** affecting the surgery prognosis were determined: **F1** - blood supply disturbance (HF, NYHA FC), **F2** - physical parameters (gender, age*, weight*, height*, body surface area*, Ketle index*, CTI*), **F3** - hemodynamic parameters (SBP*, DBP*, MBP*, BSV, HR*, BMV*, TPR*, SPR,HI*, LV stroke work*), **F4** - heart parameters (EDD*,ESD*, EDV*, ESV*, SV*, EF*, FS*, RF*, SVE*, RV*,LA*, RA*, PA*), **F5** - myocardial parameters (IVS*,LVPW*, LVMM*, sPLVWT and dPLVWT*, 2HD*), **F6** –valve morphology (calcification degree on AV, regurgitation degree on AV, MV, and TV), **F7** - valve parameters (FA and ascending aorta diameter*, AV gradients*, AO* surface, MO* surface, MV gradients*,Emv, Amv, E/A mv), **F8** - coronary blood supply parameters (blood supply type, percentage of coronary artery occlusion (LAD, DB, CA, RCA), number of planned bypass grafting). Indexed parameters, reverse values and second degree were considered in «*» variables, it has been leading to increase in prognosis efficacy (see Table 2).

№	Variable	Unit	defenition	Variable nomenclature
I Blood supply disturbance (F 1)				
1	HF		I, IIA, IIB, III	Heart failure
2	FC		I , II, III, IV	Functional class
II Physical parameters (F 2)				
1	Gender		1 - man, 2 – woman	Patient gender
2	Age*	years		Age
3	Weighr*	kg		Weight
4	Height*	cm		Height
5	BSA*	m^2	BSA= 0.007184 * Weight^0.423 * Height^0.725	Body surface area
6	Ketle index*	U	Ketle index = 10000* Weight /Height^2	Ketle index (body weight index)
7	CTI*	%		Cardiothoracic index
III Central hemodynamic parameters (F 3)				
1	SBP*	mmHg		Systolic blood pressure
2	DBP*	mmHg		Diastolic blood pressure
3	MBP*	mmHg	MBP = DBP+[(SBP - DBP)/3]	Mean blood pressure
4	PBP*	mmHg	SBP-DBP	Pulse blood pressure
5	BSV		BSV = 90,97 + 0,54 * PBP - 0,57 * DBP - 0,61*Age	Blood stroke volume by Starr (39)
6	HR*	beat per minute		Heart rate
7	CO*	l/min	CO= SV * HR / 1000	Cardiac output (blood supply)
8	TPR*	dyne*cm-5	TPR = 79,92*MBP/CO	Total peripheral resistance (59)
9	RPR		RPR = TPR /BSA	Relative peripheral resistance (110)
10	HI*	U	HI =CO /BSA	Heart index (109)
11	Asw*	U	Asw(LV) = SV*1,055*(MBP-5)*0,0136	LV stroke work (153)
12	LVMW	U	LVMW = 0,0136 * 1,055 *CO * (MBP-5)	LV minute work (157)
13	LVWI		LVWI = 0,0136 * 1,055 * HI * (MBP-5)	LV work index (160)
14	LVWSI		LVWSI = 0,0136 * 1,055 * SI * (MBP-5)	LV work stroke index (161)
15	HFi		HFi= SBP* HR /LVMM	Heart functioning index
IV Heart parameters (F4)				
1	EDD*	cm		End-diastolic dimension
2	ESD*	cm		End-systolicdimension
3	EDV*	cm^3	EDV= 7 * EDD^3 / (2.4 + EDD)	End-diastolic volume
4	ESV*	cm^3	ESV = 7 * ESD^3 / (2.4 + ESD)	End-systolic volume
5	SV*	cm^3	SV = EDV – ESV	Stroke volume
6	SI*	u	SI = SV / BSA	Stroke index (108)

7	LVEF*	%	LVEF = 100*(EDV-ESV)/EDV	Ejection fraction
8	LVFS*	%	LVSF = 100*(EDD-ESD)/EDD	Fractional shortening
9	RF	%	RF = ESV / EDV * 100	Residual fraction (55)
10	SVE*	%	SVE = EDV / ESV *100	Systolic ventricular ejection (56)
11	TC*		TC = (EDV-ESV)/(EDD-ESD)*1/ESV	Ventricular wall tensility coefficient (57)
12	RV*	cm		Right ventricle
13	LA*	cm		Left atrium
14	RA*	cm		Right atrium
15	PA*	cm		Pulmonary artery
16	PAP	mmHg		Pulmonary artery pressure
17	PA FAD	mm		PA fibrous annulus diameter
			V Myocardial function parameters (F5)	
1	dIVST*	cm		Diastolic interventricular septum thickness
2	dPLVWT*	cm		Diastolic posterior LV wall thickness
3	LVMM*	g	LVMM = 1,04 * ((EDD+VST+PLVWT)^3 - EDD^3)-13,6	LV myocardial mass
4	rsPLVWT*	U.	rsPLVWT = dPLVWT / EDD	Relative systolic posterior LV wall thickness
5	rdPLVWT*	U.	rdPLVWT = dPLVWT / ESD	Relative diastolic posterior LV wall thickness
6	2HD*	U.	2HD = (dIVST + dPLVWT)/EDD	Relative double thickness
			VI Valve morphology (F 6)	
1	AVca	score	1,2,3,4	AV calcification, degree
2	AVreg	score	1,2,3,4	AV regurgitation, degree
3	MVreg	score	1,2,3,4	MV regurgitation, degree
4	TVreg	score	1,2,3,4	TV regurgitation, degree
			VII Valve function parameters (F 7)	
1	ARD*	cm		Aortic root diameter
2	AAD *	cm		Ascending aorta diameter
3	AVppg*	mmHg		AV peak pressure gradient
4	AVmpg*	mmHg		AV mean pressure gradient
5	AVsfs	m/s		AV systolic flow speed
6	AO s*	cm^2		Aortic orifice surface area
7	E mv			MV E peak
8	A mv			MV A peak

9	E/A mv	U.	E/A mv = E mv / A mv	E/A ratio
10	MO s*	cm^2		Mitral orifice surface area
11	MV ppg	mmHg		MV peak pressure gradient
12	MV mpg	mmHg		MV mean pressure gradient
VIII Coronary blood supply parameters (F8)				
1	CVG		1-right, 2- balanced, 3- left	Blood supply type by CVG
2	LAD	%		Left anterior descending, lesion %
3	DB	%		Diagonal branch, lesion %
4	CA	%		Circumflex artery, lesion %
5	RCA	%		Right coronary artery, lesion %
6	IA	%		Intermediate artery, lesion %
7	No.of grafts	pcs		Number of grafts

Table 1. Risk factors and variables and their components

We determined that a percentage of complex factor influence on surgery prognosis - peak systolic gradient (PSG) and post-operation ejection fraction dynamics were different (Figure 1).

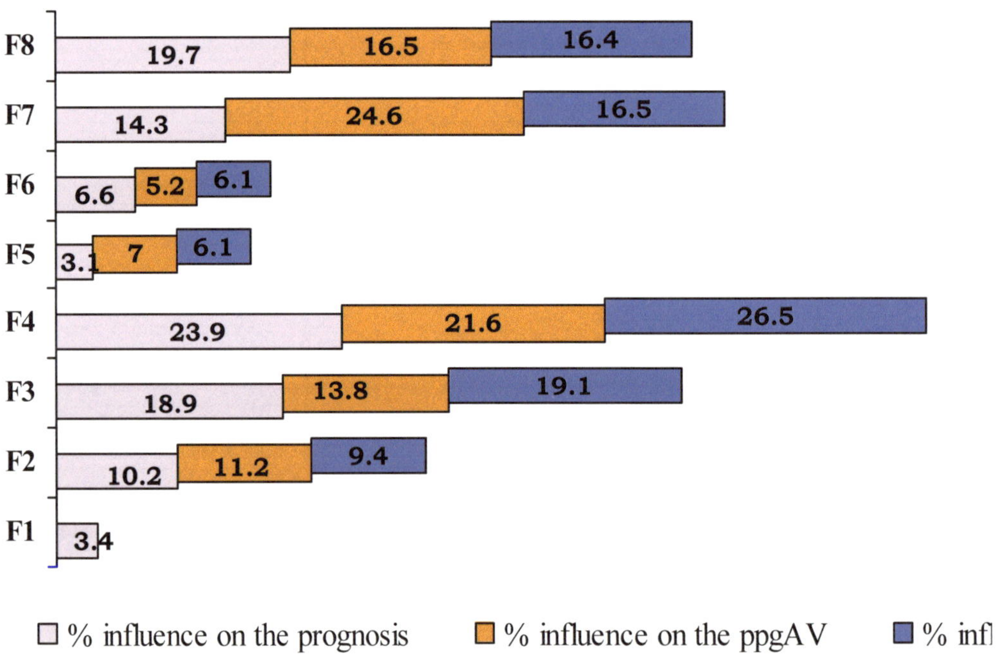

Fig. 1. Percentage of complex factor influence on prognosis, PSG, LVEF in patients suffered from valve defect combined with coronary artery lesions

Thus, heart parameters (F4) ($r=0.320$ $p<0.01$),coronary blood supply parameters (F8) ($r=0.165$ $p<0.05$), F3 ($r=0.330$ $p<0.01$), valve function parameters (F7) ($r=0.183$ $p<0.05$), and physical parameters (F2) ($r=0.223$ $p<0.05$) had greater influence on prognosis. However, valve functions (F7) (r=0.320 p<0.01), heart parameters (F4) (r=0.261 p<0.05), coronary blood supply parameters (F8) (r=0.046 p<0.05), hemodynamic parameters (F3) (r=0.284 p<0,05), and myocardial function parameters (F5)(r=0.589 p<0.001) have played greater role for peak systolic gradient (PSG). The parameters of the following factors affect changes in LV ejection fraction: heart parameters (F4) (r=0.381 p<0.01), hemodynamic parameters (F3) (r=0.332 p<0.01), coronary blood supply parameters (F8) (r=0.322 p<0.01), and valve function parameters (F7) (r=0.332 p<0.01). The positive surgery prognosis in patients with lower HF (r=-0.111) and lower NYHA FC (II, III) (r=-0.560) was higher than 80%. However, in operated patients with FC IV the surgery prognosis was less than 80%. It was noted that higher FC corresponded to lower LV EF values (r=-0.086). It means that FC IV is a high risk predictor for combined surgeries (Figure2).

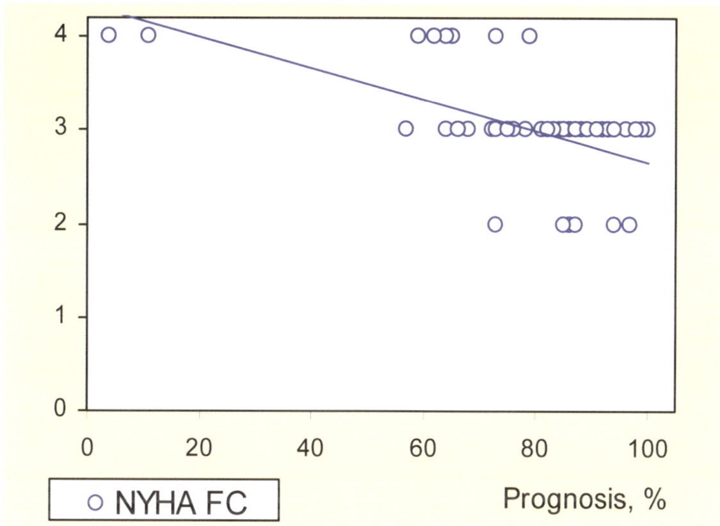

Fig. 2. Correlation between prognosis and functional class

Physical parameters (F2) suggested that PSG on AV had a trend to increase with age (r=0.264), i.e. compensated processes are progressing depending on age, although general biological and physiological processes are decreasing. However, age had no significant influence on surgery prognosis (r=-0.162). Moderate correlation between prognosis (r>0.31) and peak SPG (r>0,206) was observed when hemodynamic parameters were analyzed (F3). The correlation was direct for prognosis and reverse for SPG: e.g. in patients with CO more than 4.0 l/min surgery prognosis was higher. This parameter increased not due to HR, but due to minute volume (r=-0.215). Such pattern was observed between parameters of LV stroke work (Asw): surgery prognosis was higher if LV Asw was higher (r=0.468). But if SPG was increased, decrease in LV Asw was observed (r=-0.295). It may be concluded that increase in afterload leads to decrease in LV work efficacy (Figure 3).

If peak SPG is more than 60 mmHg, LV Asw becomes less than 100 U, and favorable surgery prognosis does not exceed 80%. If stroke work was more than 100 U, positive surgery prognosis was 80-100%. It means that in patients with coronary artery lesions in combination with aortic defect SPG ≥ 60 mmHg is one of indications for aortic valve replacement. Heart parameters (F4) had the greatest influence on surgery prognosis. Thus,

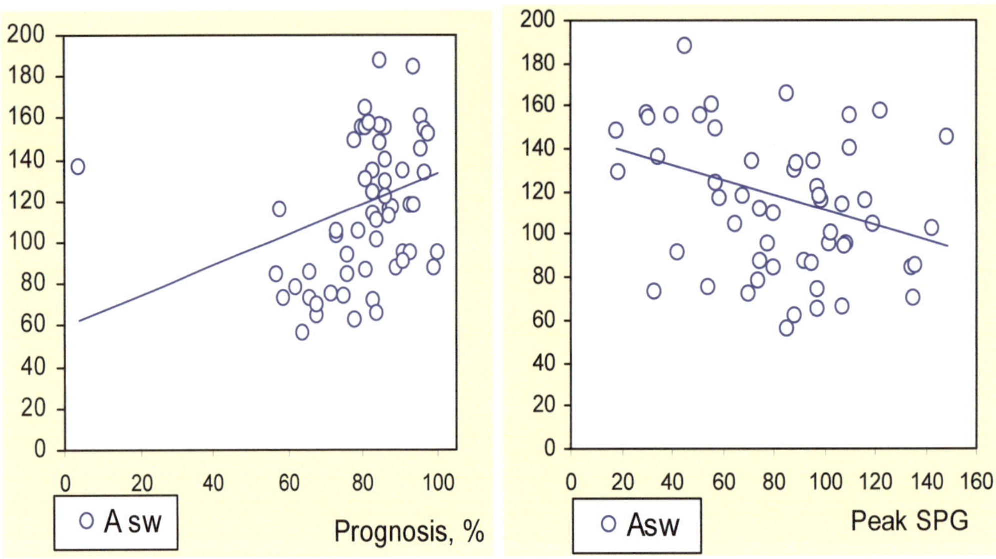

Fig. 3. Correlation between prognosis with SPG and LV stroke work

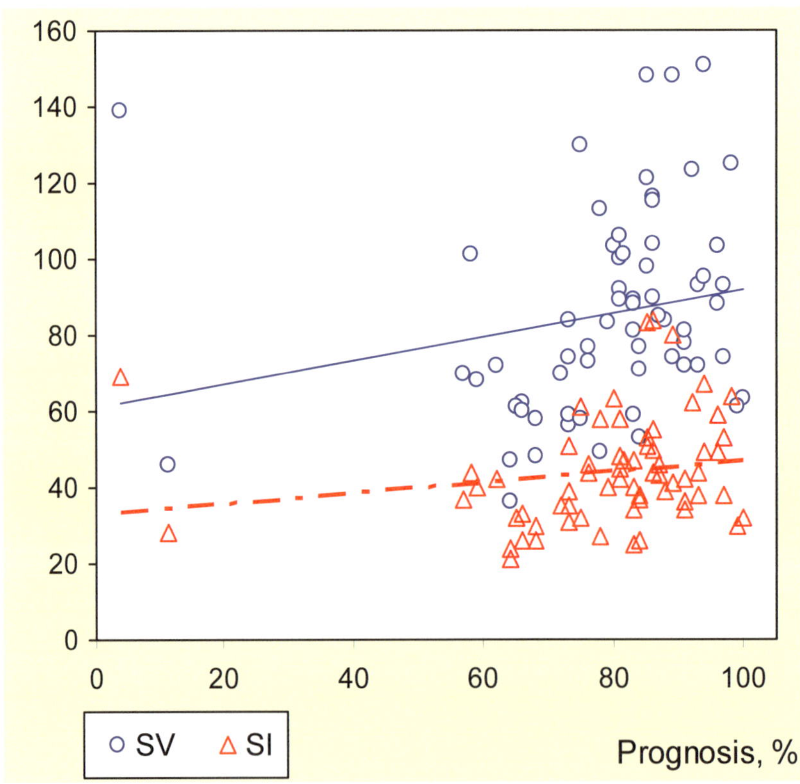

Fig. 4. Correlation between SV and SI with surgery outcome

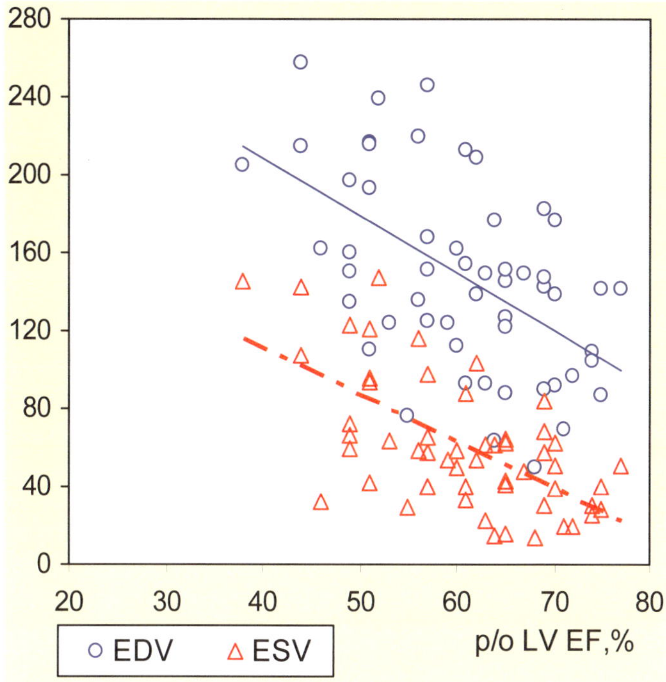

Fig. 5. Influence of EDV and ESV on LV ejection fraction

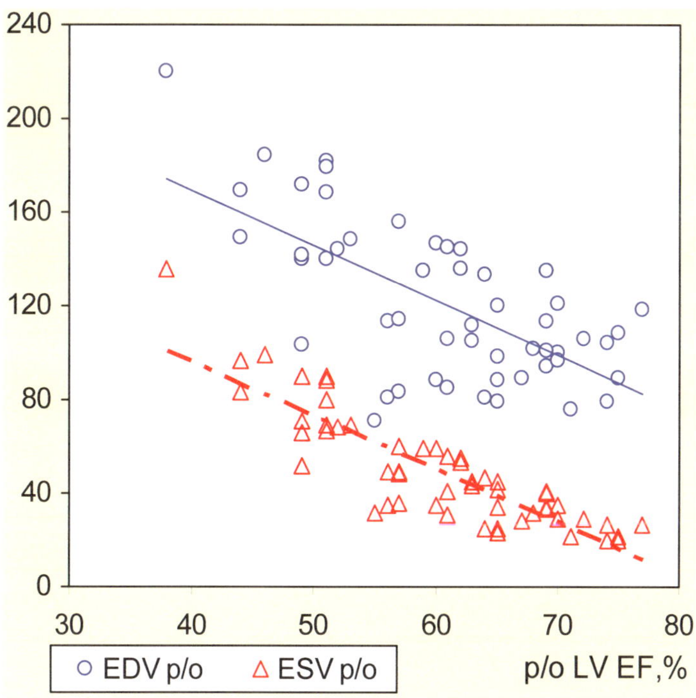

Fig. 6. Influence of p/o EDV and p/o ESV on p/o LV ejection fraction

LV parameters had direct correlation with prognosis (r>0.224) and LV EF dynamics (r> 0.598) and reverse correlation with SPG (r<-0.343). LV end-diastolic dimension (EDD) and end-diastolic volume (EDV) had a greater influence on prognosis (r=0.349 and r=0.429, respectively), than LV end-systolic dimension (ESD) and end-systolic volume (ESV) (r=0.303 and r=0.352, respectively). Even in cases when increase in LV EDD (EDV) was observed after surgery and LV ESD (ESV) was constant (or decreased), possibility of favorable surgery prognosis was increased. This relationship between EDV and ESV contributes to increase in stroke volume (SV) and suggests preservation of LV myocardial contraction. The analysis showed that increased SV (r=0.458) and stroke index (SI) (r=0.385) was associated with increased percentage of favorable prognosis. We have found that if SI was >40 ml/m2 (SV=80 ml), positive surgery prognosis was more than 80% (Figure 4).

Analysis of influence of baseline EDV and ESV on postoperative LV EF has shown that this value was greater in patients with preserved LV parameters (Figure 5), and in patients with significant reduction of LV EDV and ESV (Figure 6).

The performed analysis revealed that in patients with normal LV myocardial contractility at baseline we had good prognosis and increased LV EF after surgery. It was determined that if LV EF is higher than 50% at baseline, the positive surgery prognosis exceeds 80%. Such pattern of baseline EDV and ESV influence on LV EF dynamics was observed, if LV EF parameters obtained from calculation using the program for prognosis were analyzed. (Figure 7).

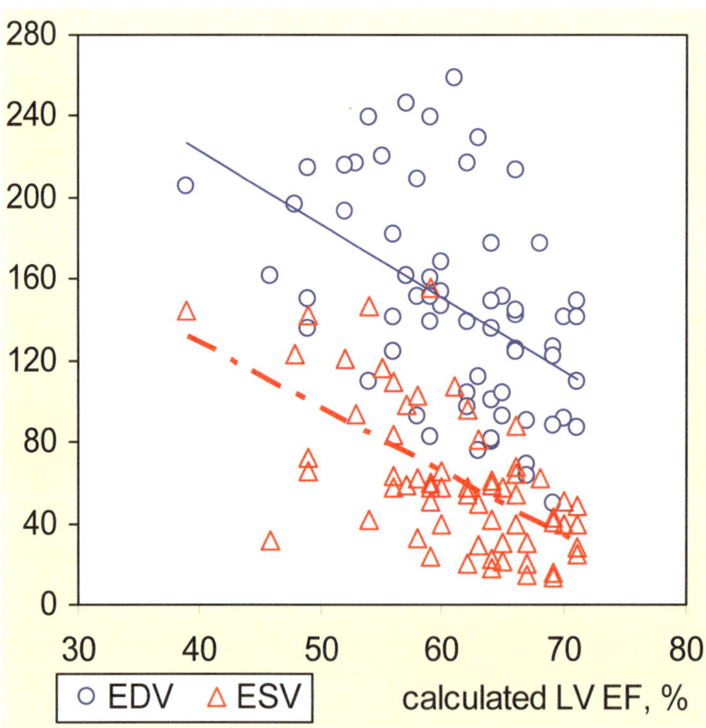

Fig. 7. Influence of baseline EDV and ESV on calculated LV EF

LV EF calculated using the program for prognosis significantly correlated with true numbers of baseline and postoperative LV EF (Figure 8).

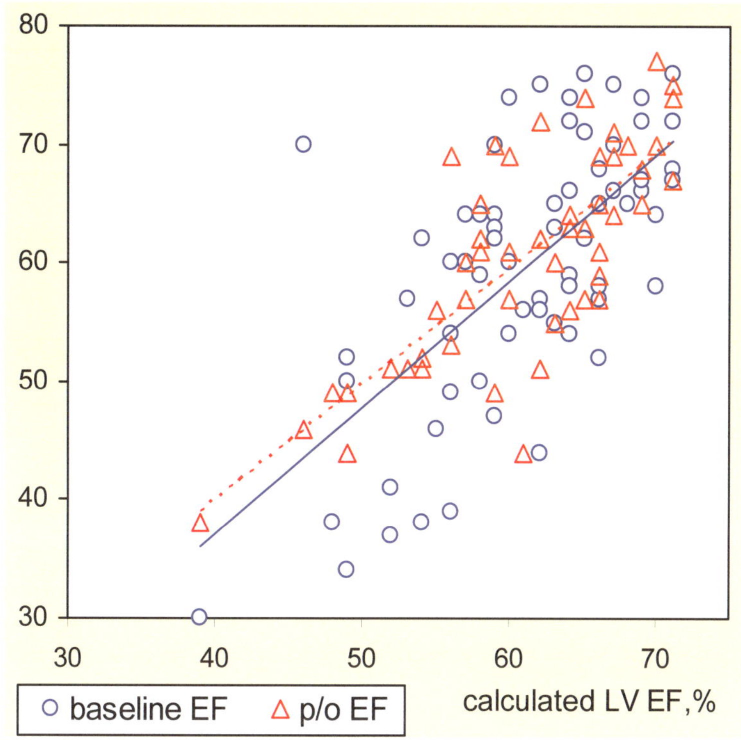

Fig. 8. Correlation of calculated LV EF with pre- and postoperative LV EF

Assessment of correlation between postoperative LV EF parameters and calculated ones using the program for surgery prognosis revealed a common pattern (trend lines had similar direction of dynamics and were approximately at the same level) (Figure 9).

Decrease in postoperative LV EF is caused by cardiopulmonary bypass, aortic occlusion, and cardioplegia through unfavorable influence on myocardial contractility in spite of coronary artery bypass grafting, procedure improving coronary blood supply, activation of hibernated myocyte.

Analysis of myocardial function parameters (F5) showed that surgery prognosis is highly affected by posterior left ventricular wall thickness (PLVWT) (r=-0.306) and to lesser extent by interventricular septum thickness (IVST) (r=-0.072). Increase in IVST leads to greater increase in peak SPG rather than PLVWT (r=0.679 and r=0.526, respectively). It can be possibly explained by appearance of additional component of LV outflow tract obstruction as a hypertrophied IVS. When thickness of IVC and PLVW ranges from 1.5 to 2.0 cm, SPG is equal to 80-120 mmHg, and positive surgery prognosis is 80-100%. However, increased dimensions of IVS and PLVW lead to decrease in percentage of favorable prognosis. Degree of ejection fraction increase was mostly related to PLVWT (r=0.433) than to IVST (r=0.265), had no relation with LV myocardial mass (r=-0.113), although increase in myocardial mass improved surgery prognosis. Thus, optimal left ventricle myocardial mass (LVMM) value was 350-600 g (200-400 g/m2) in the presence of corresponding linear parameters of LV and IVS. In these cases, positive surgery prognosis was more than 80%. Increase in ejection fraction more than 50% was postoperatively observed especially in patients with such characteristics. Analysis of valve morphology parameters (F6) revealed that significance of aortic valve calcification increases in peak SPG (r=0.448), but not affecting surgery prognosis (r=0.172). Baseline AV regurgitation also does not influence on surgery outcome (r=0.263). We can see the possible explanation of this fact is that AV calcification in the patients was mostly caused by age-related sclerosis and rheumatoid degeneration with no elements of myocardial inflammation (myocarditis) and inflammation of conduction system.

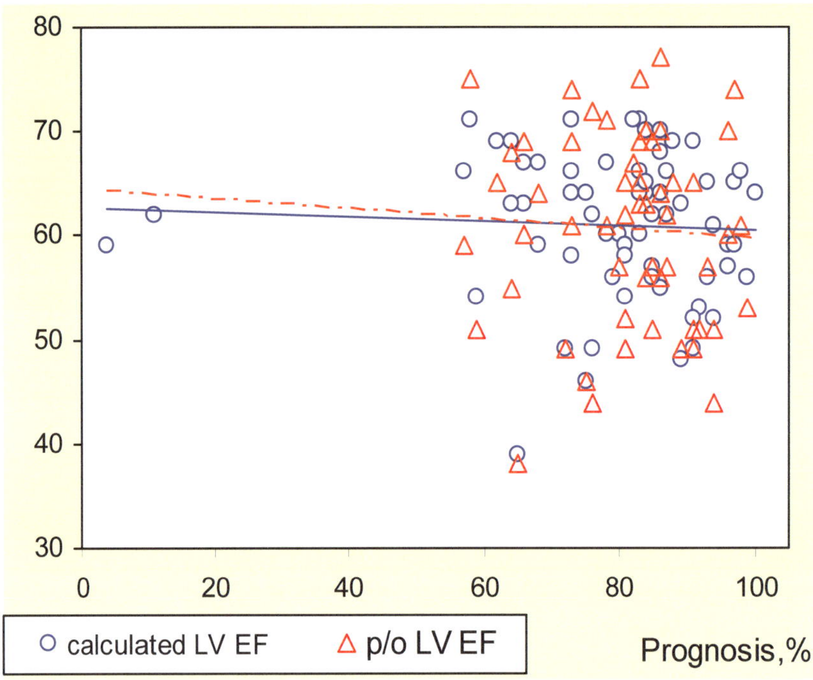

Fig. 9. Correlation between postoperative EF and calculated LV EF

Decreased ejection fraction was observed in patients who had regurgitation on MV (r=-0.377) and TV (r=-0.313) exceeding Grade I, this also resulted in impairment of surgery prognosis. Analysis of valve function parameters (F7) demonstrated that lower baseline SBG value was associated with more favorable surgery prognosis (r=-0.284). When peak SPG was less than 80 mmHg, favorable surgery prognosis ranged from 90 to 100%. Therefore, in the patients with coronary artery lesions aortic valve replacement should be performed at the early stages of defect manifestations when a systolic gradient is 60-80 mmHg. Analysis of coronary blood supply factor (F8) showed that patients with right dominance had worse surgery prognosis than patients with left dominance. Analysis demonstrated that among patients with right dominance only one artery was grafted in 41.9% patients, and 58.1% patients had two grafted arteries (35.5%) or more (22.6%). However, among patients with left dominance, one artery was grafted in 66.7% patients and only 33.3% patients had two (22.2%) or more (11.1%) grafted arteries, i.e. we see that the larger grafting volume was performed in patients with right dominance. Thus, greater number of grafts required corresponds to worse surgery prognosis (r=-0.312). Analysis of coronary artery lesions showed that significance of left descending artery (LAD) lesions, i.e. necessity of its grafting makes worse surgery prognosis (r=-0.303). It was also revealed that there is a direct correlation between grade of LAD lesion and value of mitral regurgitation (r=0.283). This suggests a significant role of LAD in coronary blood supply and it should be grafted if affected, especially in patients with combined lesion of aortic valve and coronary arteries. Our conclusions generally support the literature data. Analysis of the huge body of materials (108 687 aortic valve replacements) performed by Brown et al. in 2009 demonstrated that female gender, age above 70 years and ejection fraction less than 30% led to higher postoperative mortality, higher percentage of postoperative stroke, and prolonged duration of hospitalization.

The authors confirmed the data published by Doenst et al. in 2006 on higher incidence of stroke in women during immediate postoperative period, and did not confirmed the data on a similar percentage of mortality. Although, Doenst et al. (2006) analyzed cases of combined CABG and valve replacement (1567 patients). But this also cannot be a final conclusion (combined interventions have worse results than that of one-organ surgeries). However, Thulin and Sjogren (2000) did not demonstrate any differences in the results of simple aortic valve replacement (121 patients) and valve replacement in combination with CABG (98 patients). Some investigators apart from hemodynamic parameters pay attention on the values of laboratory tests. Thus, Florath et al. (2006) showed that elevated blood levels of glucose, creatine kinase, lactate dehydrogenase, sodium, and proteins in patients prior to aortic valve replacement and CABG (908 patients) resulted in increased postoperative mortality. Jamieson et al. demonstrated results similar to our ones (2003). Bioprosthetic valve replacement and CABG was performed in 1388 patients. The mortality rate in NYHA I-II and NYHA IV was 2% and 16%, respectively. The mortality rate in men and women was 4.6% and 13.8%, respectively. Older patients more often required repeated interventions (59 versus 52 years). Nardi et al (2009) showed that surgery prognosis was worse in patients with low ejection fraction, history of paroxysmal ventricular tachycardia, renal insufficiency, and anterior myocardial infarction prior to surgery.

4. Conclusion

Patients with aortic valve lesion combined with coronary artery lesion are a severe group for surgical treatment and require intervention at early stages of the disease. NYHA FC IV is a high-risk predictor for combined surgeries CHD + CABG. We believe that systolic gradient ≥60 mmHg in patients assigned to CABG is an indication for combined aortic valve surgery. Analysis of LV linear and volume parameters revealed that LV diastolic dimension and diastolic volume had the greatest influence on prognosis in this patient group. iEDV/iESV ratio with SI>40 ml/ m2 (SV=80 ml) is a good prognostic sign allowing to predict a prognosis of more than 80%. The optimal LVMM value was 350-600 g (200-400 g/m2) in the presence of corresponding linear parameters of LV and IVS, when a surgery prognosis was higher than 80%, and baseline LVEF was more than 50%. Appearance of functional changes in MV (regurgitation grade >1) and TV (regurgitation grade >1) is a poor prognostic factor. LAD grafting in these patients is a required intervention, even is a lesion degree is less than 70%. It allows increasing the favorable surgery percentage.

5. References

[1] Gilinov A.M., Garcia M.J. When is concomitant aortic valve replacement indicated in patients with mild to moderate stenosis undergoing coronary revascularization. Curr. Cardiol. Rep., 2005, Mar., 7 (2), 101-104

[2] Yap C.H., Sposato L., Akowuah E. et al. Contemporary results show repeat coronary artery bypass grafting remains a risk factor for operative mortality. J. Heart Valve Dis., 2007, 87, 1386-1391

[3] Urso S., Sadaba R., Greco E. et al. One-hundred aortic valve replacements in octogenarians: outcomes and risk factors for early mortality. J. Heart Valve Dis., 2007,16, 2, 139-44.

[4] Doenst T., Ivanov J., Borger M.A. et al. Sex-specific longterm outcomes after combined valve and coronary artery surgery. Ann. Thorac. Surg., 2006, 81, 1632-1636

[5] V.B. Brin, B.Ya. Zonis Circulation physiology. Rostov-on-Don University Publishing, 1984., pp. 88.

[6] Бураковский В.И., Лищук В.А., Стороженко И.Н. Применение математических моделей в клинике сердечно-сосудистой хирургии.М., 1980, стр.93-120.

[7] Yu.L. Shevchenko, N.N. Shikhverdiev, A.V. Otochkin Prognosis in heart surgery. Saint Petersburg, Piter Publishing, 1998, pp. 208.

[8] E.N. Shigan Prognostic methods and modeling in social and hygiene studies. Moscow, Meditsina, 1986. - 206 pp.

[9] Lemeshow S., Teres D., Klar J. et al. Mortality probability models (MPM II) based on an international cohort of intensive care unit patients. JAMA, 1993, 270, 2478-2486

[10] Moreno R., Miranda D.R., Matos R., Fevereiro T. Mortality after discharge from intensive care: the impact of organ system failure and nursing workload use at discharge.Intens.Care Med., 2001, 27, 999-1004

[11] Wann S., Balkhy H. Evaluation of patients after coronary artery bypass grafting. Cardiol Rev., 2009, 17, 4, 176-80

[12] Brown J.M., O;Brien S.M., Wu C. et al. Isolated aortic valve replacement in North America comprising 108,6887 patients in 10 years: changes in risks, valve types, and outcomes in the Society of Thoracic Surgeons National Database. J.Thorac. Cardiovasc. Surg., 2009, 137, 1, 82-90.

[13] Thulin L.I., Sjögren J.L. Aortic valve replacement with and without concomitant coronary artery bypass surgery in the elderly: risk factors related to long-term survival. Croat. Med. J., 2000, 41,4,406-9

[14] Florath I., Albert A., Hassanein W. et al. Current determinants of 30-day and 3-moth mortality in over 2000 aortic valve replacements: Impact of routine laboratory parameters. Eur.J.Cardiothorac.Surg., 2006, 30,5,716-21.

[15] Jamieson W.R., Burr L.H., Miyagishima R.T. et al. Re-operation for bioprosthetic aortic structural failure - risk assessment. Eur.J.Cardiothorac.Surg., 2003, 24, 6, 873-878

[16] Nardi P., Pellegrino A., Scafuri A. et al. Long-term outcome of coronary artery bypass grafting in patients wtih left ventricular dysfunction. Ann. Thorac. Surg., 2009, 87, 5, 1407-8

Part 2

Selection of Prosthesis

3

Which Valve to Who: Prosthetic Valve Selection for Aortic Valve Surgery

Bilal Kaan İnan, Mustafa Saçar,
Gökhan Önem and Ahmet Baltalarli
Kasımpaşa Military Hospital, İstanbul,
Pamukkale University, Denizli,
Turkey

1. Introduction

Harken et al. had performed the first aortic valve replacement in subcoronary position in 1960 (Harken, 1960). The "caged ball" valve used in this operation pioneered to the prosthetic valves and in the last 50 years many valve types were begun to be used. The early and long term results of the patients undergone aortic valve surgery do not depend not only the patient-related factors and the type of the surgery. The selected prosthetic valve is one of the most important factor affecting survival. According to the analysis of the multicenter randomized trials made by Hammermeister et al. involving the recent 15 years, more than one third of the deaths among the patients undergone aortic valve surgery were found to be related to the prosthetic valve (Hammermeister, 2000). The expectance from an ideal prosthetic valve is to correct the present valve pathology, to possess normal functions, to normalize patient's life standards or at least to improve it obviously, and to preserve this status during the patient's lifelong. Additionally, the implantation of the ideal prosthetic valve should be easy, the prosthetic valve should be replaced with low mortality and morbidity, should not cause a damage to the cardiovascular system, the hospitalization period should be short, the valve should be inexpensive (Rahimtoola, 2010). In spite of the whole developments in the prosthetic valve technology, the ideal prosthetic valve is not found yet, that's why the task of the surgeon is to select the prosthetic valve not depending on the nature of the disease but should be individualized to each patient.

Nowadays, the replacement alternatives for aortic valve replacement are mechanical valves, biological xenograft valves, homograft valves, autograft valves and valves implanted transapically or percutaneously which usage has increased in the recent years. Because of various advantages and disadvantages, these alternatives are prefered to each other. However, for the most appropriate valve choice, each patient should be evaluated individually. Additionally, improvements in the drug technology and risk preventing measures, due to the deceleration in the development of cardiovascular diseases, the age of the operated patients and the surviving period following the operation is increasing gradually. Cardiovascular diseases become the most important factor determining the life quality and surviving ratio in the elderly population. The main purpose of the aortic valve replacement is the improvement of life quality by prolonging the patient's life (Kolh, 2007;

Thourani, 2008). For that reason, by selecting the most appropriate valve for each patient, complications due to the valve can be decreased. Because the rate of the complications of the selected valve are affected by the age and comorbidities of the patients.

Traditionally, the most important criteria for the valve selection is the patient's age, but with the improvements in the production of prosthetic valves and fixation methods, different criteria began to come into prominence. Perforations due to the stress or dystrophic calcifications are hold to be responsible of the structural degeneration of the biological valves (Jameison, 1995). It was shown that the new generation bioprotheses are more durable and needed less reoperation in a long period (Silberman, 2008; Potter, 2005; Valfre, 2006). In addition, improvements achieved in the anticoagulant agents. The superiority of the biological valves would be limited by the technology providing patient's self-monitoring of international normalized ratio (INR) (Siebenhofer, 2004) and the development of new anticoagulant agents (Salam, 2004). These developments and innovations will be effective in the revision of the criteria in the selection of valve.

Generally, biological valves are preferred in the patients older than the age of 70 years. Besides the lower thromboembolic and hemorragic complications incidence at that age, durability of biological valves is enough for the survival of patients following aortic valve replacement (Cosgrove, 1995; Langley, 1999; Masters, 2004). Additionally, the usage of chronic anticoagulation therapy for the biological valves is not necessary as is in the mechanical valves. Generally, the mechanical valves which are more durable than the biological valves are chosen in the patients younger than the age of 60 years, because of their expected longer survival. At that age an early calcification due to the increase of the collagen degeneration and increased calcium turnover was seen in the biological valves (Gross, 1998). However, the selection of prosthetic valve is more difficult between the age 60 and 70 years. The selection of the valve can be easier by paying attention to co-morbidities. Biological valves are preferred in the patients with coronary heart disease because of the decrease in their expected survival. Additionally, generating less turbulence flow by biological valves increases the coronary by-pass graft flow (Hassanein, 2007). When a comparison is made between the biological valves, stentless biological valves are seen more advantageous in terms of coronary flow reserves. Stentless biological valves are an appropriate choice in the patients with left ventricular dysfunction in terms of postoperative recovery (Bakhtiary, 2006).

In some patients, the decision of the valve selection is unrelated to the age. Young female patients planning to become pregnant is a special patient group. In these patients, with the avoidance of an anticoagulation therapy during the pregnancy via biological valve replacement (De Santo, 2005), in experienced centers Ross procedure is offered as an alternative therapy (Bonow, 2008). Additionally, it is suggested that not only the mechanical prosthetic valves or anticoagulant agent usage, but at the same time the acceleration of the structural degeneration of biological valves is an important issue needed to be avoided during the pregnancy (Jamieson, 1988).

The pulmonary autograft procedure in patient with aortic valve disease is an alternative to the prosthetic valves and the aortic allograft. This technique was introduced in 1967 by Donald Ross (Ross, 1967). The benefits of the Ross procedure are the superior durability of the pulmonary autograft when compared to biological valves in the aortic position, the growth potential of the autograft, and avoidance of prolonged anticoagulation (Akhyari, 2009). Hence, this procedure is primarily used in young or growing patients.

Additionally, some factors provide making a decision on the valve selection regardless of the patient's age. In case of previous thromboembolism history, chronic atrial fibrillation, low ejection fraction, previously implanted valve type and intracardiac thrombus, the selection of the valve is made regardless of the patient's age. The replacement of mechanical prosthetic valves is not appropriate in the patients with low sociocultural level, exposed to frequent traumas due to occupational reasons, predisposed to bleeding, unwilling to use or is contraindicated to use anticoagulants. Biological valve options are good alternatives in these patients. In patients with small ventricle, when mitral valve replacement and aortic valve replacement are needed to be done together, and the usage of mechanical prosthesis is not appropriate due to their high profile, biological valves have to be selected for replacement.

These prosthetic valves are similar according to the perioperative mortality and immediate and long term survival (Silberman, 2008). These similar results have been shown not only for the elderly patients but also for middle aged patients (Carrier, 2001; Khan, 2001). But, during the biological valve replacement cardiopulmonary bypass time and ischemic time are longer than in those with mechanical valve replacement (Silberman, 2008) and especially stentless biologic valve implantation is more difficult in technical aspect. Thus, surgical experience and how the patients will be affected from the longer operation time are the other factors should be considered. The fact that stentless biological valves have hemodynamic advantages (Silberman, 2001), possibility of a replacement of larger sized prosthesis (Del Rizzo, 1994), better durability (Bach, 2005) and long term survival ratios (Albertucci, 1994; Westaby, 2000) in comparison with the stented biological valves, provides their preference in the young patients. The advantages of Ross procedure with respect to postoperative survival, life quality and reoperation requirement in adult patients undergone homograft and autograft aortic root replacement will provide it becoming widespread (Hammermeister, 2000; Stassano, 2009; El-Hamamsy, 2010).

Transcatheter aortic valve implantation (TAVI) recently developed and commonly used in some centers as a good alternative technique for the patients in whom the aortic valve replacement is with high risk (Cribier, 2006; Webb, 2007; Walther, 2007, Rode's-Cabau, 2010). In these patients, surgeon has to choose optimal valve and obtain the largest prosthetic valve area. TAVI has excellent hemodynamic performance. In the patients who had myocardial dysfunction, apoptosis of the cardiomyocites triggered by the ischemia, oxidative stress and inflammatory injury during the open heart surgery, could retard the postoperative recovery and improvement of myocardial functions (Anselmi, 2004, Vahasilta, 2005). In these risky patients, TAVI could protect the myocardial functions and LVEF can be increased after the intervention (Webb, 2007; Bauer, 2004; Clavel, 2009).

It was offered to choose mechanical valves in patients having chronic renal disease because of earlier degeneration by rapid calcification of biological valves. But, in ACC/AHA guideline updated in 2006, there is no recommendation for the choice of prosthetic valve type for these patients. Probably, this revision depends on new studies claimed similar results for both mechanical and biological prosthetic valve types for the patients on dialysis (Lucke, 1997; Kaplon, 2000; Herzog, 2002; Brinkman, 2002; Bonow, 2006). After these results, the criteria for the choice of valve type in the patients on dialysis shifted as those in patients without on dialysis. With holding intact parathormon, calcium, and phosphor levels at optimal levels, not only early degeneration of biological valves can be prevented but also the survival the patients on dialysis can be increased (Kazama, 2007; Kimata, 2007; Nakai, 2008). Degeneration of new generation biological valves has decreased in dialysis patients as in those non-dialysis patients with the technological improvements (Brinkman, 2002).

Because of the high mortality ratio after aortic valve replacement, measures should be taken for the prevention of infective endocarditis. Although, infective endocarditis risk after mechanical and biological valve replacement is similar in both prosthetic valve types, in case of a need for aortic valve replacement in a patient with infective endocarditis, allografts have advantages with respect to resistance to active endocarditis. But it is difficult to obtain allografts at any time and the valve durability depends on donor age, time after explantation from donor, and host immunologic response (Yacoup, 1995; Takkenberg 2002).

There are few prospective, randomized studies comparing the valve types used in aortic valve replacement. Besides, the valve types compared in these studies are limited. Large studies comparing all the prosthetic valves the autografts, mechanic valves, xenograft tissue valves will be helpful for the optimal prosthetic valve choice.

Because, the increase of durability for new generation biological valves and the decrease of the elective operations risk by the improvements of surgical techniques, the biological valves will be used widespread in the younger patients (Silberman, 2008; Bonow, 2006). We have to present this option to patients. Thus, the patients could join the decision process for the choice of the prosthetic valve type. Additionally, the patient's should learn the frequency of coagulation monitorization, the possibility for disturbed mechanical valve sound, hemorrhagic complications by using mechanical valve and reoperation caused by the structural degeneration for the biological valves.

In the patients planning to undergo aortic valve replacement, not only the patient's age but also patient's life expectancy, coagulopathy, life-style, occupation, comorbidities, anticoagulant therapy contraindication, surgeon's experience should be reviewed for the choice of the most appropriate prosthetic valve type for each person (Silberman, 2008). In this way, the best survival and improved life quality can be offered to the patient.

The factors should be kept in mind which will be given in details below:

- Patient's age
- Comorbidities
    - Chronic atrial fibrillation
    - Chronic renal failure
    - Malignancies
    - Small aortic annulus
    - Other valve diseases
    - Aortic dilatation
- Active infective endocarditis
- Young women
- Pregnancy
- Redo valve surgery

2. Patient's age

Biologic or mechanical aortic valve prostheses have been widely used in patients with aortic valve disease. The choice of prostheses remains controversial due to the higher rate of structural dysfunction with bioprosthesis and due to the risk of thromboembolism or hemorrhage releated to the anticoagulation treatment of a mechanical prosthesis. The elderly population is increasing due to increase in the human life span. Thus cardiac surgery is increasing in the elderly. In elderly patients with aortic valve replacement, early and long-term results have significantly improved due to technical optimization, better myocardial protection and postoperative management. In studies, the term elderly is often used to describe different population. Some researchers define elderly population as older than 70 years (Tseng, 1997), whereas others define elderly as being older than 65 years (Florath, 2005). Structural failure of bioprostheses are strongly related to the patient's age at valve insertion (Akins, 1998). Bioprostheses have a significantly higher rate of reoperation. Freedom from reoperation for bioprostheses is >95% at 5 years, >90% at 10 years, but <70% at 15 years. However freedom from reoperation for mechanical valves is >95% at 5 years and >90% at 15 years (Desai, 2008). Many cardiac surgeons opt patient age 70 years or older as a routine age for insertion of bioprostheses. Several studies have compared stentless and stented aortic valve bioprosthesis. Stentless aortic bioprostheses were shown to be hemodynamically superior to stented aortic bioprostheses (Borger, 2005; Walther 1999). Stentless aortic bioprostheses provide a larger effective orifice area and lower transvalvular gradients postoperatively because of the absence of a sewing ring and stent. However the implantation of the stentless valve is more difficult and is generally associated with longer myocardial ischemic time and may therefore have a higher perioperative complication rates (Borger, 2005). Choice of mechanical aortic prostheses in elderly patients is often due to different factors, including the use of anticoagulation for other diseases, less need of reoperation and preference of the patient or surgeon. In patients younger than 60 years of age, mechanical prosthesis is recommended because of prosthesis durability (Emery, 2005; Carrier, 2001). In the age between 60 and 70 years, other individual factors have to be taken into account.

Transcatheter aortic valve implantation has become a clinical reality, applied to high-risk patients who are elderly or not operative candidates. TAVI has been developed as an endovascular alternative to surgical aortic valve replacement. This technique is performed with transfemoral or transapical routes. Successful implantation rate has been found between 85% and 100% (Al-Attar, 2009; Johansson, 2011).

Homografts and autologous pulmonary valves are good alternatives for infants and childhood patients. In this method advantages like the growing ability, perfect durability, avoidance of prolonged anticoagulation, excellent hemodynamic performance, low transvalvar pressure gradient, large effective orifice area of pulmonary autologous valve are shown (Alsoufi, 2009; Gatzoulis, 1999). Complications like neoaortic failure seen in the postoperative period has decreased following the improvements in the implantation techniques of autologous pulmonary valves (David, 2000; Takkenberg, 2006), and pulmonary allograft stenosis has decreased due to appropriate usage of anti-inflammatory agents (Carr-White, 2001; Raanani, 2000). For that reason while the usage of aortic route replacement and Ross procedure are getting widespread, on the other hand it is suggested that in case of usage of pulmonary autograft the operation is complex and while during the repair of one valve pathology, two valves are jeopardized (Alexiou, 2000). It is suggested that in the childhood, metallic valves are good alternatives to Ross procedure because of their quite easier implantation, their perfect durability and hemodynamic performance (Alexiou, 2000). In the literature, late period thromboembolism and hemorrhagic complications following mechanical valve replacement in the childhood are reported in a quite low rates (Ibrahim, 1994; Champsaur, 1997; Mazzitelli, 1998; Lupinetti, 1997). The most important disadvantage of the mechanical valves in the childhood is the requirement of replacement of them with bigger size later. However, in a great majority of the childhood patients adult sized mechanical valve replacement is possible with aortoplasty technique

(Nicks, 1970). Thus, it is suggested that in this age group mechanical prosthetic valves are good alternatives of biological ones. Another alternative to Ross procedure are allografts. Allograft aortic valves do not vary in the early and late period due to hemodynamic respect (Lupinetti, 2003).

3. Comorbidities

Atrial fibrillation is the most common arrhythmia in patients undergoing aortic valve surgery (Ngaage, 2006). Many studies show that atrial fibrillation is a risk factor for decreased long-term survival (Vidaillet, 2002; Stewart, 2002). Loss of synchronous atrioventricular contraction results in ventricular dysfunction or congestive heart failure. The Framingham Study shows that stasis of blood flow in the left atrium, three- to five fold increases risk of stroke in a patient with atrial fibrillation (Wolf, 1991). Currently, acetylsalicylic acid and warfarin are approved antithrombotic agents for stroke prevention in patients with atrial fibrillation. However randomized trials are shown that antiplatelet agents are less effective than anticoagulant agents (Hart, 1999). It seems that first choice is mechanical aortic valve because of the need anticoagulant therapy in patients with chronic atrial fibrillation undergoing aortic valve surgery. Nevertheless an old patient more than 60 to 65 years who has atrial fibrillation may be preferable to insert a biologic aortic valve due to an increased risk of bleeding with anticoagulant therapy (Rahimtoola, 2003). If bleeding obliges discontinuing anticoagulant therapy, then this is a risk of thrombosis in patient with mechanical aortic valve.

Patients with chronic renal failure have a poor long-term survival secondary to their underlying renal disease. Four-year survival of patients on hemodialysis or peritoneal dialysis, regardless of whether they undergo valve replacement, is approximately 40% (Brinkman, 2002). Chronic renal failure is also a significant risk factor for increased morbidity and mortality in patients undergoing cardiac surgery (Kogan, 2008). Chronic uremia, hypertension, hyperlipidemia and increased calcium phosphate product associated with secondary hyperparathyroidism predispose to cardiac valvular abnormalities in patients with chronic renal failure. Early studies on biologic valve implantation in these patients show accelerated calcification of bioprosthetic valves (Lamberti, 1978; Monson, 1980). Therefore, mechanical valves were recommended by the ACC/AHA in patient with chronic renal failure and the guideline considered the use of biologic valves potentially harmful. (Bonow, 1998). However, current studies demonstrated that no significant survival difference between mechanical and bilologic valves (Brinkman, 2002; Thourani, 2011). Furthermore, several studies recommend biological valve instead of mechanical valve in patients on chronic dialysis (Lucke, 1997). Chronic renal failure is a known major risk factor for bleeding in patients with anticoagulant therapy (Lanefeld, 1989). These patients have also a increased risk of endocarditis due to frequent vascular access and impaired immunity (Chan, 2006). The type of aortic valve chosen for these patients should be individualized to the age of the patient and expected long-term survival. Older and patients with relative short life expectancy should be considered as candidates for biological aortic valve.

Malignant tumors is another comorbidity in patients undergoing aortic valve replacement. Currently there is no specific study investigating effects of the type of aortic valve prostheses on survival in these patients. However analyses revealed that the presence of a malignant tumor was an independent risk factor on survival after cardiac surgery (Mistiaen,

2004). Life expectancy of the patient who has malignancy has to be considered on decision for choice of prosthetic aortic valve. Biological aortic valve may be a good choice if life expectancy is about five years or less in patients with malignancy (Rahimtoola, 2010).

Aortic valve replacement is an effective therapy for patients with aortic valve pathologies, however, transvalvular gradient is almost always higher than the physiologic gradients of the aortic valve. This gradient is related to the valve size and body surface area. Severe patient-prosthesis mismatch have been found to be associated with increased early and late mortality (Rao, 2000). Aortic root enlargement procedures are an option in patients with small aortic root. However, these techniques have been found to be associated with prolonged myocardial ischemia and perioperative bleeding which is frequently seen in the elderly patients (Kunihara, 2006). Stentless biologic aortic valves or homografts seem like good choice for patients with small aortic root size at risk for patients-prosthesis mismatch (Bonow 2008). Subcoronary implantation of stentless bioprostheses has been associated with residual transvalvular gradients (Milano, 2001). Kunihara and colleagues showed that full aortic root replacement using a stentless aortic bioprostheses may be advantageous in patients with small aortic root (Kunihara, 2006). Transcatheter aortic valve implantation may be an alternative to prevent patient-prosthesis mismatch in high-risk patients (Jilaihawi, 2010). Moderate patient-prosthesis mismatch is generally well tolerated in elderly patients who have small aortic root (Takaseya, 2007). However, the effect of patient-prosthesis mismatch is more important in younger patients. New generation mechanical aortic valve which design to increase orifice area by modifying the outside geometry of the orifice housing may be an option in younger patients with small aortic root (Bach, 2002). Additionally, mechanical aortic valves which can be implanted supraannular position may be preferable in younger patients with small aortic root (Roedler, 2008). Pulmonic valve autotransplantation may be preferred to prevent patient-prosthesis mismatch and allow growth of the autograft in children (Bonow 2008). Root enlargement techniques should be considered in younger patients when a severe patient-prosthesis mismatch can not be avoided with these models of prostheses.

Whether bioprosthesis or mechanical valve in simultaneous aortic and mitral valve surgery will be associated with a better result remains under debate. There is no specific recommendation for surgical strategy of multiple valve disease in ACC/AHA practice guideline (Bonow, 2008). Caus and colleagues reported that the rate of reoperative mortality was significantly higher in patients >65 years who had double valve replacement (Caus, 1999). Hence, some surgeons recommend mechanical valves for the majority of patients in double valve replacement (Urban, 2011). However, a cohort study of 1057 patients showed that biologic valves have the best in-hospital and long-term survival in patient ≥70 years undergoing concomitant aortic and mitral valve replacement (Leavitt, 2009).

Composite graft replacement of the aortic root is a favored technique in dilatation of the ascending aorta associated with aortic valve pathologies. It is more complex than isolated aortic valve replacement. Replacement of the aortic valve and the ascending aorta with a conduit consisting of a mechanical valve and a dacron tube is generally preferred procedure. This technique has been described by Bentall and Debono in 1968 (Bentall H, 1968) and it has led to increased life expectancy for patients with Marfan syndrome. In spite of initial mortality risk is higher, long term survival has been found similar to aortic valve replacement in patients with composite mechanical valve-graft conduit aortic root replacement (Kalkat, 2007). Homografts and conduits consisting of a stented or stentless xenograft valve may be the choice especially in elderly or in patients with endocarditis.

Other option is pulmonary autograft for aortic root replacement. In the study of Akhyari and colleagues, pulmonary autograft had no advantages over composite grafts regarding mid-term morbidity and mortality in aortic position (Akhyari, 2009).

4. Active infective endocarditis

Despite advances in the diagnosis and antibiotic treatment of infective endocarditis, aortic valve endocarditis is most commonly treated surgically by valve replacement in combination with antibiotics. For patients with aortic valve endocarditis, the choice of valve between bioprostheses, homografts and mechanical prostheses remains controversial. According to the ACC/AHA guidelines for management of patients with heart valve disease, valve repair should be preferred because of the risk of infection of prosthetic materials in patients with native valve endocarditis (Bonow, 2006). There is no specific recommendation for use of particular valve prosthesis. In a randomized study, patients with aortic valve endocarditis recieving bioprostheses have been found lower 5-year survival rate than patients recieving mechanical valves and it has been found no difference between patients receiving homografts and mechanical valves (Nguyen, 2010). Wos and colleagues showed that the risk of recurrent endocarditis was higher with bioprostheses than with mechanical valves (Wos, 1996). Guerra et al also found that the risk of endocarditis reinfection is very low with mechanical valves (Guerra, 2001). Homograft seems to be good choice in severe destructive prosthetic (Musci, 2010) or native (Klieverik, 2009) valve endocarditis with aorto-ventricular dehiscence caused by abscess. Petterson et al reported that the Ross operation is an attractive option in patients with aortic valve endocarditis in all age (Petterson, 1998).

5. Prosthetic valve choice in prengnancy

Native valve diseases and prosthetic valve disfunction are still the most important surgical indications in pregnant women requiring heart surgery (Weiss, 1998). Aortic valve diseases can become more symptomatic during pregnancy. A serious aortic stenosis is seen relatively rare in pregnancy. While transvalvular gradient is below 50 mmHg the possibility of heart failure during the pregnancy and delivery is low (Oakley, 2003). In case of aortic stenosis, fetal prognosis due to growth retardation, early delivery or low birth weight is deteriorated (Hameed, 2001; Malhotra 2004). For that reason, in case of asypmtomatic aortic stenosis, with an intervention before pregnancy the becoming the situation more complex can be prevented. As long as left ventricular sistolic function is not impaired aortic insufficiency can be well tolerated during pregnancy. On the other hand severe heart insufficiency can develop in patients with acute aortic failure or low EF (Oakley, 2003). There is not enough experience about the implementation of balloon aortic valvuloplasty during pregnancy. Furthermore, a permanent solution is not provided with this approach (Siu, 1997). However, these approaches can be used as a bridge before the delivery because of the maternal and fetal mortality risk due to serious aortic stenosis and if it is required, a surgical intervention can be applied after the delivery.

It was reported that in case of a development of a valve trombosis during pregnancy in patients with a previous mechanical valve replacement a replacement can be prevented with the addition of trombolytic treatment. However, it has to be known that some complications can be seen with the trombolytic treatment, the success rate is limited, recurrences can be seen after the treatment (Elkayam2005; Roudaut 2003). As the data about this topic is limited the complication rates seen in nonpregnant patients can be taken into consideration. A surgical treatment during pregnancy can be required in patients without benefits despite medical treatments and percutaneous approaches. Although the maternal mortality is below 3% for pregnant patients undergoing CPB with aortic valve replacement, fetal loss reaches 20% (Pomini 1996). Some strategies like avoiding hypotermia, providing enough perfusion pressure are recommended in order to decrease these adverse effects of CPB. Besides that, because of the effects of cardioplegia usage like hemodilution and hyperkalemia, recently some valve operation in beating heart also are reported (Tehrani 2004). The choice of valve type for valve replacement in pregnancy is similar to the choice criteria in young women patients. In a similar way it is difficult to make a decision about the valve choice because of the degeneration risk of the biological valves in young women and the requirement of anticoagulation for the mechanical valves, the fact that the trombosis of the mechanical valves during pregnancy can be a cause of mortality, and the limited data about how the homografts are influenced during pregnancy. However, the participation of the patient in the decision process has to be provided by discussing with the pregnant patient and informating her for all of the possible complications and frequencies. During the decision besides the current pregnancy, the expectation of a new pregnacy in future is also important (Elkayam2005). On the contrary to the results of the previous studies, recent studies have demonstrated that pregnancy does not cause a deterioration or calcification in biological valves (Reimold 2003).

6. Prosthetic valve choice in young women

Especially in the developing countries valve diseases requiring a surical intervention is seen frequently in young age group due to the fact that rheumatic valve diseases are not very uncommon. Although the valve repairement is the most ideal treatment method in young age group, in case of a serious impaired structure of the valve a repairement is not always possible. In that situation valve replacement is needed. A prothesis choice is still a controverisal issue in young patients needing prosthetic valve replacement (Solymar 1991; Trimn 2007). The reason is that all of the chosed prosthetic valves have their own advantages and disadvantages. That's why the decision has to be made according to the most suitable valve alternative for the patients' characteristics. The patient has to be informed about the advantages and disadvantages of the valve types in terms of possible complications. Thereafter, the patient has to be involved in the decision process. Young women have a different situation among the patients undergoing valve surgery because of the pregnancy possibility. The fact that the bioprothesis used in young age can be exposed to early degeneration because of the rapid body metabolism or the requirement of anticoagulants in patients with preference of mechanical prosthetic valves are situations which have to be evaluated seperately. As the valve lesion present before pregnancy will become more pronounced with the pregnancy, patients can undergo a comfortable period during the pregnancy with the intervention to the valve lesion in that period. In these approaches, along with the medical treatment support, when required, balloon-plasty is the first preference. By postponding of the sugical interventions during the pregnancy, maternal and fatal risk due to the surgery is tried to be prevented. Yet if there is no benefit although the applied medical treatment and percutaneous intervention, valve repairment or valve replacement is applied surgically. The main difficulty in that stage is the choice of the valve type which will be used.

The biological grafts include heterografts, homografts and autografts. Among these prothesis, maximal clinical data exists about the porcine heterografts. Biological valves undergo some degeneration in every age and for that reason their long-term durability is influenced which results in a higher rate of valve reoperation (Brais 1985; Jamieson 2003; Gross 1998). In young patients this degeneration is seen more frequently because of the increased calcium turnover, fatigue-induced lesions and collagen degeneration, and discrete immunologic reaction (Berrebi 2001; Gross 1998; Salazar 1999; Badduke 1991; Sbarouni 1994). Additionally, in some studies it was suggested that the usage of biological valves in early periods results in increased rate of degeneration in pregnancy. Besides that, there are also studies demonstrating that the biological valves are not damaged during pregnancy due to the developments in the fixation technics of the first generation biological valves and the valve production technology (Jamieson 1995; North 1999; Salazar 1999). Interestingly, in a study showing that bioprosthesis are more rapidly degenerated during pregnancy, the survey rate of the patients with mechanical valves were found to be lower than those with biological valves (Robyn 1999). These rates were reported to be influenced by the pregnancy rate after the biological valve replacement (Lee 1994). The controversial results in different studies can be influenced by some factors like the inclusion of non-homogeneous populations, disregard of the age of patients, the time period between prosthesis implantation and gestation, and the condition of the prothesis before pregnancy, which avoids the correct evaluation of the data. Additionally, data about long-term follow up, especially in case of repeated pregnancies, is also unsufficient. Althougt there is no consensus about the influence of the pregnancy on biological valve degeneration, this possibility has to be told to the potential pregnant patient. The reason is that re-replacement is needed for the patients with degenerated biological valves. Especially the risks of such operations during pregnancy in terms of maternal and fetal prognosis has to be denoted. Fifty percent of the patients who undergone biological valve replacement in young age require a reoperation 10 years later. It means that almost all of these patients will undergo at least one re-operation during their life period (Elkayam 2005). The mortality rate following such a re-operation is reported as 3.8-8.7% (Jamieson 1995; Badduke 1991). Shaer et al. showed in their 18 years follow-up study that pregnancy has no additive contribution to the structural degeneration of biological valves. The importance of that study is that all of the patients included in the study have similar characteristic features (Fayez 2005). In studies comparing two different type heterografts used in young patients (Hancock and Carpentier-Edwards porcine bioprostheses), a structural valve deterioration in a rate of 50-70% in 10 years follow-up was demonstrated (Yum 1995; Jamieson 1988). Similarly, North et al. reported that structural valve deterioration in 10 years follow-up can be seen in high rates as 82% [preg9/5]. As it is seen the valve choice influences not only the possible complications but also the patient's survival. In a recent study about the usage of the last generation biological valves in young patients, it was shown that the valve degeneration is quite low and survival rates are distinctly high. These good results are suggested to be due to the usage of new fixation technics and the development of agents used for anti-mineralization (Carpentier 1995).

The biological valves are less thrombogenic than the mechanical valves. For that reason anticoagulation is not needed. However, tromboembolic complications due to biological valves, although rarely, are seen. They can be seen especially in the first days following valve replacement before the development of an endothelization. The annual tromboembolism risk following biological valve replacement is 0.7% (North 1999).

Patients using mechanical valves can feel uncomfortable because of the valve sounds, are more frequently asked to come for outpatient visits and need more closed monitorization with blood tests. Besides that, the mechanical prosthetic valves are not degenerated by time. The usage of anticoagulants is essential. Some physiological changes are seen with pregnancy. Fibrinogen level can increase and reach to two folds levels than normally. As factors VII, VIII, IX, and XII are increasing in the third trimestre, antritrombin II level is decreasing. Duration of pregnancy, body composition and rapid fluid shifts were demonstrated as factors influencing the coagulation system. Blood volume, viscosity, intraabdominal pressure increase and venous compression also increases (Al-Lawati AA, 2002). As there is a presence of naturally hypercoagulable state the dose of the anticoagulant treatment should be kept higher. The rate of mechanical valve trombosis reaches 14% because of this hypercoagulable state (Abbas, 2005). A maternal mortality rate of 10% is seen in these patients (Weiss BM, 1998). On the other hand, complications due to high dose anticoagulants is seen more frequently too. The superiority of the biological valves was emphasized in the retrospective evaluations of the first generation mechanicalal valves in order to avoid the complications due to high dose anticoagulants (Jamieson, 1993; Cannegieter, 1994). However, the tendency to trombosis of the mechanicalal prosthetic valves in that period was higher.
With the development of a new generation of mechanical valves, optimal anticoagulation doses were provided too. However, the usage of anticoagulants during pregnancy is still a controversial issue. Actually, as a common practice, after heparin usage in the first tremestre, warfarin treatment is used up to the expected delivery time, and then heparin is used instead again. Although there are centers accepting this procedure reliable, this subject is still a controversial subject because of the present complications (Salazar, 1996; Ismail, 1986; Pavankumar; 1988). For that reason there is no distinct concensus about the ideal anticoagulant treatment in terms of maternal and fetal prognosis. Warfarin is a good anticoagulant. But as it can pass placenta, fetal malformation, fetal loss and peripartum haemorrage can be seen in the organogenesis stage. These effects of warfarin were shown to be dose dependent [Oakley, 2003; Hanania, 2001). Although it is shown that when a 5 mg dose was not exceeded it is not a cause of embriopathy, it is known that it increases the rates of abortus. For that reason it is suggested that the embriopathy rates seen in the live births is relatively lower. Especially because of embriopathy occurring with warfarin usage between 6 and 12 weeks, a shifting heparin treatment is offered in this period (Iturbe-Alessio; 1986). As heparin is a large molecule and can not pass the placenta, negative effects on fetus is not expected. Additionally, heparin was not found to be associated with bleeding during the peripartum period (Noller, 1982; Iturbe-Alessio; 1986). For that reason warfarin treatment should be replaced with heparin treatment in the post 36 week period. A mortality rate of 1-4% is seen in the pregnant patients with mechanicalal prosthetic valves, which is more commonly due to valve thrombosis (Chan, 2000; Elkayam, 2005) The usage of heparin during pregnancy was shown to be a cause of maternal tromboemboli states like occlusive prosthetic thrombosis, including fatal events (Sbarouni, 1994; Hanania, 1994; Salazar, 1996; Oakley, 2003). The usage of low molecule weight heparins is not recommended in the pregnancy period because of the difficulty in their monitorization and titration, and their close relationship with the tromboembolic events (Iturbe-Alessio, 1986; Salazar, 1996; Meschengieser 1999). Although under current conditions warfarin seems to be more appropriate treatment method because of the reduction in maternal complications, most female patients, when they are informed, do not want to use this drug because of its fetal

effects. Moreover, even in the second trimestre, they do not want to stop heparin and go on with heparin treatment (Evans, 1997; Yinon, 2009)

Yinon et al. evaluated the usage of low molecule weight heparin and aspirin in patients with mechanicalal prosthetic valve replacement who do not want to use warfarin during pregnancy because of its embriopathy risk. The study reported that even in patients followed-up with carefull monitorization the rate of the maternal cardiac and fetal complications is high and bleeding is seen (Yinon, 2009). Additionally, non-cardiac complication rates like postpartum bleeding was found to be as high as 13%, which is higher than it is reported in the previous studies.

In order to avoid these possible complications the effect of the anticoagulation therapy during pregnancy has to be closely monitorized. It is important to identify the most important strategy by transition between warfarin and heparin in the distinct periods of pregnancy.

Homografts can be an alternative for the young women at childbearing age. There is no evident data about the possible complications of this valve not needing an anticoagulation and its generation during pregnancy (Yacoub, 1995; Waszyrowski, 1997). However, some studies in the literature gave an idea. Robyn et al. showed that less degeneration is seen after the usage of homograft in comparison with biological prosthetic valve users and less requirement of reoperation is needed (Robyn 1999). Similarly, North et al. reported in a recent study that homografts are more resistant in comparison with bioprosthetic valves in 10 years follow-up and structural valve detorioration is developed more infrequently (72% vs. 18%) (North 1999). It was shown that there was less structural failure requiring reoperation in homografts in comparison with biological grafts (Yum, 1995; Jamieson, 1988). Studies evaluating the effects of pregnancy on homografts are even more limited. Sadler et al. reported that 94% live births had eventuated in patients followed-up following homograft valve replacement and only in two patients a heart failure developed during pregnancy (Sadler, 2000). Although there are studies supporting these results, data about how the homograft are effected during pregnancy is still limited (Dyke, 2003). Prospective studies in future can suggest homografts as appropriate alternatives in young women.

Especially for young women who wants to get pregnant Ross procedure can be a good alternative because its perfect valve hemodynamics and not being thrombogenic [Al-Halees, 2002). However this opertaion is difficult in terms of technical aspect and as the operative mortality is reported as 2-13% in different studies it has to be performed in experienced centres (Rahimtoola, 2003; Takkenberg, 2002; Schmidtke 2003). Additionally, the effects of pregnancy on Ross procedure in not clear, as for homografts (Schmidtke, 2003; Dore,1997; Martin, 2003). Dore and Somerville (Dore,1997) reported in their study made with small number of patients that serious complications like mortality, trombo-embolic event or bleeding was not observed in patients who underwent Ross procedure. But, as there is not enough data for this surgical technique, its usage in young women who have potential for becoming pregnant is not still widespread.

As a conclusion, the optimal prosthetic cardiac valve for the women at childbearing age is still a controversial subject. The reason is that there is no consensus about the effects of anticoagulants and side effects in the research studies. The degenerative effects of biological valves on pregnancy is not clearly known. There are studies showing the effects of trombolytic studies even in trombosis of mechanicalal prosthetic valves. The reoperation carried out after the degeneration of biological valves was reported to be more safely performed. As it is seen, these study results give different messages. For that reason, in a process of making a choice for the prosthetic valve, a comparison should be made according to the degeneration risk of biological valves, tromboemboli due to mechanicalal prosthetic valves and bleeding complications due to anticoagulants. In summary, every patient has to be evaluated individually in order to make a desicion what is the best for her or him. (Mihaljevic, 2005). All of these results should be shared with the patient before the operation.

6.1 A valve selection for the reoperation

Sometimes a valve replacement because of valvular or non-valvular reasons is needed to be performed again. A valve replacement is made because of different reasons like the valve degeneration, calcification or valve thrombosis of the previously replaced prosthetic valve, endocarditis, dehicence, or pannus formation. In that situation, the selection of the prosthetic valve needed for the replacement should be made according to the individual characteristics. When in case of active prosthetic valve endocarditis tissue valve more resistant to infection is selected, age factor should be taken into consideration too. Especially a rapid degeneration in a patient with previously selected biological valve can be a cautionary signal that this situation can be eventuated again. A comprehensive information about the both prosthetic valve types should be given to the patient before the reoperation. Thereafter, the final decision about the valve choice should be taken together with the patient.

Recently developed percutaneous aortic valve replacement can also be appropriate alternative for the reoperation. Especially it is an appropriate alternative for the patients in whom the reoperation is riskly because of comorbid situations (Fusari, 2009). With this new approach called as "valve-in-valve", trans-catheter stent valve is implanted percutaneously in the degenerated biological valve. The early results of this tecnique are promissing, but the long period results are not still known [Gotzmann, 2011, Fusari, 2009, Ye, 2007). At the same time, it should not be forgotten that complications like occlusion of the coronary ostiums, endocarditis, embolization of the prosthesis, iatrogenic aortic dissection can be seen (Tay, 2011; Kukucka, 2011; Carnero-Alcázar 2010).

7. References

Abbas AE, Lester SJ & Connolly H. (2005). Pregnancy and the cardiovascular system. *Int J Cardiol* 98:179–189.

Akins CW, Buckley MJ, Daggett WM et al. (1998). Risk of reoperative valve replacement for failed mitral and aortic bioprostheses. *Ann Thorac Surg* 65:1545-1552.

Akhyari P, Bara C, Kofidis T, Khaladj N, Haverich A & Klima U. (2009). Aortic root and ascending aortic replacement. Bentall or Ross Procedure? *In Heart J* 50:47-57.

Al-Attar N, Himbert D, Descoutures F et al. (2009). Transcatheter Aortic Valve Implantation: Selection Strategy Is Crucial for Outcome. *Ann Thorac Surg* 87:1757-1763.

Albertucci M, Wong K, Petrou M, et al. (1994). The use of unstented homograft valves for aortic valve reoperations: Review of a twenty-three-year experience. *J Thorac Cardiovasc Surg* 107:152-161.

Alexiou C, McDonald A, Langley SM, Dalrymple-Hay MJ, Haw MP & Monro JL. (2000). Aortic valve replacement in children: are mechanical prostheses a good option? *Eur J Cardiothorac Surg* 17:125-133.

Al-Halees Z, Pieters F, Qadoura F, Shahid M, Al-Amri M & Al-Fadley F. (2002). The Ross procedure is the procedure of choice for congenital aortic valve disease. *J Thorac Cardiovasc Surg* 123:437- 441.

Al-Lawati AA, Venkitraman M, Al-Delaime T & Valliathu J. (2002). Pregnancy and mechanical heart valves replacement; dilemma of anticoagulation. *Eur J Cardiothorac Surg*. 22:223–227.

Alsoufi B, Manlhiot C, McCrindle BW, Canver CC, Sallehuddin A, Al-Oufi S, Joufan M & Al-Halees Z. (2009) Aortic and mitral valve replacement in children: is there any role for biologic and bioprosthetic substitutes? *Eur J Cardiothorac Surg* 36:84-90.

Anselmi A, Abbate A, Girola F, Nasso G, Biondi-Zoccai GG, Possati G & Gaudino M. (2004). Myocardial ischemia, stunning, inflammation, and apoptosis during cardiac surgery: a review of evidence. *Eur J Cardiothorac Surg* 25:304–311.

Bach, DS, Sakwa MP, Goldbach M, Petracek MR, Emery RW & Mohr FW. (2002). Hemodynamics and early clinical performance of the St. Jude medical regent mechanical aortic valve. *Ann Thorac Surg* 74:2003-2009.

Bach DS, Kon ND, Dumesnil JG, et al. (2005). Ten year outcome after aortic valve replacement with the Freestyle stentless bioprosthesis. *Ann Thorac Surg* 80:480-487.

Badduke BR, Jamieson WR, Miyagishima RT, et al. (1991). Pregnancy and childbearing in a population with biologic valvular prostheses. *J Thorac Cardiovasc Surg* 102:179-186.

Bakhtiary F, Schiemann M, Dzemali O, et al. (2006). Stentless bioprostheses improve postoperative coronary flow more than stented prostheses after valve replacement for aortic stenosis. *J Thorac Cardiovasc Surg* 131:883-888.

Bauer F, Eltchaninoff H, Tron C, et al. (2004). Acute improvement in global and regional left ventricular systolic function after percutaneous heart valve implantation in patients with symptomatic aortic stenosis. *Circulation* 110: 1473–1476.

Ben Ismail M, Abid F, Trabeisi S, Tarktak M, Fekih M. (1986). Cardiac valve prostheses, and pregnancy anticoagulation. *Br Heart J* 55:101–105.

Bentall H, De Bono A. (1968). A Technique for complete replacement of the ascending aorta. *Thorax* 23:338-339.

Berrebi AJ, Carpentier SM, Phan KP, Nguyen VP, Chauvaud SM & Carpentier A. (2001). Results of up to 9 years of high-temperature-fixed valvular bioprostheses in a young population. *Ann Thorac Surg* 71(5 Suppl.):S353—355.

Bonow RO, Carabello BA, deLeon AC Jr, et al. (1998). Guidelines for the management of patients with valvular heart disease: executive summary. A report of the American College of Cardiology / American Heart Association Task Force on Practice Guidelines. *Circulation* 98:1949–1984.

Bonow RO, Carabello BA, Chatterjee K, et al. (2006). ACC/AHA2006 practice guidelines for the management of patients with valvular heart disease: Executive summary: A report of the American College of Cardiology/American Heart Association Task Force on Practice Guidelines. *J Am Coll Cardiol* 48:598-675.

Bonow RO, Carabello B, Chatterjee K, et al. (2006). ACC/AHA 2006 guidelines for the management of patients with valvular heart disease: a report of the American College of Cardiology/American Heart Association Task Force on Practice Guidelines (writing committee to revise the 1998 Guidelines for the Management of Patients With Valvular Heart Disease): developed in collaboration with the Society of Cardiovascular Anesthesiologists: endorsed by the Society for Cardiovascular

Angiography and Interventions and the Society of Thoracic Surgeons. *Circulation* 114:e84–231.

Bonow RO, Carabello BA, Chatterjee K, et al. (2008). 2008 Focused update incorporated into the ACC/AHA 2006 Guidelines for management of patients with valvular heart disease. A report of the American College of Cardiology/American Heart Association Task Force on Practice Guidelines (Writing Committee to revise the 1998 guidelines for management of patients with valvular heart desease). Endorsed by the Society of Cardiovascular Anesthesiologists, Society for Cardiovascular Anjiography and Interventions, and Society of Thoracic Surgeons. J Am Coll Cardiol 52:e1-142.

Borger MA, Carson SM, Ivanov J et al. (2005). Stentless Aortic Valves are Hemodynamically Superior to Stented Valves During Mid-Term Follow-Up: A Large Retrospective Study. *Ann Thorac Surg* 80:2180-2185.

Brais M, Bedard P, Goldstein W, et al. (1985). Ionescu-Shiley pericardial xenografts and follow up of up to 6 years. *Ann Thorac Surg* 39:105-111.

Brinkman WT, Williams WH, Guyton RA, Jones EL & Craver JM. (2002). Valve replacement in patients on chronic dialysis: Implications for valve prosthesis selection. *Ann Thorac Surg* 74:37-42.

Cannegieter SC, Rosendaal FR & Briet E. (1994). Thromboembolic and bleeding complications in patients with mechanical heart valve prostheses. *Circulation* 89:635- 641.

Carnero-Alcázar M, Maroto Castellanos LC, Carnicer JC & Rodríguez Hernández JE. (2010). Transapical aortic valve prosthetic endocarditis. *Interact Cardiovasc Thorac Surg* 11(3):252-253.

Carpentier SM, Carpentier AF, Chen L, Shen M, Quintero LJ & Witzel TH. (1995). Calcium mitigation in bioprosthetic tissues by iron pretreatment: the challenge of iron leaching. *Ann Thorac Surg* 60:S332–S338.

Carrier M, Pellerin M, Perrault LP et al. (2001). Aortic Valve Replacement With Mechanical and Biologic Prostheses in Middle-Aged Patients. *Ann Thorac Surg* 71:S253-256.

Carr-White GS, Kilner PJ, Hon JK, Rutledge T, Edwards S, Burman ED, Pennell DJ & Yacoub MH. (2001). Incidence, location, pathology, and significance of pulmonary homograft stenosis after the Ross operation. *Circulation* 104 (12 Suppl 1):I16-20.

Caus T, Albertini JN, Chi Y, Collart F, Monties JR & Mesana T. Multiple valve replacement increases the risk of reoperation for structural degeneration of bioprostheses. *J Heart Valve Dis* 8:376-383.

Champsaur G, Robin J, Tronc F, Curtil A, Ninet J, Sassolas F, Vedrinne C & Bozio A. (1997). Mechanical valve in aortic position is a valid option in children and adolescents. *Eur J Cardiothorac Surg* 11:117-122.

Chan V, Jamieson E, Fleisher AG, Denmark D, Chan F & Germann E. (2006). Valve replacement surgery in end-stage renal failure: Mechanical prostheses versus bioprostheses. *Ann Thorac Surg* 81:857-862.

Chan WS, Anand S & Ginsberg JS. (2000). Anticoagulation of pregnant women with mechanical heart valves: a systematic review of the literature. *Arch Intern Med* 160:191–196.

Clavel MA, Webb JG, Pibarot P, et al. (2009). Comparison of the hemodynamic performance of percutaneous and surgical bioprostheses for the treatment of severe aortic stenosis. *J Am Coll Cardiol* 53:1883–1891.

Cosgrove DM, Lytle BW, Taylor PC, et al. (1995). The Carpentier-Edwards pericardial aortic valve. Ten-year results. *J Thorac Cardiovasc Surg* 110:651-662.

Cribier A, Eltchaninoff H, Tron C, et al. (2006). Treatment of calcific aortic stenosis with the percutaneous heart valve: mid-term follow-up from the initial feasibility studies: the French experience. *J Am Coll Cardiol* 47:1214–1223.

David TE, Omran A, Ivanov J, Armstrong S, de Sa MP, Sonnenberg B & Webb G. (2000). Dilation of the pulmonary autograft after the Ross procedure. *J Thorac Cardiovasc Surg* 119:210-220.

De Santo LS, Romano G, Della Corte A, et al. (2005). Mitral mechanical replacement in young rheumatic women: analysis of long-term survival, valve-related complications, and pregnancy outcomes over a 3707-patient-year follow-up. *J Thorac Cardiovasc Surg* 130:13-19.

Del Rizzo DI, Goldman BS, Joyner CP, et al. (1994). Initial clinical experience with the Toronto stentless porcine valve. *J Card Surg* 9:379-385.

Desai MD, Christakis GT. (2008). Bioprosthetic Aortic Valve Replacement: Stented Pericardial and Porcine Valves, In: *Cardiac Surgery in the Adult,* Cohn LH. pp. 877, McGraw-Hill Companies, New York.

Dore A & Sommerville J. (1997). Pregnancy in patients with pulmonary autograft valve replacement. *Eur Heart J* 18:1659–1662.

Dyke & Igic. (2003). Management of Prosthetic Heart Valve Anticoagulation in Pregnancy. *ACC Current Journal Review* 17-22.

El-Hamamsy I, Eryigit Z, Stevens LM, et al. (2010). Long-term outcomes after autograft versus homograft aortic root replacement in adults with aortic valve disease: a randomised controlled trial. *Lancet* 376:524-531.

Elkayam U. (2005). Valvular heart disease and pregnancy. Part II: Prosthetic valves. *J Am Coll Cardiol* 46:403–410.

El SF, Hassan W, Latroche B, et al. (2005). Pregnancy has no effect on the rate of structural deterioration of bioprosthetic valves: Long-term 18-year follow up results. *J Heart Valve Dis* 14:481-485.

Emery RW, Krogh CC, Arom KV et al. (2005). The St. Jude Medical Cardiac Valve Prosthesis: A 25-Year Experience With Single Valve Replacement. *Ann Thorac Surg* 79:776-783.

Florath I, Albert A, Rosendahl U, Alexander T, Ennker IC & Ennker J. (2005). Mid term outcome and quality of life after aortic valve replacement in elderly people: mechanical versus stentless biological valves. *Heart* 91:1023–1029.

Fusari M, Alamanni F, Bona V, et al. (2009). Transcatheter aortic valve implantation in the operating room: early experience. *J Cardiovasc Med (Hagerstown)* 10(5):383-393.

Gatzoulis MA. (1999). Ross procedure: the treatment of choice for aortic valve disease? *Int J Cardiol* 71:205-206.

Gotzmann M, Bojara W, Lindstaedt M, et al. (2011). One-year results of transcatheter aortic valve implantation in severe symptomatic aortic valve stenosis. *Am J Cardiol* 107(11):1687-1692.

Gross C, Klima U, Mair R & Brücke P. (1998). Aortic homografts versus mechanical valves in aortic valve replacement in young patients: a retrospective study. *Ann Thorac Surg* 66(6 Suppl):S194-S197.

Guerra JM, Tornos MP, Permanyer-Miralda G, et al. (2001). Long term results of mechanical prostheses for treatment of active infective endocarditis. Heart 86:63-68.

Hameed A, Karaalp IS, Tummala PP, et al. (2001). The effect of valvular heart disease on maternal and fetal outcome during pregnancy. *J Am Coll Cardiol* 37:893–899.

Hammermeister K, Sethi GK, Henderson WG, Grover FL, Oprian C & Rahimtoola SH. (2000). Outcomes 15 years after valve replacement with a mechanical versus a bioprosthetic valve: Final report of the veterans affairs randomized trial. *J Am Coll Cardiol* 36:1152-1158.

Hanania G. (2001). Management of anticoagulants during pregnancy. *Heart* 86:125–126.

Hanania G, Thomas D, Michel PL, et al. (1994). Pregnancy and prosthetic heart valves: a French cooperative retrospective study of 155 cases. *Eur Heart J* 15:1651–1658.

Harken DE, Soroff HS, Taylor WJ, et al. Partial and complete prostheses in aortic insufficiency. (1960). *J Thorac Cardiovasc Surg* 40:744-762.

Hart RG, Benavente O, McBride R & Pearce LA. (1999). Antithrombotic therapy to prevent stroke in patients with atrial fibrillation: a meta-analysis. *Ann Intern Med* 131: 492-501.

Hassanein W, Albert A, Florath I, Hegazy YY, Rosendahl U, Bauer S & Ennker J. (2007). Concomitant aortic valve replacement and coronary bypass: the effect of valve type on the blood flow in bypass grafts. *Eur J Cardiothorac Surg* 31:391-396.

Herzog CA, Ma JZ & Collins AJ. (2002). Long-term survival of dialysis patients in the United States with prosthetic heart valves: should ACC/AHA practice guidelines on valve selection be modified? *Circulation* 105:1336–41.

Ibrahim M, Cleland J, O'Kane H, Gladstone D, Mullholland C & Craig B. (1994). St Jude Medical prosthesis in children. *J Thorac Cardiovasc Surg* 108:52-56.

Iturbe-Alessio I, Fonseca MC, Mutchinik O, Santos MA, Zajarias A & Salazar E. Risks of anticoagulant therapy in pregnant women with artificial heart valves. *N Engl J Med* 1986;315:1390-1393.

Jamieson WR. (1993). Modern cardiac valve devices: bioprostheses and mechanical prostheses: state of the art. *J Card Surg* 8:89 –98.

Jamieson WRE, Burr LH, Miyagishima RT, et al. (2003). Reoperation for bioprosthetic aortic structural failure risk assessment. *Eur J Cardiothorac Surg* 24:873-878.

Jamieson WRE, Miller DC, Akims CW, et al. (1995). Pregnancy and bioprostheses: influence of structural valve deterioration. *Ann Thorac Surg* 60 Suppl:S282–S287.

Jamieson WR, Burr LH, Miyagishima RT, et al. (1995). Structural deterioration in Carpentier-Edwards standard and supraannular porcine bioprostheses. *Ann Thorac Surg* 60(2 Suppl):S241-247.

Jamieson WRE, Rosado LJ, Munro AI, et al. (1988). Carpentier-Edwards standard porcine bioprostheses: primary tissue failure (structure valve deterioration) by age groups. *Ann Thorac Surg* 46:155- 162.

Jilaihawi H, Chin D, Spyt T, et al. (2010). Prosthesis-patient mismatch after transcatheter aortic valve implantation with th Medtronic-Corevalve bioprosthesis. *Eur Heart J* 31:857-864.

Johansson M, Nozohoor S, Kimblad PO, Harnek J, Olivecrona GK & Sjögren J. (2011). Transapical Versus Transfemoral Aortic Valve Implantation: A Comparison of Survival and Safety. *Ann Thorac Surg* 91:57-63.

Kalkat MS, Edwards MB, Taylor KM & Bonser RS. (2007). Composite aortic valve graft replacement. Mortality outcomes in a national registry. *Circulation* 116(Suppl I): I-301-I-306.

Kaplon RJ, Cosgrove DM, Gillinov AM, Lytle BW, Blackstone EH & Smedira NG. (2000). Cardiac valve replacement in patients on dialysis: Infl uence of prosthesis on survival. *Ann Thorac Surg* 70:438–441.

Kazama JJ. (2007). Japanese Society of Dialysis Therapy treatment guidelines for secondary hyperparathyroidism. *Ther Apher Dial* 11(suppl 1):S44–47.

Khan SS, Trento A, DeRobertis M, et al. (2001). Twenty-year comparison of tissue and mechanical valve replacement. *J Thorac Cardiovasc Surg* 122):257-269.

Kimata N, Miwa N, Otsubo S, et al. (2007). Achievement of the Japanese Society for Dialysis Therapy guideline targets for mineral metabolism measures: One Japanese university center result. *Ther Apher Dial* 11(suppl 1):S62–66.

Klieverik LMA, Yacoup MH, Edwards S, et al. Surgical treatment of actice native aortic valve endocarditis with allografts and mechanical prostheses. *Ann Thorac Surg* 88:1814-1821.

Kogan A, Medalion B, Kornowski R, et al. (2008). Cardiac surgery in patients on chronic hemodialysis: short and long-term survival. *Thorac Cardiovasc Surg* 56:123–127.

Kolh P, Kerzmann A, Honore C, Comte L & Limet R. (2007). Aortic valve surgery in octogenarians: predictive factors for operative and long-term results. *Eur J Cardiothorac Surg* 31:600-606.

Kukucka M, Pasic M, Dreysse S & Hetzer R. (2011). Delayed subtotal coronary obstruction after transapical aortic valve implantation. *Interact Cardiovasc Thorac Surg* 12(1):57-60.

Kunihara T, Schmidt K, Glombitza P, Dzindzibadze V, Lausberg H & Schafers HJ. (2006). Root replacement using stentless valves in the small aortic root: A propensity score analysis. 82:1379-1384.

Lamberti JJ, Wainer BH, Fisher KA, Karunaratne HB & Al- Sadir J. (1978). Calcific stenosis of the porcine heterograft. Ann Thorac Surg 28:28–32.

Lanefeld CS & Goldman L. (1989). Major bleeding in outpatients treated with warfarin: incidence and prediction by factors known at the start of outpatient therapy. *Am J Med* 87:147–152.

Langley SM, McGuirk SP, Chaudhry MA, Livesey SA, Ross JK & Monro JL. (1999). Twenty-year follow-up of aortic valve replacement with antibiotic sterilized homografts in 200 patients. Semin Thorac Cardiovasc Surg 11(4 Suppl 1):28-34.

Leavitt BJ, Baribeau YR, DiScipio AW, et al. (2009). Outcomes of patients of undergoing concomitant aortic and mitral valve surgery in Northern New England. Circulation 120(suppl 1):S155-S162.

Lee CW, Wu CC, Lin PY, Hsieh FJ & Chen HY. (1994). Pregnancy following cardiac prosthetic valve replacement. *Obstet Gynecol* 83:353– 6.

Lucke JC, Samy RN, Atkins BZ, et al. (1997). Results of valve replacement with mechanical and biological prosthesis in chronic renal dialysis patients. *Ann Thorac Surg* 64:129-132.

Lupinetti F, Warner J, Jones TK & Herndon P. (1997). Comparison of human tissues and mechanical prostheses for aortic valve replacement in children. *Circulation* 96:321-325.

Lupinetti FM, Duncan BW, Lewin M, Dyamenahalli U & Rosenthal GL. (2003). Comparison of autograft and allograft aortic valve replacement in children. *J Thorac Cardiovasc Surg* 126:240-246.

Malhotra M, Sharma JB, Tripathii R, Arora P & Arora R. (2004). Maternal and fetal outcome in valvular heart disease. *Int J Gynaecol Obstet* 84:11–16.

Martin TC, Idahosa V, Ogunbiyi A, Fevrier-Roberts G & Winter A. (2003). Successful pregnancy and delivery after pulmonary autograft operation (Ross procedure) for rheumatic aortic valve insufficiency. *West Indian Med J* 52:62– 64.

Masters RG, Haddad M, Pipe AL, Veinot JP & Mesana T. (2004). Clinical outcomes with the Hancock II bioprosthetic valve. *Ann Thorac Surg* 78:832-836.

Mazzitelli D, Guenther T, Schreiber C, Wottke M, Michel J & Meisner H. (1998). Aortic valve replacement in children: are we on the right track? *Eur J Cardiothorac Surg* 13:565-571.

Meschengieser SS, Fondevila CG, Santarelli MT & Lazzari MA. (1999). Anticoagulation in pregnant women with mechanical heart valve prostheses. *Heart* 82:23-26.

Mihaljevic T, Paul S, Leacche M, Rawn JD, Cohn LH & Byrne JG. (2005). Valve replacement in women of childbearing age: influences on mother, fetus and neonate. *J Heart Valve Dis* 151-1577.

Milano AD, Blanzola C, Mecozzi G, D'Alfanzo A, De Carlo M, Nardi C & Bartolotti U. (2001). Hemodynamic performance of stented and stentless aortic bioprostheses. *Ann Thorac Surg* 72:33-38.

Mistiaen WP, Cauwelaert PV, Muylaert P, Wuyts F, Harrisson F & Bortier H. (2004). Effects of prior malignancy on survival after cardiac surgery. *Ann Thorac Surg* 77:1593-1597.

Monson BK, Wickstrom PH, Haglin JJ, Francis G, Comty CM & Helseth MK. (1980). Cardiac operation and end stage renal disease. Ann Thorac Surg 30:267–272.

Musci M, Hübler M, Amiri A, et al. (2010). Surgical treatment for active infective prosthetic valve endocarditis: 22-year single-centre experience. Eur J Cardiothorac Surg 38:528-538.

Nakai S, Akiba T, Kazama J, et al. (2008). Effects of serum calcium, phosphorus, and intact parathyroid hormone levels on survival in chronic hemodialysis patients in Japan. *Ther Apher Dial* 12: 49–54.

Ngaage AL, Schaff HV, Barnes SA et al. (2006). Prognostic implications of preoperative atrial fibrillation in patients undergoing aortic valve replacement: Is there an argument for concomitant arrhythmia surgery? *Ann Thorac Surg 82:1392-1399.*

Nguyen DT, Delahaye F, Obadia JF, et al. (2010). Aortic valve replacement for active endocarditis: 5-year survival comparison of bioprostheses, homografts and mechanical prostheses. *Eur J Cardiothorac Surg* 37:1025-1032.

Nicks R, Cartmill T & Bernstein L. (1970). Hypoplasia of the aortic root. *Thorax* 25:339-346.

North RA, Sadler L, Stewart AW, McCowan LM, Kerr AR & White HD. 1999. Long-term survival and valve-related complications in young women with cardiac valve replacements. *Circulation* 99:2669–2676.

Oakley C, Child A, Iung B, Presbitero P & Tornos P. (2003). Task Force on the management of cardiovascular diseases during pregnancy of the European Society of Cardiology. Expert consensus document on management of cardiovascular diseases during pregnancy. *Eur Heart J* 24:761–781.

Pavankumar P, Venugopal P, Kaul U, Lyer KS, Sas B & Sampathkumar A. (1988). Pregnancy in patients with prosthetic cardiac valves - a 10 year experience. *Scand J Thorac Cardiovasc Surg* 22:19–22.

Petterson G, Tingleff J & Joyce FS. (1998). Treatment of aortic valve endocarditis with the Ross operation. *Eur J Cardiothorac Surg* 13:678-684.

Pomini F, Mercogliano D, Cavalletti C, et al. (1996). Cardiopulmonary bypass in pregnancy. *Ann Thorac Surg* 61:259-268.

Potter DD, Sundt TM 3rd, Zehr KJ, et al. (2005). Operative risk of reoperative aortic valve replacement. *J Thorac Cardiovasc Surg* 129:94-103.

Raanani E, Yau TM, David TE, Dellgren G, Sonnenberg BD & Omran A. (2000) Risk factors for late pulmonary homograft stenosis after the Ross procedure. *Ann Thorac Surg* 70:1953-1957.

Rahimtoola SH. (2003). Choice of prosthetic heart valve in adults. *J Am Coll Cardiol* 41:893-904.

Rahimtoola SH. (2010). Choice of prosthetic heart valve in adults. An Update. *J Am Coll Cardiol* 55:2413-2426.

Rao V, Jamieson WR, Ivanov J, Armstrong S & David TE. (2000). Prosthesis-patient mismatch affects survival after aortic valve replacement. *Circulation* 102(19 Suppl 3):III5-9.

Reimold SC & Rutherford JD. (2003). Valvular heart disease in pregnancy. *N Engl J Med* 349:52–59.

Rode´s-Cabau J, Webb JG, Cheung A, et al. (2010). Transcatheter aortic valve implantation for the treatment of severe symptomatic aortic stenosis in patients at very high or prohibitive surgical risk: acute and late outcomes of the multicenter Canadian experience. *J Am Coll Cardiol* 55:1080–1090.

Roedler S, Czerny M, Neuhauser J, et al. (2008). Mechanical aortic valve prostheses in the small aortic root: Top Hat versus standard CarbomMedics aortic valve. *Ann Thorac Surg* 86:64-70.

Ross DN. (1967). Replacement of aortic and mitral valves with a pulmonary autograft. Lancet 2:956-958.

Roudaut R, Lafitte S, Roudaut MF, et al. (2003). Fibrinolysis of mechanical prosthetic valve thrombosis: a single-center study of 127 cases. *J Am Coll Cardiol* 41: 653–658.

Sadler L, McCowan L, White H, et al. (2000). Pregnancy outcomes and cardiac complications in women with mechanical bioprosthetic and homografts valves. *BJOG* 107:245–253.

Salam AM & Al-Mousa EN. (2004). The therapeutic potential of ximelagatran to become the anticoagulant of choice in medicine: a review of recently completed clinical trials. *Expert Opin Pharmacother* 5:1423-1430.

Salazar E, Espinola N, Roman L & Casanova JM. (1999). Effect of pregnancy on the duration of bovine pericardial bioprostheses. *Am Heart J* 137:714-720.

Salazar E, Iziguirre R, Verdego J & Mutchinick O. (1996). Failure of adjusted doses of subcutaneous heparin to prevent thrombo-embolic phenomena in pregnant patients with mechanical cardiac valve prostheses. *J Am Coll Cardiol* 27:1698–1703.

Sbarouni E & Oakley CM. (1994). Outcome of pregnancy in women with valve prostheses. *Br Heart J* 71:196-201.

Schmidtke C, Stierle U, Sievers HH & Graf B. (2003). The Ross procedure (pulmonary autograft) as an alternative for aortic valve replacement. *Dtsch Med Wochenschr* 128:1759–1764.

Siebenhofer A, Berghold A & Sawicki PT. (2004). Systematic review of studies of self-management of oral anticoagulation. *Thromb Haemost* 91:225-32.

Silberman S, Shaheen J, Merin O, et al. (2001). Exercise hemodynamics of aortic prostheses: Comparison between stentless bioprostheses and mechanical valves. *Ann Thorac Surg* 72:1217-1221.

Silberman S, Oren A, Dotan M, Merin O, Fink D, Deeb M & Bitran D. (2008). Aortic valve replacement: choice between mechanical valves and bioprostheses. *J Card Surg* 23:299-306.

Siu SC, Sermer M, Harrison DA, et al. (1997). Risk and predictors for pregnancy-related complications in women with heart disease. *Circulation* 96:2789–2794.

Solymar L, Rao PS, Mardini MK, Fawzy ME & Guinn G. (1991). Prosthetic valves in children and adolescents. *Am Heart J* 121(2 Pt.1):557-568.

Stassano P, Di Tommaso L Monaco M, et al. (2009). Aortic valve replacement: a prospective randomized evaluation of mechanical versus biological valves in patients ages 55 to 70 years, *J Am Coll Cardiol* 54;1862–1868.

Stewart S, Hart CL, Hole DJ & McMurray JJ. (2002). A populationbased study of the long-term risks associated with atrial fibrillation: 20-year follow-up of the Renfrew/Paisley study. Am J Med 113:359–364.

Takaseya T, Kawara T, Tokunaga S, Kohno M, Oishi Y & Morita S. (2007). Aortic valve replacement with 17-mm St. Jude medical prostheses for a small aortic root in elderly patients. Ann Thorac Surg 83:2050-2053.

Takkenberg JJ, Dossche KM, Hazekamp MG, et al. (2002). Report of the Dutch experience with the Ross procedure in 343 patients. *Eur J Cardio Thorac Surg* 22:70 –77.

Takkenberg JJ, van Herwerden LA, Eijkemans MJ, Bekkers JA & Bogers AJ. (2002). Evolution of allograft aortic valve replacement over 13 years: results of 275 procedures. *Eur J Cardiothorac Surg* 21:683-691.

Takkeberg JJ, van Herwerden LA, Galema TW, Bekkers JA, Kleyburg-Linkers VE, Eijkemans MJ & Bogers AJ. (2006). Serial echocardiographic assessment of neo-aortic regurgitation and root dimensions after the modified Ross procedure. *J Heart Valve Dis* 15:100-106.

Tay EL, Gurvitch R, Wijeysinghe N, et al. (2011). Outcome of patients after transcatheter aortic valve embolization. *JACC Cardiovasc Interv* 4(2):228-34.

Tehrani H, Masroor S, Lombardi P, Rosenkranz E & Salerno T. (2004). Beating heart aortic valvereplacement in a pregnant patient. *J Card Surg* 19:57-58.

Thourani VH, Myung R, Kilgo P, et al. (2008). Long-term outcomes after isolated aortic valve replacement in octogenarians: a modern perspective. *Ann Thorac Surg* 86:1458-1464.

Thourani VH, Sarin EL, Keeling WB, et al. (2011). Long-term survival for patients with preoperative renal failure undergoing bioprosthetic or mechanical valve replacement. *Ann Thorac Surg* 91:1127-1134.

Trimn J, Hung L & Rahimtoola SH. (2007). Prosthetic heart valves and pregnancy, In: *Heart Disease in Pregnancy,* Oakley C, Warnes C. pp:104 –121, Blackwell Publishers, London.

Tseng E, Lee C, Cameron DE et al. (1997). Aortic valve replacement in the elderly: risk factors and long term results. Ann Surg 225:793- 804.

Urban M, Pirk J, Turek D & Netuka I. (2011). In patients with concomitant aortic and mitral valve disease is aortic valve replacement with mitral valve repair superior to double valve replacement? *Interact Cardiovasc Thorac Surg* 12:238-242.

Vahasilta T, Saraste A, Kito V, et al. (2005). Malmberg M, Kiss J, Kentala E, Kallojoki M, Savunen T. Cardiomyocyte apoptosis after antegrade and retrograde cardioplegia. *Ann Thorac Surg* 80:2229–2234.

Valfrè C, Rizzoli G, Zussa C, et al. (2006). Clinical results of Hancock II versus Hancock Standard at long-term follow-up. *J Thorac Cardiovasc Surg* 132:595-601.

Vidaillet H, Granada JF, Chyou PH, et al. (2002) A populationbased study of mortality among patients with atrial fibrillation or flutter. *Am J Med* 113:365–370.

Walther T, Falk V, Langebartels G, Kruger M, et al. (1999). Prospectively randomized evaluation of stentless versus conventional biological aortic valves: impact on early regression of left ventricular hypertrophy. *Circulation* 100(suppl 19):II6 -10.

Walther T, Simon P, Dewey T, et al. (2007). Transapical minimally invasive aortic valve implantation: multicenter experience. *Circulation* 116(suppl 11):I-240–I-245.

Waszyrowski T, Kasprzak JD, Krzeminska-Pakula M, Dziatkowiak A & Zaslonka J. (1997). Early and long-term outcome of aortic valve replacement with homograft vs mechanical prosthesis: 8-year follow-up study. *Clin Cardiol* 20:843- 848.

Weiss BM, von Segesser LK, Alon E, et al. (1998). Outcome of cardiovasc surgery and pregnancy: a systematic review of the period 1984–1996. *Am J Obstet Gynecol* 179:1643–1653.

Webb JG, Pasupati S, Humphries K, et al. (2007). Percutaneous transarterial aortic valve replacement in selected high-risk patients with aortic stenosis. *Circulation* 116:755–763.

Westaby S, Horton M, Jin XY, et al. (2000). Survival advantage of stentless aortic bioprostheses. *Ann Thorac Surg* 70:785-791.

Wolf PA, Abbott RD & Kannel WB. (1991). Atrial fibrillation as an independent risk factor for stroke: The Framingham Study. *Stroke* 22:983-988.

Wos S, Jasinski M, Bachowski R, et al. (1996). Results of mechanical prosthetic valve replacement in active valcular endocarditis. *J Cardiovasc Surg (Torino)* 37:29-32.

Yacoub M, Rasmi NR, Sundt TM, et al. (1995). Fourteen-year experience with homovital homografts for aortic valve replacement. *J Thorac Cardiovasc Surg* 110:186 -193.

Ye J, Cheung A, Lichtenstein SV, et al. (2007). Six-month outcome of transapical transcatheter aortic valve implantation in the initial seven patients. *Eur J Cardiothorac Surg* 31(1):16-21.

Yinon Y, Siu SC, Warshafsky C, et al. (2009). Silversides CK. Use of low molecular weight heparin in pregnant women with mechanical heart valves. *Am J Cardiol* 1;104(9):1259-1263.

Yum Kl, Miller DC, Moore KA, et al. (1995). Durability of the Hancock MO bioprostheses compared with the standard aortic valve bioprostheses. *Ann Thorac Surg* 60 Suppl:S221- S228.

4

Prosthetic Aortic Valves: A Surgical and Bioengineering Approach

Dimosthenis Mavrilas[1], Efstratios Apostolakis[2] and Petros Koutsoukos[3]
[1]*Mechanical Engineering & Aer/tics, University of Patras,*
[2]*School of Medicine, University of Ioannina,*
[3]*Chemical Engineering, University of Patras,*
Greece

1. Introduction

The need for replacement of damaged or malfunctioning organs or tissues in the human body has led through intense and innovative research during the past century to the development of materials and devices which are compatible with living tissues. Materials' compatibility consists in their capability to be accepted by the body when implanted and in contact with other tissues and body fluids. These materials, known as biomaterials, are the fundamental tools for engineering implantable devices dedicated to function in a specific way that substitutes corresponding function of the tissues or organs replaced due to malfunction, in synergism with the surrounding biological environment. Bone fracture healing by the incorporation of plates was known as early as the beginning of the century. Implants to replace heart valves and hip joints have been reported in the early 60s (Park & Lakes, 1992). Among the problems recorded when the first implants were employed were corrosion, mechanical failure and rejection by the body. The latter remains the main problem in the development of novel biomaterials which can be used as implants. Biomaterials now play a major role in replacing or improving the function of every major body system (skeletal, circulatory, nervous, etc.). Commonly employed implants include orthopedic devices such as total knee and hip joint replacements, spinal implants, and bone fixators; cardiac implants such as artificial heart valves and pacemakers; soft tissue implants such as breast implants and injectable collagen for soft tissue augmentation; and dental implants to replace teeth/root systems and bony tissue in the oral cavity.

When a man-made material is placed in the human body, tissue reacts to the implant in a variety of ways depending on the material type and function. The mechanism of tissue attachment depends on the tissue response to the implant surface. In general, materials can be placed into three classes that represent the tissue response they elicit: inert, bioresorbable, and bioactive. **Inert materials** such as titanium and alumina (Al_2O_3) are nearly chemically inert in the body and exhibit minimal chemical interaction with adjacent tissue. A fibrous tissue capsule will normally form around inert implants. Tissue attachment with inert materials can be through tissue growth into surface irregularities, by bone cement, or by press fitting into a defect. This morphological fixation is not ideal for the long-term stability of permanent implants and often becomes a problem with orthopedic and dental implant applications. **Bioresorbable materials**, such as tricalcium phosphate and polylacticpolyglycolic acid copolymers, are designed to be slowly degraded under the biological-biochemical action of the living organism in bioresorbable products (like water, ions of electrolytes or CO_2), replaced by living tissue (such as bone or soft tissues in tissue engineering) or liberating drugs, as in drug-delivery applications. **Bioactive materials** bond to surrounding tissues (like bone or soft tissues) through a time-dependent, kinetic modification of the surface triggered by their contact and function after implantation with parts of living organism. In particular, ion-exchange reactions or ion incorporation into the crystal lattice between the bioactive implant and the surrounding body fluids results in the formation of a biologically active interface layer on the implant surface responsible for the relatively strong interfacial bonding.

1.1 Anatomy of the normal aortic valve

The aortic valve (figure 1) is composed of three components: the annulus, the cusps or leaflets and the commissures. The annulus of the valve, in contrast to this of atrioventricular valves, does not located at the same level. Here, the annulus consists of ventriculo-arterial junction and is oriented in a curvilinear, semilunar fashion. It consists of three almost semicircular dense fibrous collagen structures forming three scallops, the whole encircling the ventriculo-aortic junction like a coronet. The three aortic leaflets are folds of endocardium with a central lamina fibrosa, which is locally thickened. Each leaflet is attached to the aortic wall (its upper part) and to the left ventricle (its lowest part or nadir of

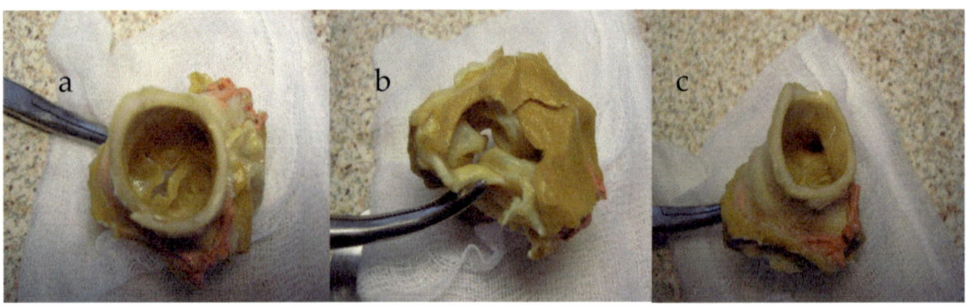

Fig. 1. Anatomy of aortic valve construct. a. View from aorta & b. from left ventricle. c: View from aorta, showing leaflet junction, sinus of Valsalva and coronary ostium. Pictures are from a porcine aortic valve, of similar anatomy with human aortic valve

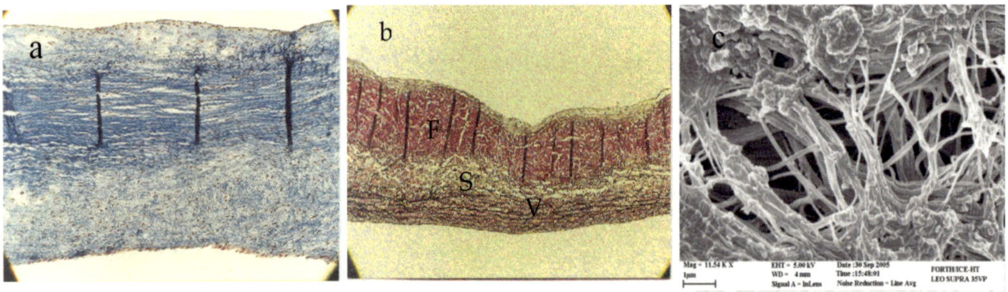

Fig. 2. Histological sections (a and b) and SEM microphotograph (c) of valvular leaflet tissue, demonstrating its multilaminate, 3D fiber reinforced composite structure, make it suitable for the complicated leaflet movements during valve function. F: Fibrosa, S: Spongiosa & V: Ventricularis

the leaflet). Leaflets are multilaminate composite tissue structures of 3 layers (Figure 2.): the ventricularis, composed of elastin- rich fibers aligned in a radial direction, perpendicular to the leaflet margin, the fibrosa, on the aortic side of the leaflet, comprising primarily fibroblasts and collagen fibers arranged circumferentially, parallel to the leaflet margin and the spongiosa, a layer of loose connective tissue at the base of the leaflet, between the fibrosa and ventricularis, composed of fibroblasts, mesenchymal cells, and a glycosaminoglycan (GAG) rich organic matrix. This composite tissue structure provides tensile strength and pliability to the leaflets for decades of repetitive motion per minute (Freeman & Otto, 2005). The aortic surface of each leaflet is rougher than its ventricular surface.

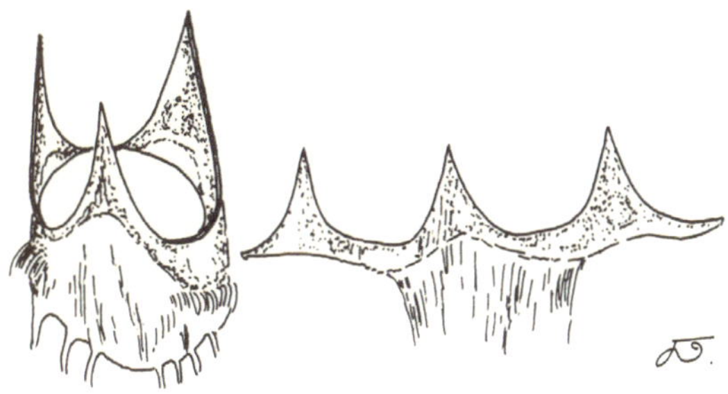

Fig. 3. Schematic representation of the three aortic valve commissures in natural and open configuration (acknowledged art work by G. Athanassiou)

The commissures (figure 3) form tall, peaked spaces between the attachments of neighbouring cusps, and reach the so-called aortic sino-tubular junction. The latter is a ridge, called also "supraortic ridge" that separates the sinus and tubular portions of the ascending aorta (Malouf et al., 2008). The commissure between the right and non-coronary (or posterior) aortic leaflet overlies the membranous septum and corresponds to that laid between the anterior and septal leaflets of the tricuspid valve (Malouf et al., 2008). The commissure between the right and left aortic leaflet contacts its corresponding pulmonary ones and overlies the infundibular septum. Finally, the intervalvular fibrosa, at the commissure between the left and non-coronary aortic leaflet, fuses the aortic valve to the anterior mitral leaflet (Edwards, 1996; Malouf et al., 2008).

1.2 Physiology of the normal aortic valve

During left ventricular systole, the systolic pressure inside rises exceeding the aortic pressure and the aortic valve is passively opened. Blood, ejected by the left ventricle (LV) pushes the aortic cusps upward and away from the centre of the aortic lumen. During this phase of cardiac cycle, the major opening diameter of the aortic valve is about equal to that of the ascending aorta at the level of sino-tubular junction (Stewart et al., 1998). In fact, the relatively inaccurate measurements of LV and intraaortic pressure during left ventricular catheterization show that there is no clinically significant gradient across the normal aortic valve. This measurement is curious because it suggests that blood does not travel down a pressure gradient during ejection. If flow out of the LV and through the outflow tract and the aortic valve was simply frictional, then a pressure gradient should needed between the LV and ascending aorta to obtain blood flow, according to the low of the physics: Q(flow)=Pressure Gradient/Resistance. However, this assumption does not hold when considering pulsatile blood flow in large vessels such as the aorta, since the inertia and momentum of the blood ejected from the LV is much more important than resistance. In fact, it has been experimentally shown that at the first 40% of the ejection phase, during blood acceleration, small pressure gradients (about 10 mmHg) are observed between LV and aorta (Hall & Julian, 1989). This small gradient persists for about 45% of the ejection after which the gradient reverses as forward blood flow is decelerated.

The fibrous wall of the sinuses of Valsalva (figure 1) at the nadirs of annular scallops is not extensible in contrast to their upper parts (at the level of commissures) where it produces its biggest increase of aortic radius, about 16% in the peak of systole, due to the fibro-elastic composition of the aortic wall (Williams et al., 1989). During this phase the commissures move apart, making the fully open orifice triangular, the free margins of the aortic leaflets becoming almost straight lines between commissures. However, they do not flatten against the sinus wall, which is an important factor for the subsequent valve closure (Williams et al., 1989). Most of the blood ejected during systole is directed to the ascending aorta while a small volume enters into the sinuses of Valsalva. Valve geometry in the sinus region produces vortical blood flow at systole, which helps to coronary perfusion, maintain the triangular "mid-position" of the leaflets and probably initiate their re-approximation at the end of systole. During diastole, the three aortic leaflets fall passively towards the centre of the aortic lumen and, under the pressure of the supravalvular blood column they hermetically contact each other along lines of coaptation. Therefore during diastole the three normal aortic leaflets, such as the yacht-sails, support the entire intraaortic blood column and prevent its partial regurgitation into the left ventricle. Experiments have shown that only 4% of blood ejected during systole regurgitates through the centre of the valve during diastole. In the absence of sinuses of Valsalva the regurgitant blood may be increased up to 23% (Williams et al., 1989).

1.3 The diseased stenotic aortic valve

Normal aortic valve histology and anatomy may be changed under pathologic conditions with corresponding alterations in its normal physiological function. Age-related changes in fibromuscular skeleton of the heart include myxomatous degeneration and collagen infiltration, called aortic valve sclerosis. This sclerosis is observed in as many as 30% of elderly people, namely in 25% of people 65 to 74 years of age and in 48% of people older than 84 years (Freeman & Otto, 2005; Otto et al., 1999; Stewart et al., 1997). Histopathologic studies of aortic sclerosis show focal subendothelial plaquelike lesions on the aortic side of the leaflet that extend to the adjacent fibrosa layer. Similarities to atherosclerosis are present in these lesions, with prominent accumulation of "atherogenic" lipoproteins, including LDL and lipoprotein(a), evidence of LDL oxidation, an inflammatory cell infiltrate and microscopic calcification (Olsson et al., 1999; Otto et al., 1999; Wallby et al, 2002). The initiation of these lesions is possibly due to increased mechanical or decreased shear stress, similar to that seen in early atherosclerotic lesions (Freeman & Otto, 2005). Of note, these changes are more prominent on the aortic surface of the leaflets where the mechanical stress of the aortic valve is highest, especially in the flexion area near the attachment to the aortic root. Shear stress across the endothelium of the non-coronary cusp is lower than the left and right coronary cusps because of the absence of diastolic coronary flow, which likely explains why the non-coronary cusp is often the first cusp affected (Freeman & Otto, 2005).

Other age-related changes become in the valve, in the aortic wall, as well as in the myocardium. The central nodules on the cusps and the closure lines become more prominent. At the same time the Valsalva's sinuses are stretched, the diameter of the supra-

aortic ridge increased and the surface area and mass of the aortic leaflets also increased (Hall & Julian, 1989). In the 6th and 7th decades the fibrosa of the leaflet begins to calcify, first at the point of attachment to the aortic wall, which is where maximum flexion occurs. This calcification may gradually extend throughout the valve, limiting the valve's opening. Occasionally, the calcified leaflets may develop local ulcerations and thrombus formations (Otto et al., 1999; Schwartz & Zipes, 2005). Of course, in the cases of the rheumatic disease the course of chronic inflammatory disease produce the above-mentioned changes (calcification, thickening of the leaflets, fusion of commissures, local ulcerations, sub-endothelial atherosclerotic plaques, etc.) much earlier.
In normal adults, the area of the aortic valve orifice is 2.6 to 3.5 cm^2. Experimental studies have suggested that the aortic orifice must be reduced to approximately one quarter of this in order to diminish significantly the cardiac output. A reduction in this area to 1 cm^2 is associated with a rise in left ventricular systolic pressure and a pressure drop across the aortic valve (Hall & Julian, 1989). Aortic stenosis is generally considered to be critical when the systolic pressure difference across the valve exceeds 50 mmHg in the presence of a normal cardiac output or if the effective aortic orifice is less than 0.4 cm^2 (Hall & Julian, 1989). According to Rahimtoola, the aortic valve area has to be reduced by about 50% of normal before a measurable gradient can be demonstrated (Rahimtoola, 2004). When a pressure gradient develops between LV and aorta LV pressure is increased, ventricular wall stress increased contributing to development of myocardial hypertrophy and the LV function impairs. A diastolic dysfunction is caused of a combination of impaired myocardial relaxation during diastolic phase and increased myocardial stiffness (Hess et al., 1993). Patients with severe LV hypertrophy may exhibit LV diastolic dysfunction, which consequently may produce the syndrome of clinical heart failure with symptoms of paroxysmal nocturnal dyspnea, orthopnea or even pulmonary oedema, even if the systolic LV function is normal (Rahimtoola, 2004).
Prospective studies on the rate of hemodynamic progression in patients diagnosed with aortic stenosis documented an increasing rate of aortic jet velocity, in average 0.3 m/s per year, with an increase in mean trans-aortic pressure gradient of 7 mm Hg per year and a decrease in aortic valve area of 0.1 cm^2 per year (Brener et al., 1995; Faggiano et al., 1996; Freeman & Otto, 2005). During this later course, for the cases of symptomatic aortic stenosis or of the asymptomatic with significant (> 50 mmHg) trans-valvular mean gradient, surgical management is indicated.

1.4 The surgical management of the stenotic aortic valve

There are four options for the management of the severe calcific aortic stenosis: the balloon aortic valvuloplasty, the "open" aortic valve commissurotomy, the percutaneous aortic valve implantation, and the "classic" aortic valve replacement.
At **balloon aortic valvuloplasty** (BAV), a ballon-catheter is introduced after a femoral artery puncture and retrograde till the left ventricle (Diethrich, 1993; Smedira et al., 1993). Inflation of the balloon within the aortic orifice can stretch the calcified annulus, fracture calcified areas and dissect the fused commissures. Disadvantages of the method, as the risk of stroke and increase of pre-existent valve regurgitation (Cormier & Vahanian, 1992) are controversial to increase of effective orifice area. An overall 65% survival and 40% free of death or re-operation over 1-year survival has been reported (Davidson et al., 1990). However, no beneficial effect on long-term clinical outcome demonstrated due to significant residual obstruction from leaflet thickening and annular calcification, resulted in severe re-stenosis

typically occurred within months (Bonow et al., 1998; Cormier & Vahanian, 1992; Freeman & Otto, 2005; Smedira et al., 1993).
The **"open" aortic valvulotomy**, performed rarely, usually during another open heart operation, is based on the -by a scalpel- commissurotomy of the fused commissure (-s). Because of the excessive calcification and rigidity of the leaflets, a central postoperative insufficiency is anticipated. The main indication is the case of congenital aortic stenosis with one or two congenitally fused commissures. In fact, in young patients, if the valve is pliable, mobile, and free of calcification, simple commissurotomy may be feasible. The operative mortality in these cases does not exceed 1% (Rahimtoola, 2004).
The impetus for the development of **percutaneous or transcatheter aortic valve replacement** (PAVI or TAVI) lies in the need for an intervention that is more durable than balloon aortic valvuloplasty and that can be used in patients who are too risk for the "classic" aortic valve replacement. The basic concept is based on the use of an outer expandable stent (scaffold) to resist the rigidity of the calcified aortic annulus and native leaflets (Davidson & Baim, 2008). In the inner surface of this stent three appropriately prepared pericardial or porcine leaflets are fixed constituting –after full expansion of the stent- a well functioning valvular prosthesis. The first implantation in the human being was done in France since 1992 by Cribier et al. (Cribier et al., 2002). The introduction of the catheter bearing the valved-stent requires direct femoral or iliac artery access, while in a few cases with stenotic iliac arteries the catheter is introduced through the apex of the left ventricle (transapical introduction), after a left anterior thoracotomy. The results of this method after more than 10 years of application are encouraged. Procedural mortality is 2-3%, one-month survival about 88% and the 1-year is ranged 65 to 78% (Bosmans et al., 2011).
Finally, **the aortic valve replacement** is the "classical" surgical treatment of calcific aortic stenosis, especially for the elderly. During this method, the three calcified leaflets of the valve are resected, as well as the calcific deposits of the annulus. Then, sutures are passed circumferentially through the annulus and the sewing ring of the prosthesis. Finally, the sutures are tied down in the native annulus. Aortic valve replacement by using 3rd-generation prosthetic valves –mechanical or biological- obtains excellent early and late outcomes with low mortality and morbidity. Recent surgical series report operative mortality rates for aortic valve replacement as low as 1%, increasing to 9% in higher-risk patients. Long-term survival after valve replacement is 80% at 3 years, with an age-corrected survival postoperatively that is nearly normalized (Freeman & Otto, 2005; Rahimtoola, 2010). Significant postoperative morbidity, such as thromboembolism, hemorrhagic complications from anticoagulation, prosthetic valve dysfunction, and endocarditis, are rare and occur at a rate of 2% to 3% per year (Rahimtoola, 2010).

2. Aortic valve prostheses: The parallel evolution of mechanical & bioprosthetic valves

Cardiac valve prostheses are devices designed and constructed properly to assure unidirectional blood flow. Like the natural cardiac valves, they work passively, due to pressure difference across their structure, with parts able to be moved between two positions: open position, when blood circulates, as in the case of aortic valves from left ventricle to the aorta during myocardial contraction (systolic phase) and closed position, when blood circulation stops (during the diastolic phase for the aortic valve). From a mechanical point of view, cardiac valves work as common one-way valves of hydraulic systems. Despite their simple working principle, the design and orthotopic surgical implantation of cardiac valves was not possible till the development of extracorporeal blood circulation devices, introduced by Gibbon (Gibbon, 1954), by which blood circulation was maintained during open heart surgical procedures. Two main types of prosthetic heart valves are available: Mechanical (MHV) and biological or bioprosthetic (BHV) heart valves. MHVs in general composed of two main parts: One non-moving, which is sutured properly in the anatomic region of the failed, surgically excised, natural valve, in the interior region of which a second, moving part is included, passively guided by pressure difference changes between the inlet and outlet regions around it. The main difference is on the type of the moving part (occluder): The ball type and the disk type valves. For each of the two basic constructions many different designs and materials were used and a great branch of technology was developed. In a near parallel approach, BHVs, based on mimicking the design and function of natural heart valves were developed and applied. Although they simply were made of animal derived valves of proper size and structure, like porcine aortic valves, after biochemical treatment for removing antigenic factors, different designs have been introduced nowadays using combinations of artificial and natural derived biomaterials.

2.1 Evolution of mechanical heart valve prostheses

Different surgical operations were approached before extracorporeal circulation by implantation of artificial valve designs in peripheral vessels, like that of Hufnagel & Harvey in 1952 (Hufnagel & Harvey, 1953), when an aortic valve, made by a combination of biologically inert materials (a lucite® tube-like design with a mobile spherical poppet inside) was implanted in the descending thoracic aorta of a patient with a significant aortic insufficiency. However, it was at end of 50s when a caged ball type MHV was introduced. This design, in its final appearance, consists of a metallic ring with a soft material in its perimeter for stable suturing on surrounding soft tissues without blood leakage through the suturing line. A cage design, usually a three metal struts, is welded in the ring into which a ball made of silicon or other polymeric material is moved from the closed position, where it is pushed in touch with the ring, to the open once where it is attached the top of the cage (figure 4a). Starr and co-workers began in 1960 (their first report appeared in 1963) (Starr et al., 1963) to implant the caged ball aortic prosthesis in the orthotopic position with many of these prostheses remained well functioning for up to 40 years (Shiono et al., 2005). Major problems with these initial so-called "ball valves" were the compromised hemodynamic performance (small effective orifice area, big size of the sewing ring, turbulent flow) and the thromboembolic complications (high-grade haemolysis, thrombosis). For the last reason, all these valves required intense anticoagulation therapy (Ezekowitz, 2002).

To find a solution in these problems, after a substitution of ball with a disk type occluder (caged disk valves) to achieve less moving mass and reducing the valve height inside the aortic root, the second-generation of prosthetic valves, the so-called "tilting-disk valve", was developed in 1968 (Emery et al., 2008) (figure 4b). Tilting disk valves were the result of evolution in MHV technology towards reduction of whole volume, occluder mass and surface area projected vertical to the blood flow axis, maximizing of opening angle of the disk and designed the disk shape so as to approach a near physiological central flow velocity profile. Haemocompatibily was also improved by a minimization of the blood

contact area, material coating with biocompatible compounds (like pyrolitic carbon) and appropriate disk morphology for smoother blood flow around it. The most usable models were the Björk-Shiley and the Medronic Hall type. The main problems with these valves were the rare rupture of metal strut supporting disk movement and subsequent embolisation by the disk, non-axial flow, even in the models of Björk-Shiley with disk opening angle of 72°. Due to the excessive turbulent flow through the two orifices of the valve (a small and a bigger), a high-grade of haemolysis in patients was reported. However, good long-term results characterized that type of MHV (Oxenham et al., 2003).
The 3rd generation of mechanical valves was appeared in 1977 with the introduction of the St. Jude Medical (SJM) bileaflet valve coated with pyrolitic carbon (Emery et al., 2008; Gott et al., 2003). Over the following decades, the dramatic step of bileaflet prostheses nearly obviated the use of all other kinds of mechanical valves in all over the world (Emery et al., 2008). In fact, the low-profile SJM valve demonstrated low rates of thomboembolism, low trans-valvular gradients, low grade of haemolysis and minimal valvular insufficiency (Chambers et al., 2005; Gott et al., 2003; Walther et al., 2000). Out of the SJM valve, several other 3rd generation models were introduced such as the ATS Medical Prosthesis, the Sulzer CarboMedics , the On-X prosthesis and the Sorin prosthetic valve, all of them with similar haemodynamic and clinical outcomes (Chambers et al., 2005; Walther et al., 2000). Since the introduction of this 3rd generation of the valves and till over 2.1 million of these models have been implanted all over the world. In the meantime, many useful changes in valve design have been made in the new models. There are many changes on the effective flow orifice area, on the shape of the leaflets (straight, convex or concave), on the pivot style, on the angle of orientation of the leaflets (from 72° to 90°), on the sewing-ring etc. (Chambers et al., 2005; Gelsomino et al., 2002; Gott et al., 2003; Walther et al., 2000).

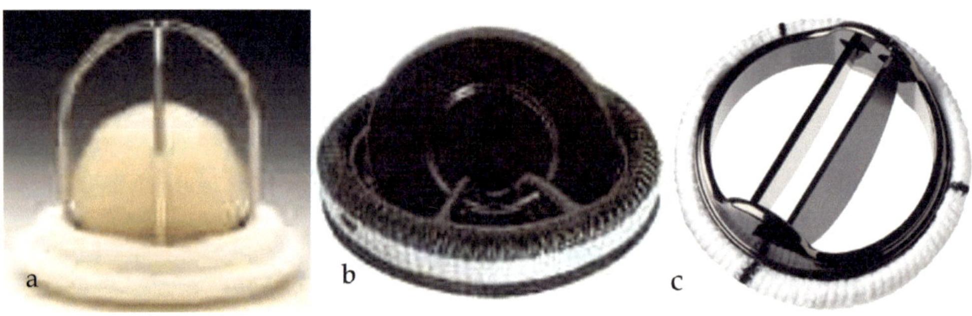

Fig. 4. Three generations of mechanical heart valves: a. caged ball, b. tilting disk & c. bileaflet mechanical heart valves

2.2 Evolution of bioprosthetic heart valves

Heart valve transplantation is the substitution of the diseased heart valves with healthy living heart valves (valves transplanted from genetically similar donors-homologous valves), including auto transplantation (the substitution of the aortic valve with the pulmonary valve and the later with a prosthetic non-living valve - the Ross procedure). Murray in 1956 demonstrated that human aortic valves from cadavers could be used as a valve transplant in the descending thoracic aorta in patients with aortic insufficiency (Murray, 1956). Based on this research Kerwin and co-workers six years later reported their first clinical applications in patients, with one of them having 6-year follow-up (Kerwin et al., 1962). The first orthotopic insertion of homograft valve was performed in 1962 by Barratt-Boyes (Barratt-Boyes, 1964). The introduction of other biological valves began in 1967 when Senning used pieces of fascia lata of the patient for replacement of the diseased aortic valve (Senning, 1967; Ionescu & Ross, 1969).

Xenograft or heterograft valves, animal derived heart valves or BHVs made from different animal derived tissues are alternatives, offering the advantage of been prepared much prior the operation, available in different sizes and designs. BHVs include a variety of heart valve replacement using as substitutes heart valves of different orientations and technologies. Among different types, porcine aortic and bovine pericardial xenograft BHVs has been established as valve substitutes. Porcine aortic valves, after a treatment for removing excess fatty and aortic wall tissue and part of septal myocardial tissue from valve leaflets are imposed in biochemical preparation, aimed in removing antigenic factors (valve cells) and stabilize the remaining acellular valve tissue against enzyme reactions by different chemical compounds. Formaldehyde was first used for porcine valve fixation (Angel, 1972), substituted later by glutaraldehyde because of its ability for double-edge cross linking of collagen molecules (Woodroof, 1972), resulted in better longevity of valves. The stabilized tissue valve is sutured in specially designed frames composed of aortic ring and three commissures. A metallic or polymeric frame is used as a skeleton, covered with biocompatible textiles (like Teflon® or Dacron®) onto which the valve tissue is sutured with permanent sutures).

Improvement of BHV function was achieved with the use of different membranous soft tissues for the construction of valve leaflets and suturing them in similar artificial frames like that of the porcine valves. Percutaneous tissue was used for that scope; however, pericardial tissue from different animals was finally used alternatively. Pericardial tissue is a big membrane enclosing the heart. Its histology is similar to heart valve leaflets with respect of its composition of collagen and elastin fiber networks in different layers inside an amorhous organic matrix of glycosaminoglycans (GAGs), proteoglycanes (PGs), and other proteins. Extracellular water solution of electrolytes and soluble proteins compose 65-70% of the tissue mass weight. Cells, like fibroblast, epithelial, muscle cells and other types are present. Despite these similarities with other soft tissues, including heart valve leaflets, fibber structure of bovine pericardium is quite different. Fibber orientation in valve leaflets is specified for supporting their motion and strengthening mechanical stress developed during valve function. The different anatomic position and function of pericardial tissue resulted in a different fibber orientation, varied across its surface. For this reason special attention is given in selection criteria of specific regions from the whole pericardial membrane for better suitability to function as heart valve leaflets (Simionescu et al., 1993). The benefits from the use of pericardial tissue (especially bovine ones, which is the standard selection last years) instead of porcine valves were better opening area of the valve, coaptation of the valve leaflets and flexibility in design of valve anatomic configuration. However, similar problems with porcine BHVs, tissue deterioration and calcification still remain.

The first xenograft valve, a stent-mounted porcine aortic valve was implanted by Binet et al. in 1965 (Binet et al., 1965), while the glutaraldehyde-preserved stent-mounted porcine valves were introduced by Carpentier et al., in 1967 (Carpentier et al., 1969). Over the past 40 years, advances in tissue fixation (bovine pericardium and porcine aortic valves) methodologies and chemical treatments to prevent calcification, have yielded improvements in the longevity of bioprostheses.

Like the mechanical valves, the development of biologic valves is characterized by the appearance of first-, second-, and third-generation prostheses. **First-generation** bioprostheses were preserved with high-pressure fixation. They include the Medtronic Hancock Standard, and the Carpentier-Edwards Standard valves, both porcine prostheses. **Second-generation** prostheses are treated with low-, or zero-pressure fixation. Pericardial prostheses include the Carpentier-Edwards Perimount, and the Pericarbon Sorin prostheses. Porcine prostheses include the Medtronic Hancock II, the Medtronic Intact, and the Carpentier-Edwards Supraannular prostheses. In the third-generation prostheses were included all valves with zero-, or low-pressure fixation, decellularization of animal tissues and simultaneous anti-mineralization processes (e.g. a-amino oleic acid) to reduce material fatigue and calcification. In these models the stents have become gradually thinner and flexible, the profile much lower and the effective orifice area larger. Porcine prostheses include the Medtronic Mosaic, and the St. Jude Medical Epic valve. Pericardial prostheses include the Carpentier-Edwards Magna and the Mitroflow Pericardial valve.

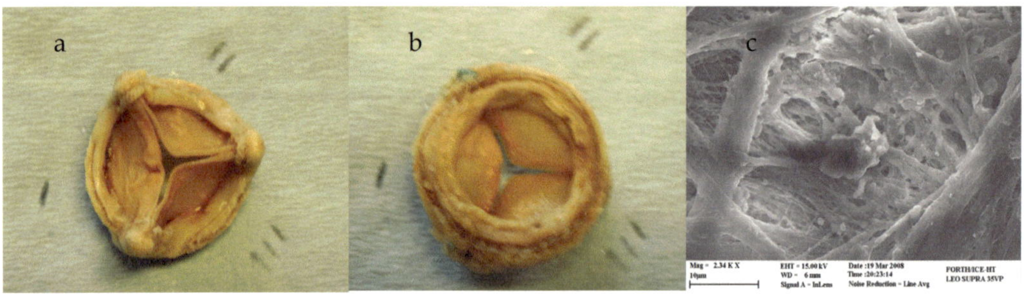

Fig. 5. Pericardial bioprosthetic heart valve explanted due to severe calcification. A: aortic side, b: ventricular side, c: SEM micrograph of the same valve demonstrating calcific crystals deposited implemented with leaflet tissue fibber network

2.3 Comparison of MHV with BHV replacement

Aortic valve replacement by using a mechanical prosthetic valve is not indicated for all patients suffered from aortic valve stenosis. Generally, the two main advantages of the mechanical valves are the absence of degeneration (long-term rigidity) and the larger effective flow orifice, both contributing to better long-term outcomes. In fact, according to many studies followed over time frames, freedom from all-valve related events and from the risk of reoperation were improved in patients with mechanical valve prostheses as compared to those with biologic prostheses (Ezekowitz, 2002; Gott et al., 2003). On the other hand, the main disadvantage of mechanical valves is the obligatory need for long-life anticoagulation (Ezekowitz, 2002). The use of porcine BHVs resulted in a better function in patient circulatory system, improving failed valve insufficiency due to stenosis or regurgitation of diseased natural valves. A central blood flow with a near physiological velocity profile, low pressure gradient across the valve, near physiological leaflet movements and no need for long term anticoagulation therapy were the benefits of their use. However, porcine BHVs longevity remains limited, mainly because of calcification of valve leaflets. Calcific crystal deposits are gradually developed in valve leaflets caused stiffening and incompetence in their moving ability and valve dysfunction due to stenosis or regurgitation. BHV calcification is more often in younger patients, for which MHVs are the gold standard in heart valve replacement.

Valve type	Advantages	Disadvantages
Mechanical 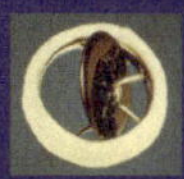	• Longevity • Easy implantation • Variety of size-designs • Availability	• Non physiological geometry - hemodynamic • Chronic anticoagulation therapy • Risk of thromboembolism • Regular medical examinations
Bioprosthetic 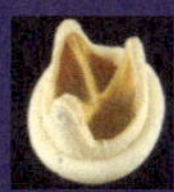	• Physiological anatomy - hemodynamic • Minimize anticoagulation therapy • Availability	• Tissue deterioration • Calcification • Undesirable host reactions
Living grafts	• Ideal anatomy - hemodynamic • Physiological remodeling • Minimal anticoagulation therapy	• Tissue deterioration • Calcification • Minimal availability • Undesirable immunologic reactions

Table 1. Comparison of different types of heart valve substitutes

A mechanical valve prosthesis is recommended to patients having valve re-operation, regardless of the nature of the first operation, as the risk of the second operation is significantly higher (Gelsomino et al., 2002; Potter et al., 2005). The most debated age for making decision according the selection of type of prosthesis is the decade between 60 and 70 years. The final decision is dependent on other parameters, which have to be taken into account, like the existence of atrial fibrillation, chronic renal failure, cerebrovascular disease, history of gastrointestinal bleeding, contraindication to oral anticoagulants, etc. (Emery et al., 2002).
In 1962, D. Harken summarized the 10 important characteristics that an ideal heartc valve must satisfy:

1. Not propagate emboli.
2. Be chemically inert and not damage blood elements.
3. Offer no resistance to physiological flows.
4. Close promptly (less than 0.05 second).
5. Remain closed during the appropriate phase of the cardiac cycle.
6. Lasting physical and geometric features.
7. Be inserted in a physiological site, generally the normal anatomical site.
8. Be capable of permanent fixation.
9. Not annoy the patient.
10. Be technically practical to insert (Harken et al., 1962).

After a near 50 years of evolution today's mechanical or biological valve do not satisfy all those requirements.

3. Biomechanics of heart valve prostheses

During their motion natural valve leaflets imposed to different mechanical loading and corresponding stress fields. Mechanical bending is developed during opening especially at sites near their attachments to valvular ring, while shear stress is gradually developed at their sides faced blood flow. A near parabolic velocity profile is produced in fully developed central axial blood flow across the valve which fast stabilizes leaflets in a position parallel to its axis. Upon starting of closing phase of the valves a reverse leaflet movement is performed with changing stress fields applied to their structure, till the closing position during which these membranous tissues, supported at their sites of attachment on valvular rings and their coaptation areas, are imposed in surface tensile loading, while obstructing blood backflow and big pressure differences between their sides. As a result of all these different mechanical loadings imposed, leaflet tissue is remodelled in a multilaminate, anisotropic (see diagram in figure 6) reinforced composite biomaterial, demonstrating a structure of multilayered 3D collagen and elastin fibrous networks, integrated and moved into an amorphous organic protein matrix, filled with cells and extracellular water, electrolytes and soluble proteins of low molecular weight. This tissue structure, different in individual valve leaflets, is specifically able to function at the specific anatomic position. Been in a different position, like, for example, from pulmonary artery to aorta as in Ross procedure, tissue remodelling started to make the pulmonary valve leaflets able to resist higher mechanical loading in aortic position, compared with that of pulmonary circulation.

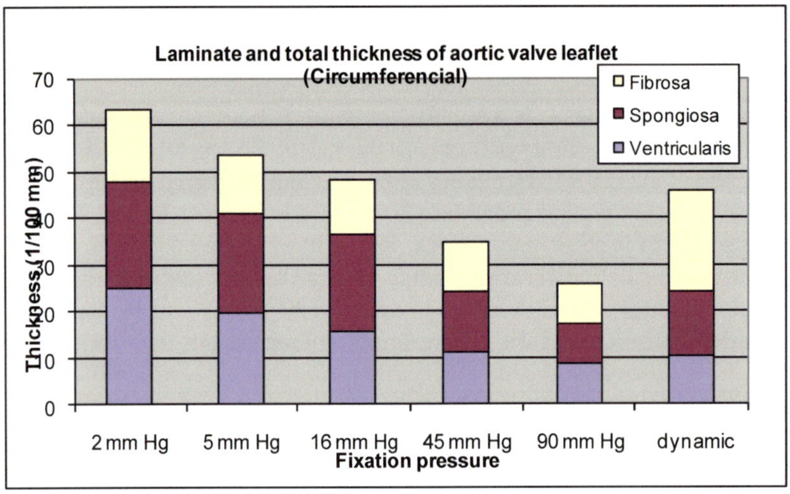

Fig. 6. Diagram (from measurements in histological sections) of the laminate and total leaflet thickness changed under different pressure levels applied during their fixation with glutaraldehyde. In dynamic mode, the valve was under normal function during fixation. Anisotropic deformation of the different tissue laminates is demonstrated as pressure increases

Natural heart valve leaflets exhibit non linear viscoelastic mechanical behaviour under mechanical loading (figure 7a). A similar mechanical behaviour is demonstrated by tissue heart valves of all species, as well all membranous soft tissues. Chemical modification of bioprosthetic heart valves, needed for removing antigenic factors and stabilization against enzyme biodegradation, resulted in significant stiffening of leaflet tissue compared with its natural state, as demonstrated by increase of high (collagen) modulus (figure 7b).

Other viscoelastic mechanical parameters of valve leaflet tissue, like low (elastin) modulus (the slope of the first linear part of the loading stress-strain curve (fig. 7a)) and relaxation index may also changed, although hysteresis, another viscoelastic characteristic of membranous soft tissues (defined as the ratio of dissipated to the loading energy in every loading-unloading cycle) demonstrating energy dissipation inside the tissue during cyclic deformation, measured at 20/35% of loading energy depending on cyclic frequency seems to be unchanged after chemical modification.

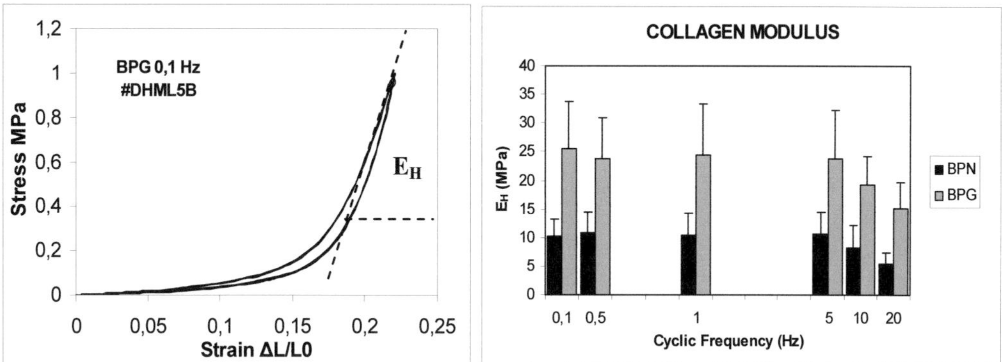

(a) (b)

Fig. 7. (a) Typical stress-strain diagram of a pericardial tissue under uniaxial tensile cyclic loading 0.1 Hz demonstrating non linear mechanical behaviour. E_H is the characteristic high (collagen) modulus, the tangential modulus of the second linear phase. (b) Collagen modulus of fresh natural (BPN) and glutaraldehyde treated (BPG) bovine pericardial tissue (mean ± SE) at different cyclic loading rates

4. Heart valve calcification

Pathology of natural heart valve calcification causes valve dysfunction (stenosis, regurgitation, tissue rupture). A lot of possible aetiologies and mechanisms seem to be implemented in its initiation and development in human body tissues. Chronic pathologies, infections, metabolism, long term drag therapies and age related tissue degeneration, as well biochemical compounds involved in the structure of implanted biomaterials may contribute in different ways in growth of different types of calcium phosphate crystals from ions of electrolytes diluted in biological fluids, that finally deposited in valve tissue structure (Gross, 2003; Schoen & Levy, 2005). However, despite the complicated aetiologies and mechanisms of tissue calcification, crystal growth is basically a physicochemical process of calcium and phosphate ion crystallization under certain physicochemical conditions that may be satisfied during the function of a living organism.

4.1 Biomineralization: Physicochemical background

Calcium phosphate deposition on implants may result from the presence of high phosphorus levels in the biological fluids in contact with the implanted surface. Due to their very low solubility products, a number of phosphate scale minerals may form in aqueous supersaturated solutions. In the order of decreasing solubility, they are listed in the following table 2. At high solution supersaturations it is possible that a number of precursor phases may be formed, depending on the solution pH, which finally transform into the thermodynamically more stable HAP, in accordance to Ostwald's rule of stages which predicts that the least stable phase having the highest solubility is formed preferentially during a stepwise precipitation process. It is well established that kinetic factors may be more important in determining the nature and, hence, the characteristics of the solid deposits formed during the precipitation process than the respective equilibrium consideration complications that may arise from the formation of mixed solid phases, caused of the overgrowth of one crystalline phase over another.

Solid Phase	**Abbrev.**	**Formula**	**Therm.Solub. Product**
Dicalcium phosphate dihydrate	DCPD	$CaHPO_4.2H_2O$	$1.87x10^{-7}$(mol L^{-1})*
Dicalcium phosphate anhydrous	DCPA	$CaHPO_4$	$9.2x10^{-7}$ (mol L^{-1})*
β.Tricalcium phosphate	TCP	$Ca_3(PO_4)_2$	$2.8x10^{-9}$ (mol L^{-1})**
Octacalcium phosphate	OCP	$Ca_8H_2(PO_4)_6.5H_2O$	$2.5x10^{-99}$(mol L^{-1})***
Hydroxyapatite	HAP	$Ca_{10}(PO_4)_6(OH)_6$	$5.5x10^{-118}$ (mol L^{-1})****
Defect Apatites		$Ca_{10-x}(HPO_4)_x(PO_4)_{6-x}(OH)_{2-x}$ ($o \leq x \leq 2$)	

Table 2. Calcium phosphate crystalline phases, formulae and corresponding thermodynamic solubility products. *(Hench & Wilson, 1991), **(Eanes et al., 1965), ***(LeGeros et al., 1975), ****(Betts & Posner, 1974)

The tendency for a particular calcium phosphate phase to form in supersaturated aqueous media may be determined from the solubility phase diagrams such as the diagram shown in figure 8. It has been reported that when calcium phosphate is precipitated from highly supersaturated solutions forms an unstable precursor phase. This phase is characterized by the absence of peaks in the powder x-ray diffraction pattern and is known as the amorphous calcium phosphate (ACP). The composition of ACP appears to depend upon the precipitation conditions and is usually formed in supersaturated solutions at pH >7.0 (Betts & Posner, 1974; Eanes et al., 1965; LeGeros et al., 1975; Newesely, 1966). In slightly acidic calcium phosphate solutions the monoclinic DCPD is formed (Bets & Posner, 1974; Brown & Lehr, 1959). OCP is formed by the hydrolysis of DCPD in solutions of pH 5-6 and may also be precipitated heterogeneously upon TCP (Brown et al., 1957). HAP is the thermodynamically most stable phase and often, when precipitated in the presence of foreign ions, substitution of calcium, phosphate and/or hydroxyls by some of these ions take place. Thus, substitutions of OH^- by F^- or Cl^- ions, of the phosphate by sulfate and carbonate and of the calcium by Sr^{2+}, Mg^{2+} and Na^+ ions have been reported (Heughebaert et al., 1983; Legeros R.Z & Legeros J.P., 1984; Moreno & Varughese, 1981; Nathan, 1984).
A considerable amount of the work done for the identification of calcium phosphate minerals which precipitates spontaneously has been based on the stoichiometric molar ratio of calcium to phosphate calculated from the respective changes in the solutions. This ratio has been found in several cases to be 1.45±0.05 which is considerably lower than the value of 1.67 corresponding to HAP which is generally implied as the precipitating mineral. A number of different precursor phases have been postulated to be formed including TCP (Montel et al., 1981; Narasaraju & Phebe, 1996; Walton et al., 1967), OCP (Eanes & Posner, 1968, Posner, 1969) and DCPD (Furedi-Milhofer et al., 1976). On the basis of the analysis of the induction times preceding the spontaneous precipitation of calcium phosphate, it was concluded that at high solution supersaturations the initially forming ACP was converted into an apatitic mineral through an OCP precursor phase formation (Fransis & Webb, 1971).

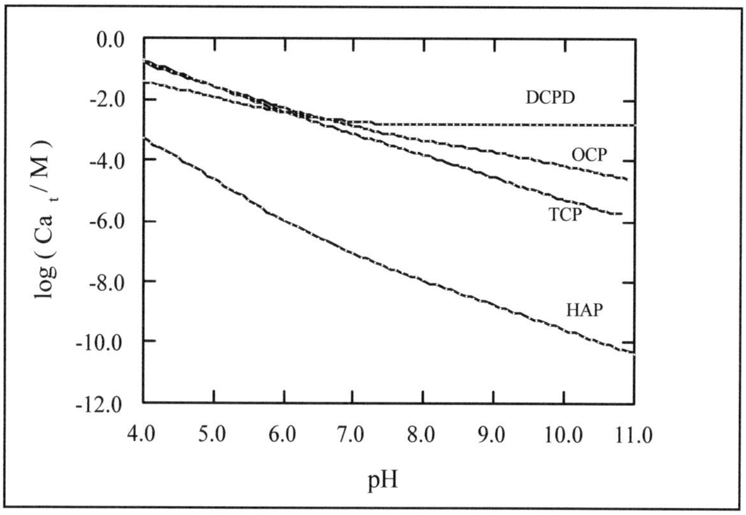

Fig. 8. Solubility isothems for calcium phosphate phases at 25°C, Ionic strength 0.1M NaCl

Spontaneous precipitation investigations have been faced with the problem that at high supersaturations the ACP forming initially results in a rapid decrease of the calcium and phosphate ion activities which fall bellow the values needed for the spontaneous formation of other calcium phosphate phases. A careful analysis of the precipitation of calcium phosphate over the pH range 5.0-8.0 suggested that the limiting ion activity product for ACP was constant as expected for a discrete mineral phase. Moreover it has also been shown that the presence of magnesium in the precipitation medium promoted the formation of DCPD at the expense of ACP (Feenstra & de Bruyn, 1979; Posner et al., 1984).

The driving force for the formation of a solid phase in a continuous aqueous phase is the solution supersaturation which can be developed in many ways including temperature fluctuation, pH change, mixing of incompatible waters, increasing the concentration by evaporation or solid dissolution etc. Although supersaturation is the driving force for the formation of a salt, the exact values in which precipitation occurs are quite different from salt to salt and as a rule, the degree of supersaturation needed for a sparingly soluble salt is orders of magnitude higher than the corresponding value for a soluble salt. For sparingly soluble salts $M_{v+}A_{v-}$ the supersaturation ratio, S, is defined as:

$$S = \left\{ \frac{\left(a_{M^{m+}}\right)_s^{\nu+} \left(\alpha_{A^{a-}}\right)_s^{\nu-}}{\left(a_{M^{m+}}\right)_\infty^{\nu+} \left(a_{A^{a-}}\right)_\infty^{\nu-}} \right\} = \left(\frac{IP}{K_s^{\,o}}\right)^{1/\nu} \tag{1}$$

where subscripts s and ∞ refer to solution and equilibrium conditions respectively, a denote the activities of the respective ions and $\nu_{+}+\nu_{-}=\nu$. IP and $K_s^{\,o}$ are the ion products in the supersaturated solution and at equilibrium respectively.

The fundamental driving force for the formation of a salt from a supersaturated solution is the difference in chemical potential of the solute in the supersaturated solution from the respective value at equilibrium:

$$\Delta\mu = \mu_\infty - \mu_s \tag{2}$$

Since the chemical potential is expressed in terms of the standard potential and the activity, a, of the solute:

$$\mu = \mu^o + RT \ln a \tag{3}$$

where R and T are the gas constant and the absolute temperature respectively. Substitution of eq. (3) to eq.(2) gives for the driving force for solid deposition (Mullin, 1993):

$$\frac{\Delta\mu}{RT} = \ln\left(\frac{a_s}{a_\infty}\right) = \ln S \tag{4}$$

For electrolyte solutions the mean ionic activity is taken:

$$a = a_{\pm}^{\ \nu}(\nu = \nu_+ + \nu_-) \tag{5}$$

and

$$\frac{\Delta\mu}{RT} = \ln\left(\frac{\alpha_{\pm,s}}{\alpha_{\pm,\infty}}\right)^{\frac{1}{\nu}} = \ln S \tag{6}$$

4.2 Crystal growth in heart valves

Degeneration of the leaflet tissue, together with calcification constitutes the principal reasons for bioprosthetic valve failure (Schoen et al., 1992). Calcification consists as already mentioned in the formation of sparingly soluble salts of calcium phosphate due to the presence of high levels of calcium and phosphate in blood serum (Schneck, 1995). Although the calcific deposits consist of apatitic calcium phosphate (HAP containing mainly carbonate, fluoride, magnesium and sodium) the formation of transient precursor phases such as DCPD and OCP is possible, as in vitro studies have shown (Brown et al., 1957; Heughebaert et al., 1983; Moreno & Varughese, 1981). The formation of calcium phosphates on porcine heart valves to a percentage of 30-50% is responsible for their dysfunction after 12-15 years due to stenosis or insufficiency (Narasaraju & Rao, 1979).

Despite the fact that the thermodynamic driving force in blood serum for nucleation and growth is sufficiently high for the homogeneous formation of calcium phosphates, the process is believed to be heterogeneous as dead cell remnants, lipids or degenerative collagen fragments may provide active sites for heterogeneous nucleation. Chemical treatment of porcine and pericardial bioprosthetic valves with glutaraldehyde is considered as one of the main causes of valve calcification (Hammersmeister et al., 1993; Schoen & Levy, 1992). Despite intensive research of the past few decades, the mechanism of initiation and development of calcific deposits on tissues in contact with blood is still poorly understood. As a result the development and production of biological valves resistant to calcification is still a major challenge (Grabenwoger et al., 1996; Schoen et al, 1987). Biological, chemical and mechanical factors seem to play a significant role in the kinetics of the process of calcification (Zipkin, 1970).

4.3 Models of heart valve calcification

Heart valve calcification is a slow process, difficult to be studied in vivo in humans. Various animal models, like the rat subcutaneous implantation, have been used for simulation of biological environment but in accelerated process conditions, in order to study calcification mechanisms. In vitro calcification models have also proposed. These models have the advantage of studying the role of isolated or group of parameters that may contribute in calcification. Both models are very useful especially as pre-screening methods for studying the efficacy of various anticalcification treatments proposed (Bailey et al., 2004; Gross, 2003; Kapolos et al., 1997; Krings et al., 2009; Schoen & Levy, 2005).

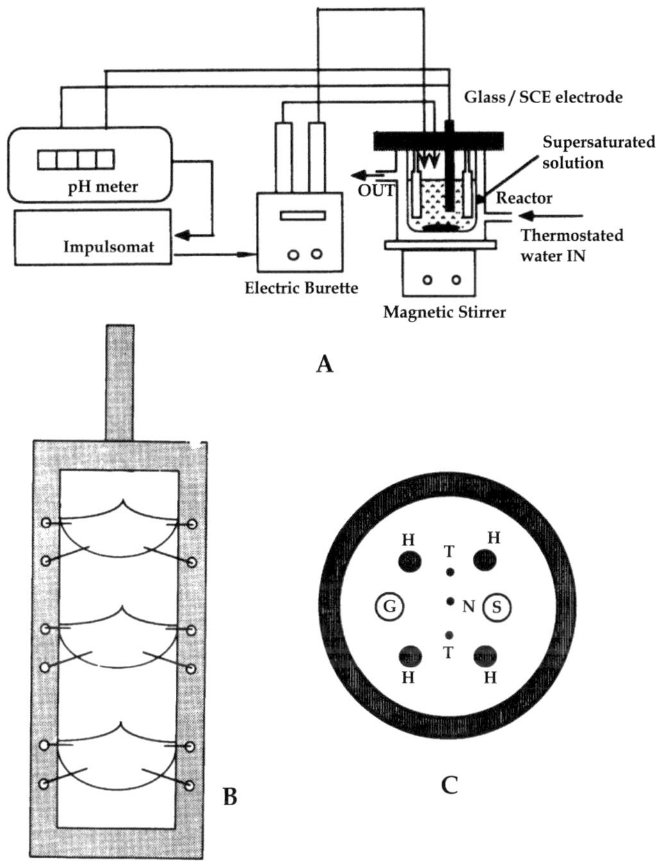

Fig. 9. Experimental set-up for the quantitative investigation of the calcification of heart valves in vitro. (A) Automatic titrator apparatus (B) Mounting of heart valves (C) Lid of the reactor (Kapolos et al., 1997)

The use of various model experimental procedures has resulted in the suggestion that the calcification is initiated at the matrix vesicles (Anderson, 1983; Wuthier, 1982), by acid phospholipids (Boskey, 1981; Boskey & Posner, 1977) or by heterogeneous nucleation of various calcium phosphate phases in the body fluids considered as aqueous solutions supersaturated with respect to the salts formed (Kim & Trump, 1975; Dallas et al., 1989;, Schoen et al., 1985; Brown et al., 1988; Grott et al., 1992). Despite intensive research, it seems that there is no agreement on the mechanism of formation of calcific deposits. As a result, the evaluations of bioprosthetic materials used for cardiac valve replacements are often met with not unfounded criticism. One of the most successful experimental models presented, which is appropriate for the in vitro investigation of mineralization processes is the constant supersaturation model introduced and further developed by Nancollas and co-workers (Thomson & Nancollas, 1978; Amzad et al., 1978). This methodology allows for the solution supersaturation to be kept constant by the addition of titrant solutions. The concentrations of the reagents in these solutions are calculated so that full replacement of the precipitated mass is ensured. In the case of tests performed on the mineralization of heart valves the rates obtained from this system were proportional to the solution's supersaturation.

An in vitro model, based in the constant supersaturation model was introduced in 1997 in our laboratories for the investigation of heart valve calcification in vitro. The experimental set-up is shown in figure 9. Porcine aortic heart valves, treated with glutaraldehyde were sutured on Plexiglas® frames to be kept in flat position during stirring. The frames were immersed in supersaturated solution with respect to calcium and phosphate ions in near physiological concentrations, at 37°C. Solution's pH drop, associated with initiation of crystal growth deposited out of solution, triggered titrant addition with movement of computer controlled syringe pumps.

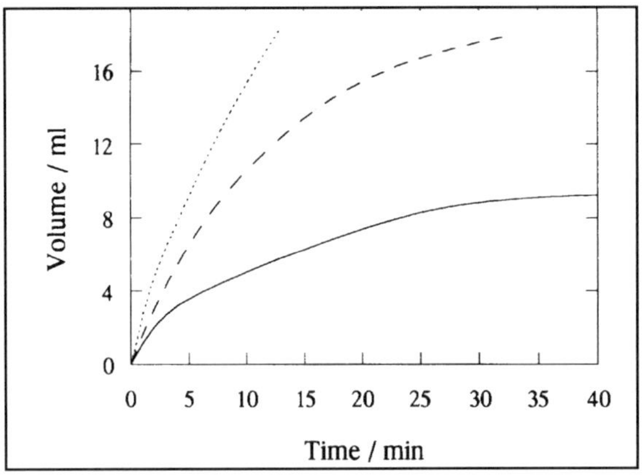

Fig. 10. Titrant addition for maintaining constant supersaturation during the course of mineralization of artificial heart valves. The rates were increased with increasing solution supersaturation (σ=0.72 , 1.09, 1.25 from the lower to the upper curve respectively)

Figure 10 presents experimental recordings of titrant volume added with time, in order to maintain solution's supersaturation constant. The signal from a pH drop sensitive device resulted from the growth of calcium phosphate crystals precipitated out of the solution, triggered titrant addition in small time steps. The diagrams correspond to different solution supersaturations. The mineral phase deposited on the glutaraldehyde treated porcine valves was identified as OCP, hydrolysed partially to HAP. The extent of hydrolysis was larger at the lower supersaturations, while at higher supersaturations with respect to OCP, this phase was stabilized, as may be seen in the scanning electron micrographs shown in figure11a-c. The characteristic plate like crystals are clearly seen in figure 11b.The rates, calculated from the titrants addition rates and normalized per unit geometric surface area of the exposed valves, were fitted to the semi empirical equation:

$$R_g = k_g f(S)\sigma^n \tag{7}$$

where k_g is the rate constant for crystal growth, *f(S)* a function of the total number of the growth sites available and *n* the apparent order of the crystal growth process. Logarithmic plots according to eq.7 yielded the kinetics shown in figure 12. The practical implications of this finding is that the deposition of the mineral phase on the membrane matrix is controlled by the diffusion of the growth units on the OCP nuclei been formed.

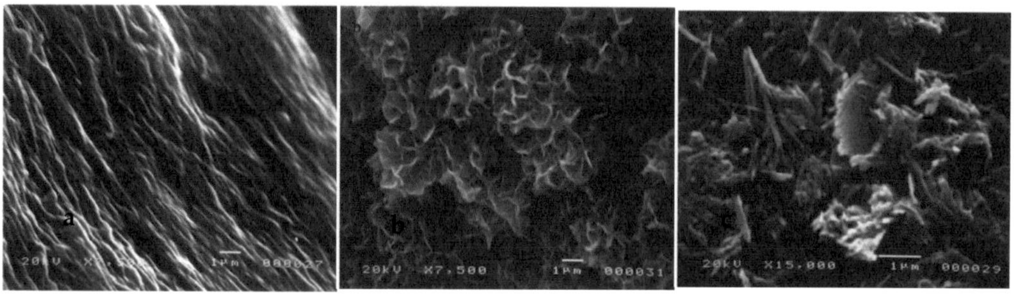

Fig. 11. Scanning electron micrographs of : (a) surface of the valves (b) OCP deposited on the valves at higher relative supersaturation and (c) OCP+HAP on valves at low relative supersaturation

Possible strategies aiming at the retardation of the calcification process should therefore rely on the alteration of the surfaces so as to make surface integration more difficult. An additional feature revealed by the kinetics plots at constant supersaturation (figure 12) is that the glutaraldehyde treated porcine valves are substrates favoring the mineral nucleation and growth.

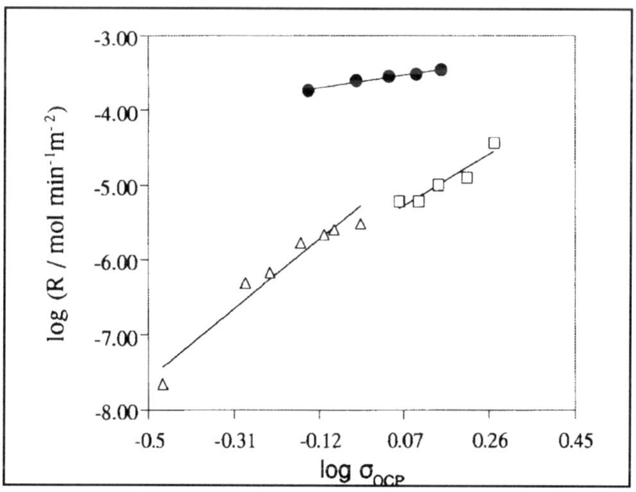

Fig. 12. Logarithm of the rate of OCP formation on glutaraldeyde treated porcine valves (black circles) as a function of the relative solution supersaturation; pH 7.4, 37° C, 0.15M NaCl. Open squares and triangles refer to literature results. Experiments performed in our laboratory with the same methodology on fresh, untreated porcine valves have shown that these tissues failed to induce any formation of calcium phosphate deposits although they were kept in the mineralizing solution for as long as four days

Comparison with data obtained for OCP synthetic crystals (Tomazic et al., 1989) and collagen of various types (Heughebaert & Nancollas, 1984; Combes, 1996) showed that glutaraldehyde treated porcine valves accelerated the formation of OCP. The significantly larger value of the rate constant suggested that in this case the number of active sites is not possibly a function of the available surface area. Structural factors on a molecular level should also be considered. Calcium phosphate crystal growth and crystal phases transformations obtained from the results of our in vitro model have been well correlated with similar results obtained from microscopic examinations, chemical analysis and spectrophotometric characterization of crystal phases on samples from calcified natural and bioprosthetic heart valves (Mikroulis et al., 2002). From the composition, the morphology and the size of the developed crystals their nature was determined by comparison with reference synthetic calcium phosphate phases. With this technique it was possible to determine the morphology of CDs developed at the internal sites of the tissue at high magnifications. It seems that in cases of natural heart valves the CDs are mixture of HAP ($Ca:PO_4$=1.67) and OCP ($Ca:PO_4$=1.33), while in bioprosthetic CDs the percentage of OCP is higher than of native in which the ratio $Ca:PO_4$ (1,82) is close to the $Ca:PO_4$ composition of mature physiological biomineral in bone (1,75).
As an overall conclusion from combined studies examined CDs from calcified valve leaflets in vitro, in animal models and in vivo, a model of development of calcification by crystal growth through the formation of precursor phases, which are gradually hydrolyzed in smaller in size, thermodynamically more stable crystal formations may be introduced. According to this, initiation of calcification may be supposed to take place in sites of heterogenous nucleation, formed in different tissue deficiencies, together with local changes in already highly supersaturated body fluids. This model can be very useful in the introduction of anticalcification therapies or techniques for better biomaterials.

5. Conclusion

Heart valve calcification is still a serious complication for a great number of patients, especially in economical active ages and the elderly. Although anticalcification therapies and procedures have been introduced for valve repair, valve replacement, especially that of aortic and mitral valves is the last choice. Unfortunately, till today there is no "ideal" aortic valve prosthesis. The latter would be easy to be implanted, possess long-term durability, would have no thrombogenicity, maximum effective orifice area, without haemolysis, "resistant" to infective endocarditis, and produce minima noise (Birkmeyer et al., 2000). Currently, available options for the patient include mechanical valve, stented or stentless biologic heterograft valves, allograft valves and pulmonary autograft valves. For the selection between mechanical and biologic valve the surgeon should balance the risks and benefits of each model. The mechanical valve has a long-term durability (till 35-40 years), but on the other hand its thrombogenicity is high, 2-4% per year. In addition, the administered anticoagulation has a significantly increased risk of bleeding. The biologic valve has an increased risk of degeneration, as its durability lasts not more than 10-12 years after implantation (Siddiqui et al., 2009). After this time, a significant regurgitation demands its replacement with an increased operative mortality in comparison to the initial implantation (about two-fold higher). On the other hand, the thrombogenicity of the biologic valve is lower than of mechanical ones, about 1% per year (Puvimanasinghe et al., 2003). Analyses based on mathematical models of data suggest that the selection of 3rd-generation biologic valve for patients at about 60 years of age derive improved life expectancy and event-free expectancy regardless of the need for concomitant coronary artery surgery (Birkmeyer et al., 2000). Of course, for special patient groups the indications should be changed. Patients who do need a long-term anticoagulation such as those with chronic atrial fibrillation, intracardiac thrombus, history of thromboembolic events, hypercoagulable state or low ejection fraction, should receive a mechanical valve regardless of age. In the contrary, patients with contraindication to anticoagulants, with bleeding disorders, women of child-bearing age, should receive a biologic valve (Bonow et al., 2006). Patients with chronic renal failure have a higher risk of earlier bioprosthetic valve degeneration, and also an increased incidence of anticoagulation-related complications. For that reason, the current ACC/AHA guidelines (2006) do not recommend the routine use of a mechanical prosthesis (Bonow et al., 2006).

6. The future: Tissue engineering (TE)

Artificial devices designed and manufactured for mid and long term implantation in patients has to satisfy quality criteria of biocompatibility and function during all implantation time expected. This time period is varied, from a few months, for temporary used prostheses, like some orthopaedic fixation plaques and screws, to long life function, as in the case of prosthetic heart valves. Despite of their evolution and future trends, even if medical technology could make implants satisfying that criteria, prosthetic devices made of, in its best, biologically inert biomaterials cannot meet a serious clinical problem: they cannot follow changes in patient's body from the time of implantation to end of their expected life. In other words, they cannot grow up and remodelled with patient. Tissue engineering is a recent technological approach in the construction of artificial implants that can be gradually remodelled into the patient in real living tissue and organs, following regeneration and auto repair capabilities similar to that of the other natural patient body components (Kretlow & Mikos, 2008; Zilla et al., 2008). Attempts for the construction of TE implants are spread to different tissues and organs, like dermal parches, cartilage, bone and cardiovascular implants and TE or hybrid organs like pancreas or liver. Design and construction of cardiovascular TE implants, like heart valves and blood vessels, is still a challenge because of numerous worldwide needs and the severity of possible failure.

As a general rule TE valves composed of two groups of biomaterials. One group is composing the scaffold, a structure having the morphology of natural heart valves, usually a biodegradable flexible composite synthetic membrane of a polymeric fibber network embedded in amorphous organic matrix. Different structure of valve parts like valve ring, wall stent and leaflets give to the synthetic valve mechanical strength and flexibility identical to function like natural heart valves. However, scaffolds have a temporary role as, in addition and in parallel with their normal physiological function as heart valves, they may have the ability to support cell adhesion in their structure. Different cells, like fibroblasts, smooth muscle cells and endothelia may adhere, proliferate, stimulated and function into the scaffold valve structure to produce different tissue components that will synergy to compose suitable valvular tissue. Some of these valve cells are transported into scaffold material prior implantation, followed by in vitro cell culture and parallel mechanical valve function in special designed devices, bioreactors. A hybrid structure of synthetic and living biomaterials is made in vitro, which by implantation in the living organism is expected to continue remodelling into real living tissue and organ. As the final form, a natural living heart valve, without any synthetic scaffold components is expected to replace the fully biodegraded initially implanted heart valve device (Flanangan & Pandit, 2003; Ye et al., 2000; Jockenhoevel et al., 2001). Key factors for succession of such an approach are:

- Biocompatibility and mechanical function of scaffold.
- Rate and products of biodegradation.
- Functionalization of scaffold to enhance cell adhesion.
- Selection of initial cell population suitable for in vitro cell culture. Non differentiated cells, like bone marrow or umbilical cord derived stem cells, seem to be advantageous in responding to biochemical environment and stimulation in bioreactors, towards differentiation to cells needed for the in vitro synthesis of initial components of valvular tissue.

Understanding of cell-biomaterial-biomechanics interaction needs a multidisciplinary synergism in order to result in successful TE valve, avoiding possible future undesirable side effects, like valve failure or carcinogenesis.

7. References

Amjad Z, Koutsoukos P.G., Tomson M.B. & Nancollas G.H. (1978). The growth of hydroxyapatite from solution. A new constant composition method. *J.Dent. Res.*Vol. 57,pp.909-910.

Anderson H.C. (1983). Calcific diseases. A concept. *Arch. Pathol. Lab. Med.* Vol.107, pp.341-348.

Angell W.W, Bush W.S. & Iben B.A. (1972). Formalin preservation of porcine heterografts. In *Biological tissue in heart valve replacemen,*. Ionescu M.I., Ross D.N. & Wooler G.H., Ch.23;pp.543-552, Butterworths London.

Barratt-Boyes B.G. (1964). Homograft aortic valve replacement in aortic incompetence and stenosis. *Thorax* Vol. 19;pp.129-131.

Binet J., Duran C., Carpentier A. & Langlois J. (1965). Heterologous aortic valve transplantation. *Lancet* Vol.286; pp.1275.

Birkmeyer N., Birkmeyer J., Tosteson A. et al. (2000). Prosthetic valve type for patients undergoing aortic valve replacement: a decision analysis. *Ann Thorac Surg*, Vol.70;pp.1946-1962.

Betts F. & Posner A.S. (1974). An X-ray radial distribution study of amorphous calcium phosphate. *Mater. Res. Bull.*, Vol.9;pp.907-914.

Boskey A.L. & Posner A.S. (1977). The role of synthetic and bone extracted Ca-phospholipid-phosphate complexes in hydroxyapatite formation. *Calcif. Tissue Res.* Vol.18;pp.155-160.

Boskey A.L. (1981) Current concepts of the physiology and biochemistry of calcification. *Clin. Orthop.* Vol.157;pp.225-238 .

Bosmans J., Kefer J., De Bruyne B. et al. (2011). Procedural, 30-day and one year outcome following CoreValve or Edwards transcatheter aortic valve implantation: results of the Belgian national registry. *Interactive CardioVascular and Thoracic Surgery.* Vol.12(5);pp.762-767.

Bonow R.O., Carabello B., de Leon A.C.Jr. et al. (1998).ACC/AHA guidelines for the management of patients with valvular heart disease: a report of the American

College of Cardiology/ American Heart Association Task Force on Practice Guidelines (Committee on Management of Patients With Valvular Heart Disease). *JACC* Vol.32;pp.1486 -1588.

Brener S.J., Duffy C., Thomas J.D. et al. (1995). Progression of aortic stenosis in 394 patients: relation to changes in myocardial and mitral valve dysfunction. *J Am Coll Cardiol.* Vol.25:pp.305-310.

Brown W.E., Lehr J.R., Smith J.P. & Frazier A.W. (1957). Crystallography of octacalcium phosphate, *J. Amer. Chem. Soc.* Vol.79;pp.5318-5319.

Brown W.E., Edelman N. & Tomazic B. (1988). Octacalcium phosphate as a precursor in biomineral formation. *Adv. Dent. Res.* Vol.1;pp.306-312 .

Carpentier A., Lemaigre G., Robert L. et al. (1969). Biological factors affecting long-term results of valvular heterografts. *J Thorac Cardiovasc Surg* Vol.58;pp.467-483.

Chambers J., Roxburgh J., Blauth C. et al. (2005). A randomized comparison of the MCRI On-X and Carbomedics Top Hat bileaflet mechanical replacement aortic valves: early postoperative hemoduynamic function and clinical events. *J Thorac Cardiovasc Surg* Vol.130;pp. 759-764.

Combes C. (1996). Croissance Cristalline de phosphates de calcium sur des substrats d' interet biologiques: Le titane et le Collagène, *Thèse,* pp.55-60. INPT, Toulouse, France.

Cormier B, & Vahanian A. (1992). Indications and outcome of valvuloplasty. *Curr Opin Cardiol* Vol.7;pp.222-226.

Cribier A., Elchaninoff H., Bash A. et al. (2002). Percutaneous transcatheter implantation of an aortic valve prosthesis for calcific aortic stenosis: First human case description. *Circulation* Vol.106;pp.3006-3008.

Dalas E., Ioannou P.V. & Koutsoukos P.G. (1989). Effect of fatty acyl and cation content of cardiolipins on in vitro calcification. *Langmuir,*Vol.5;pp.157-160.

Davidson M. & Baim D. (2008). Percutaneous aortic valve interventions. In *Cardiac Surgery in the Adult,* Cohn L. pp.963-968. 3rd Edition, Mc Graw Hill Medical, New York-Chicago-San Francisco.

Davidson C.J., Harrison J.K.., Leithe M.E. et al. (1990). Failure of aortic balloon valvuloplasty to result in sustained clinical improvement in patients with depressed left ventricular function. *Am J Cardiol,* Vol.65;pp.72-77.

Diethrich E. (1993). The treatment of aortic stenosis: is valvuloplasty ever an alternative to surgery? *J Interv Cardiol,*Vol.3;pp.7-13.

Eanes E.A., Gillessen I.H. & Posmer A.S. (1965). Intermediate stages in the precipitation of hydroxyapatite. *Nature,* Vol.208;pp.365-367.

Eanes E.D. & Posner A.S. (1968). Alkaline earth intermediate phases in the basic solution preparation of phosphates. *Calcif. Tiss. Res.,* Vol.2;pp.38-48.

Edwards W. (1996). Applied anatomy of the heart. In: *Mayo Clinic Practice of Cardiology,* Giuliani E., Gersh B., McGoon M., Hayes D. & Schaff H., pp. 466-468. 3rd Ed, Mosby St. Louis-Baltimore-Boston.

Emery R., Arom K., Kshetry V. et al. (2002). Decision making in the choice of heart valve for replacement in patients aged 60-70 years: twenty-year follow-up of the St. Jude Medical aortic valve prostheses. *J Heart Valve Dis,* Vol.11; (Suppl 1);pp.S37-S44.

Emery R., Krogh C., Jones D. et al. (2004). Five-year follow-up of the ATS mechanical heart valve. *J Heart Valve Dis,* Vol.13;pp.231-236.

Emery R., Emery A., Knutsen A. et al. (2008). Aortic valve replacement with a mechanical cardiac valve prosthesis. In: *Cardiac Surgery in the Adult.* Cohn L. pp.841-854. 3rd Edition, Mc Graw Hill Medical, New York-Chicago-San Francisco.

Ezekowitz M. (2002) Anticoagulation management of valve replacement patients. *J Heart Valve Dis,* Vol.11, (suppl1);pp.S56-S60.

Faggiano P., Aurigemma G.P., Rusconi C. et al. (1996). Progression of valvular AS in adults: literature review and clinical implications. *Am Heart J,* Vol.132;pp.408 –417.

Feenstra T.P. & de Bruyn P.L. (1979). Formation of calcium phosphates in moderately Supersaturated Solutions. *J. Phys. Chem.,* Vol.83;pp.475-479.

Flanangan T.C. & Pandit A. (2003). Living artificial heart valve alternatives: A review. *European Cells and Materials,* Vol.6;pp.28-45.

Francis M.D. & Webb N.C. (1971). Hydroxyapatite Formation from a Hydrated calcium Monohydrogen Phosphate Precursor. *Calcif. Tissue Res.,* Vol.6;pp.335-342.

Freeman R. & Otto C. (2005). Spectrum of Calcific Aortic Valve Disease: Pathogenesis, Disease Progression, and Treatment Strategies. *Circulation,* Vol.111;pp.3316-3326.

Furedi-Milhofer H., Brecevic L. & Purgaric B. (1976). Crystal growth and phase transformation in the precipitation of calcium phosphates, *Faraday Discussions Chem. Soc.,* Vol.61;pp.184-190.

Gelsomino S., Morocutti G., Da Col P. et al. (2002). Preliminary experience with the St. Jude Medical Regent mechanical heart valve in the aortic position: early in vivo hemodynamic results. *Ann Thorac Surg,* Vol.73pp.1830-1836.

Gibbon J.H. Jr. (1954). Application of a mechanical heart and lung apparatus to cardiac surgery. *Minn Med,* Vol.37;pp.171-185.

Gott V., Alejo D. & Cameron D. (2003). Mechanical heart valves: 50 years of evolution. *Ann Thorac Surg,* Vol.76;pp.S2230-S2239.

Grabenwoger M., Sider J., Fitzal F. et al. (1996). Impact of Glutaraldehyde on Calcification of Pericardial Bioprosthetic Heart Valve Material. *Ann Thomac Surg,* Vol.62;pp.772-777.

Gross J.M. (2003). Calcification of bioprosthetic heart valves and its assessment. *J Thorac Cardiovasc Surg,* Vol. 125;pp.S6-S8.

Grott T.P., Chih P., Dorsey L.M.A. et al. (1992). Calcificationof Porcine valves: A successful new method of antimineralization. *Ann Thorac Surg,* Vol.53;pp.207-216.

Hall R. & Julian D. (1989). *Diseases of the cardiac valves.* Churchill Livingstone, Edinburgh-London-Melbourne-New York.

Hammermeister K.E., Sethi G.K., Henderson W.G. et al. (1993). A comparison of outcomes in men 11 years after heart-valve replacement with a mechanical valve or bioprosthesis. *New Engl. J Med,* Vol.328;pp.189-1296.

Harken D.E., Taylor W.J., Lefemine A.A. et al., (1962). Aortic valve replacement with a caged ball valve. *American Journal of Cardiology,* Vol.9(2);pp.292-299.

Hench L.L. & Wilson J. (1991). Bioceramics. *Materials Research Society Bulletin,* Vol.16(9);pp. 62-74.

Hess O., Villari B. & Krayenbuehl H. (1993). Diastolic dysfunction in aortic stenosis. *Circulation,* Vol.87 (Suppl IV);pp.73-76.

Heughebaert J.C., Zawacki S.J. & Nancollas G.H. (1983). *J. Crystal Growth,*. Vol.63; pp.83-90.

Heughebaert J.C. & Nancollas G.H. (1984). Kinetics of crystallization of octacalcium phosphate. *J. Phys. Chem,* Vol. 88;pp.2478-2481.

Hufnagel C.A. & Harvey W.P. (1953). Surgical correction of aortic insufficiency. *Bull Georgetown U Med Cenert;* Vol.6;pp.60-61.

Ionescu M. & Ross D. (1969). Heart-valve replacement with autologous fascia lata. *Lancet,* Vol.2;pp.335-338.

Jockenhoevel S., Zund G., Hoerstrup S.P. et al. (2001). Fibrin gel - advantages of a new scaffold in cardiovascular tissue engineering. *European Journal of Cardio-thoracic Surgery,* Vol.19;pp.424-430.

Kapolos J., Mavrilas D., Missirlis Y.F. & Koutsoukos P. G. (1997). Model experimental system for investigation of heart valve calcification in vitro. *J Biomed Mater Res (Appl Biomater),* Vol.38;pp.183-190.

Kretlow J.D. & Mikos A.G. (2008). 2007 AlChE Alpha Chi Sigma Award: From material to tissue: Biomaterial development, scaffold fabrication, and tissue engineering. *AIChE J.* Vol.54(12);pp.3048-3067.

Kim K.M. & Trump B.F. (1975). Amorphous calcium phosphate precipitations in human aortic valve. *Calcif. Tissue Res,* Vol.18;pp.155-160.

Krings M., Kanellopoulou D., Koutsoukos P.G. et al. (2009). Development of a new combined test setup for accelerated dynamic pH-controlled in vitro calcification of porcine heart valves. *Int J Artif Organs,* Vol.32;pp.794-801.

LeGeros R.Z., Shirra W.P., Mirawite M.A. & LeGeros J.P., (1975). In: *Physico-Chimie et Cristallographie des Apatites d' Interêt Biologique,* CNRS, Colloque Internationaux, Paris.

LeGeros R.Z. & LeGeros J.P. (1984). Phosphate minerals in human tissues, In: *Phosphate Minerals,* Nriagu J.O., Moore P.B.,pp. 351-385, Springer Velag, Berlin Heidelberg.

Malouf J., Edwards W., Tajik J. & Seward J. (2008). Functional anatomy of the heart. In: *Hurst' s The Heart,* Fuster V., O'Rourke R., Walsh R. & Poole-Wilson P. pp.61-63. 12th Edition, McGraw Hill, New York-Chicago-San Fransisco.

Mikroulis D., Mavrilas D., Kapolos J. et al. (2002). Physicochemical and Microscopical study of Calcific Deposits from Natural and Bioprosthetic heart Valves. Comparison and implications for mineralization mechanism. *J Mater Sci: Mater Med.* Vol.13;pp. 885-889.

Moreno E.C. & Varughese K.J. (1981). Crystal growth of apatites from dilute solutions, *J. Crystal Growth,* Vol.53;pp.20-30.

Montel G., Bonel G., Heughebaert J.C. et al. (1981). New Concepts in the Composition, Crystallization and Growth of the Mineral Component of Calcified Tissue. *J. Crystal Growth,* Vol.53;pp.74-99.

Mullin J.W. (1993). *Crystallization,* pp.118-122. 3rd Ed. Butterworth-Heinemann, Oxford.

Murray G. (1956). Homologous aortic valve segment transplant as surgical treatment for aortic and mitral insufficiency. *Angiology,* Vol.7;pp.466-471.

Narasaraju T.S.B. & Phebe D.E. (1996). Some physico-chemical aspects of hydroxyapatite, *J. Mater. Science,* Vol.31;pp.1-21.

Narasaraju T.S.B, Rao K.K. & Rai U.S. (1979). Determination of solubility products of hydroxylapatite, chloroapatite and their solid solutions. *Canad. J.Chem.,* Vol.57;pp. 1919-1922.

Nathan Y. (1984). The mineralogy and geochemistry of phosphorites. In: *Phosphate Minerals,* Nriagu J.O. &, Moore P.B. pp. 275-291, Springer Verlag, Berlin Heidelberg.

Newesely H. (1966). Changes in Crystal types of low solubility calcium phosphates in of accompanying ions. *Arch. Oral Biol. Sp.* Suppl., 6;pp.174 .

Olsson M., Thyberg J. & Nilsson J. (1999). Presence of oxidized low density lipoprotein in nonrheumatic stenotic aortic valves. *Arterioscler Thromb Vasc Biol.* Vol.19;pp.1218-1222.

Otto C., Lind B., Kitzman D. et al. (1999). Association of aortic-valve sclerosis with cardiovascular mortality and morbidity in the elderly. *N Engl J Med,* Vol.341;pp. 142-147.

Oxenham H., Bloomfield P., Wheatley D. et al. (2003). Twenty-year comparison of a Bjork-Shilley mechanical heart valve with porcine bioprostheses. *Heart* Vol.89;pp.715.

Park J.B. & Lakes R.S. (1992). *Biomaterials: An Introduction.* Chapter 1;pp.4. Plenum Press, NY.

Posner A.S. (1969). Crystal Chemistry of Bone Mineral. *Physiol. Rev.,* Vol.49;pp.760-792.

Posner A.S., Blumenthal N.C. & Betts F. (1984). Chemistry and structure of precipitated hydroxyapatites. In: *Phosphate Minerals,* Nriagu J.O. & Moore P.B., pp. 330-350. Springer Verlag, Berlin Heidelberg.

Potter D., Sundt T., Zehr K. et al. (2005). Operative risk of reoperative aortic valve replacement. *J Thorac Cardiovasc Surg,* Vol.129;pp.94-103.

Puvimanasinghe J., Takkenberg J., Eijkemans M., et al. (2003). Choice of a mechanical valve or a bioprosthesis for AVR: does CABG matter? *Eur J Cardiothorac Surg* Vol.23;pp.688-695.

Rahimtoola S. (2004). Aortic valve disease. In: *Hurst's The Heart,* Fuster V., Wayne Alexander R.O., Rourke R., et al. pp.1644-1645. 11th Edition, Mac Graw Hill Medical Publishing Division, New York-Chicago-San Francisco.

Rahimtoola S. (2010). Choice of prosthetic heart valve in adults. *JACC* Vol.55;pp.2413-2426.

Schoen F.J., Levy B.J., Nelson A.C. et al. (1985). Onset and progression of experimental bioprosthetic heart valve calcification. *Lab. Invest.* Vol.52;pp.523-532.

Shoen F.J., Kujovich J.L., Webb C.L. & Levy R.J. (1987). Chemically determined mineral content of explanted porcine valve bioprostheses. Correlation with radiographic assessment of calcification and clinical data. *Circulation* Vol.76;pp.1061-1066.

Schoen F.J., Harasaki H., Kim K.H. et al. (1988). Biomaterial associated calcification: pathology, mechanisms and strategies of prevention. *J. Biomed Mater Res: Appl Biomater* Vol.22;pp.11-36.

Schoen F.J., Levy R.J. & Piehler H.R. (1992). Pathological considerations in replacement cardiac valves. *Cardiovasc. Pathol.* Vol.1;pp.29-52.

Schoen F.J. & Levy R.J. (1992). Heart valve biorpostheses antimineralization. *Eur J Cardiothorac Surg* Vol.6 (suppl 1);pp.91-94.

Schoen F.J. & Levy R.J. (2005). Calcification of tissue heart valve substitutes: Progress toward understanding and prevention. *Ann Thorac Surg,* Vol.79;pp.1072-1080.

Schwartz J. & Zipes D. (2005). Cardiovascular disease in the elderly. In: *Braunwald's Heart Disease,* Zipes D., Libby P., O. Bonow R. & Braunwald E. pp.1944. 7th Edition, Elsevier Saunders, Philadelphia, Penn.

Schneck D.J. (1995). An outline of cardiovascular structure and function in: *The Biomedical Engineering Handbook,* Bronzino J.D. pp 3-14, CRC Press Boca Raton, Fla.

Senning A. (1967). Fascia lata replacement of aortic valves. *J Thorac Cardiovasc Surg* Vol.54;pp.465-470.

Shiono M., Sezai Y., Sezai A., et al. (2005). Long-term results of the cloth-covered Starr-Edwards ball valve. *Ann Thorac Surg* Vol.80;pp.204.

Siddiqui R., Abraham J., Butany J. (2009). Bioprosthetic heart valves: modes of failure. *Histopathology* Vol.55pp.135-44.

Simionescu, D., Simionescu, A., Deac, R. (1993). Mapping of glutaraldehyde-treated bovine pericardium and tissue selection for bioprosthetic heart valves. *J Biomed Mater Res* Vol.27;pp.697-704.

Smedira N., Ports T., Merrick S., et al. (1993). Balloon aortic valvuloplasty as a bridge to aortic valve replacement in critically patients. *Ann Thorac Surg,* Vol.55;pp.914.

Starr A., Edwards W., McCord M. et al. (1963). Aortic replacement. *Circulation* Vol.27;pp.779.

Stewart B.F., Siscovick D., Lind B.K. et al. (1997). Clinical factors associated with calcific aortic valve disease: Cardiovascular Health Study. *J Am Coll Cardiol.* Vol.29;pp.630 - 634.

Stewart W. (1998). Intraoperative echocardiography. In: *Textbook of Cardiovascular Medicine,* Topol E. pp.1497-1525. Lippincott-Raven: Philladelphia.

Tomazic B.B., Brown W.E. & Schoen F.J. (1989). Physicochemical characterization of bioprosthetic heart valve calcific deposits. *Calcified Tissue Int.* Vol.46;pp.S94.

Tomson M.B. & Nancollas G.H. (1978). Mineralization kinetics: a constant composition approach, *Science,* Vol.200;pp.1059-1060.

Wallby L., Janerot-Sjoberg B., Steffensen T. et al. (2002). T lymphocyte infiltration in non-rheumatic aortic stenosis: a comparative descriptive study between tricuspid and bicuspid aortic valves. *Heart.* Vol.88;pp.348 -351.

Walther T., Falk V., Tiggers R. et al. (2000). Comparison of On-X and SJM HP bileaflet aortic valves. *J Heart Valve Dis* Vol.9;pp.403-407.

Walton A.G., Badin W.J., Furedi, H. & Schwarz A. (1967). Nucleation of calcium phosphate from solution. *Canad. J. Chem.,* Vol.45;pp.2696-2701.

Williams P., Warwick R., Dyson M. & Bannister L. (1989). *Gray's Anatomy,* 37th Edition, Churchill Livingstone, Edinburg-London-Melbourne and New York.

Woodroof A.E. (1972). The chemistry and biology of aldehyde treated tissue heart valve xenografts. In: *Biological tissue in heart valve replacement,* Ionescu M.I., Ross D.N. & Wooler G.H.,Ch.10;pp.347-362. Butterworths London.

Wuthier R.E. (1982). A review of the primary mechanism of endochondrial calcification with special emphasis on the role of cells, mitochondria and matrix vesicles. *Clin.Orthopad,* Vol.169;pp.219-252.

Ye Q., Zund G., Benedikt P. et al. (2000). Fibrin gel as a three dimensional matrix in cardiovascular tissue engineering. *European Journal of Cardio-thoracic Surgery,* Vol.17;pp.587-591.

Zilla P., Brink J., Human P & Bezuidenhout D. (2008). Prosthetic heart valves: Catering for the few. *Biomaterials,* Vol. 29;pp.385-406.

Zipkin I. (1970). The inorganic composition of bones and teeth. In: Biological Calcification: Cellular and Molecular Aspects, Schraer H. pp.69-103, Appleton Century Crofts, New York.

Part 3

Aortic Root Replacement

5

Valve-Sparing Aortic Root Replacement and Aortic Valve Repair

William Y. Shi, Michael O' Keefe and George Matalanis
Department of Cardiac Surgery, Austin Hospital, University of Melbourne, Melbourne, Australia

1. Introduction

The impetus behind preservation of the native aortic valve derives from the desire to avoid the inherent shortcomings of prosthetic valves. These include the requirement for long term anticoagulation in the case of mechanical valves, and tissue degeneration with the need for re-operations with bioprostheses. Aortic valve preservation in the setting of aortic root dilatation is technically challenging, however potentially rewarding if these benefits can be achieved. This enthusiasm for aortic valve preservation must of course be tempered by the potential risks of residual or recurrent significant aortic regurgitation and subsequent complex re-operations associated with repair failures.
Appreciation of the complex three-dimensional anatomy of the normal aortic root and how it changes in pathological states is essential to facilitate reconstruction.

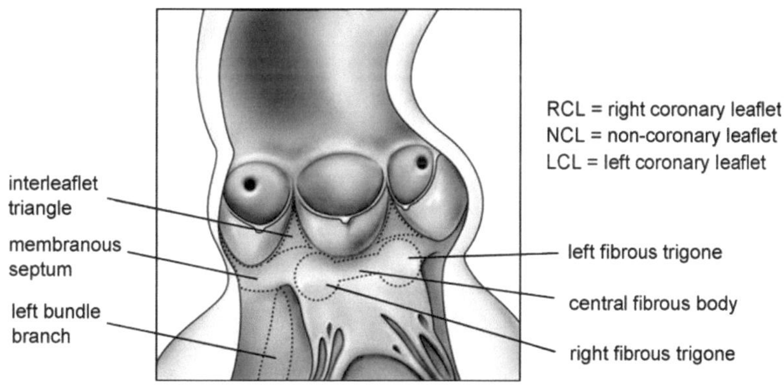

Reprinted from Heart, Lung and Circulation, 2004;13 Suppl 3, Matalanis G, Valve sparing aortic root repairs--an anatomical approach. S13-18., Copyright (2004), with permission from Elsevier

Fig. 1. The aortic valves, leaflets and adjacent aortic root structures, which participate in normal aortic valve function

2. Aortic root anatomy

The aortic valve's function is dependant upon its leaflets, the sinotubular junction (STJ), aortic sinuses and annulus, which together constitute the aortic root. Important geometric relationships exist between several of the aortic root dimensions [1-3].

In clinical practice the aortic annulus is defined as the superior most aspect of the left ventricular outflow tract (LVOT) which connects the aortic cusps and sinuses to the left ventricle. The annulus' perimeter consists of fibrous (55%) and muscular (45%) components. Of the two, the fibrous component is the one that tends to dilate first in aneurysmal disease.

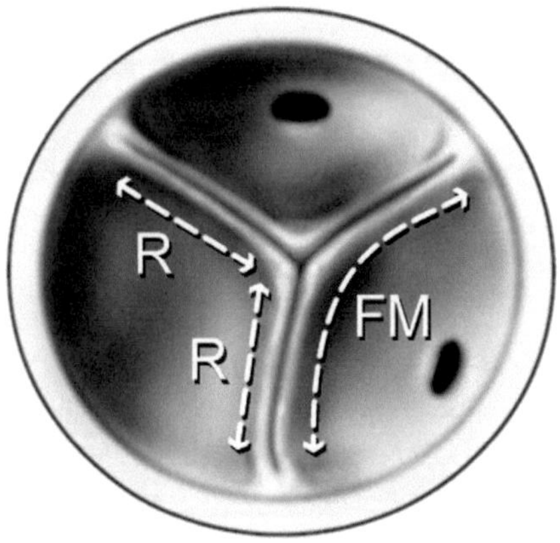

Reprinted from Heart, Lung and Circulation, 2004;13 Suppl 3, Matalanis G, Valve sparing aortic root repairs--an anatomical approach. S13-18., Copyright (2004), with permission from Elsevier

Fig. 2. Dimensions of the aortic valve cusps, whereby R is the radius of the STJ and FM represents the length of the valve cusp free margin

For a trileaflet valve to be competent in the closed position, while not be stenotic in the open position, the length of the free margin (FM) must geometrically be equivalent to the diameter at the STJ (Fig. 2):

Valve in Closed position

$\mathbf{FM} \approx 2 \times R$ (Radius of STJ)
$\mathbf{FM} \approx D$ (Diameter of STJ) .... ①

Valve in Open position

In order for the valve to hug the perimeter of the STJ in the open position, the circumference of the STJ (C) must be equivalent to the total length FM of the "n" leaflets combined:

$C \approx \mathbf{FM} \times n$; and thus
$\mathbf{FM} \approx C/n$ .... ②
Combining ① and ② we get:
$\mathbf{D} \approx C/n$
From basic geometry we know that $C = D \times \pi$, therefore:
$\mathbf{D} \approx (D \times \pi)/n$
$\pi \approx n$
since $\pi \approx 3$
hence $\mathbf{n} \approx 3$
ie. trileaflet design works best

Table 1. Why a trileaflet valve is ideal geometric design

Therefore the ideal number of cusps whereby the valve will neither be incompetent nor stenotic is three (trileaflet). By similar arguments, we can understand how if a bileaflet valve is to open properly (i.e. not be stenotic) it will have redundant FM in the closed position, and thus prolapse and become incompetent. On the other hand, if the bileaflet valve is to close properly (i.e. with no prolapse), it will have a smaller diameter than the STJ in the open position and therefore be stenotic.

We can also derive the geometrically ideal FM length in relation to the length of the line of valve attachment.

The line of attachment of the leaflet is approximately a semicircle. Thus in the open position with the free margin of the leaflet hugging the line joining the 2 adjacent commissures, the FM approximates the diameter of the semicircle. Therefore,

$$\textbf{Base} \approx \pi/2 \times \text{FM} \approx 1.5 \times \text{FM}$$

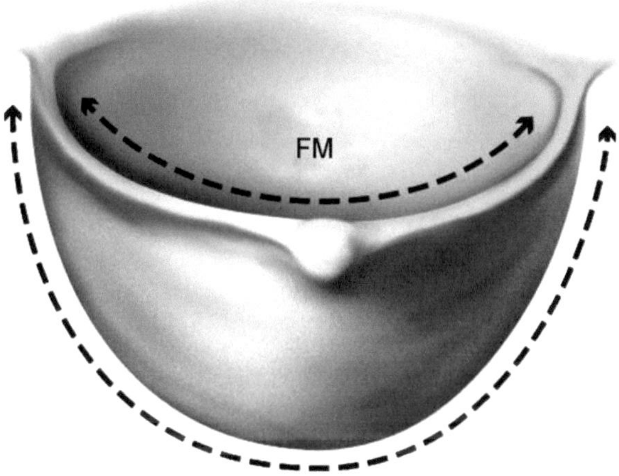

Reprinted from Heart, Lung and Circulation, 2004;13 Suppl 3, Matalanis G, Valve sparing aortic root repairs--an anatomical approach. S13-18., Copyright (2004), with permission from Elsevier

Fig. 3. The relationship between the base and free margin lengths - base ≈ 1.5 x FM

There are three aortic sinuses corresponding to the respective leaflets. These sinuses play an important role in minimising leaflet stress and strain [4] by helping to evenly distribute the diastolic pressure load across the leaflets and the sinus wall through the formation of a relatively spherical shape together with the valve cusps.

A spherical surface is the shape that gives the minimal surface area for a given volume, thus minimising the stress forces on the leaflets in diastole.

In systole, the sinuses allow the development of eddy currents, which prevent contact between leaflet and aortic wall (Fig. 4). This may also keep the leaflets away from the coronary ostia, however this is not likely to be a major factor as the majority of coronary flow occurs during diastole. In late systole, these currents help the leaflets drift towards the centre, such that they are in contact immediately prior to the onset of diastole [5]. This results in closure prior to the reversal of pressure difference across the valve, thus abolishing early diastolic reguritation.

It has been shown that increased stiffness of the aortic sinuses in advanced age and atherosclerosis contributes towards valve degeneration [6]. With reduced sinus compliance, leaflets may be more inclined to abruptly contact the aortic wall upon opening causing valve damage, while the delay in eddie current formation, with subsequent delay in valve closure may increase the regurgitant volume [3].

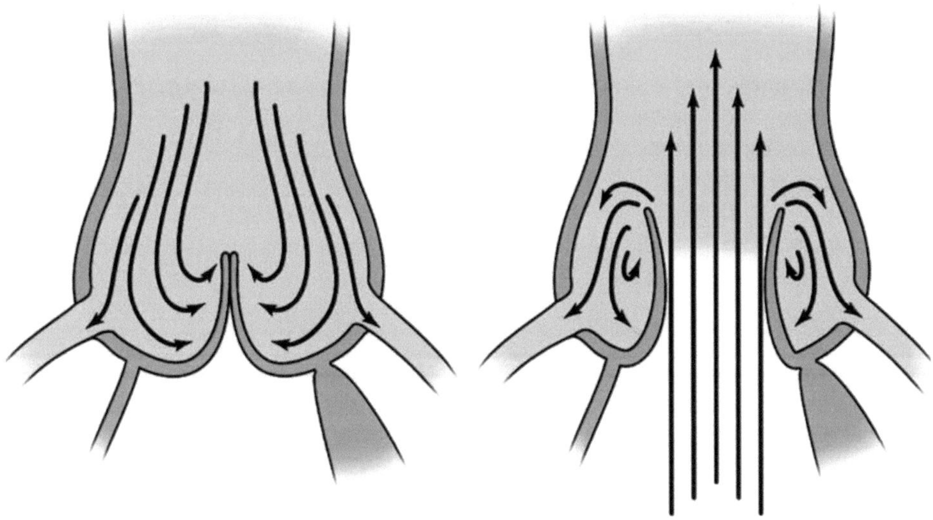

Reprinted from Heart, Lung and Circulation, 2004;13 Suppl 3, Matalanis G, Valve sparing aortic root repairs--an anatomical approach. S13-18., Copyright (2004), with permission from Elsevier

Fig. 4. The aortic sinuses form an integral part of the normal aortic valve function both in diastole and systole

3. Aortic root pathology

This chapter will focus primarily on aortic valve regurgitation, the most common cause of which is aortic root dilatation. Even in patients with an intact aortic root, dilatation of the ascending aorta may result in aortic regurgitation secondary to sinotubular junction dilatation. Age-related aortic dilatation is the most common cause of aortic dilatation. With age, degenerative changes in collagen and elastin leads to weakness and dilatation of the aortic wall. A genetic component also exists, whereby up to 15% of first-degree relatives to those with aortic aneurysms being affected.

Dilatation of the aorta is common in patients with Marfan's syndrome. Here, a defect in the glycoprotein fibrillin-1 results in cystic medical degeneration in the aortic wall, predisposing individuals to aortic dilatation. These patients are usually younger, and the aortic sinuses are the first to dilate, followed by the sinotubular junction and eventually the aortic annulus, result in leaflet prolapse and regurgitation. Loeys-Dietz syndrome is connective tissue disorder, it results from mutations in the genetic coding of transforming growth factor beta 1, which leads to aortic dilatation. Type IV Ehler Danlos syndrome is a deficiency in type III collagen, again increasing the risk of developing aneurysms of the aorta.

Additional causes for aortic aneurysms include arteritis (Giant Cell, Takayasu's, Kawasaki), infection (syphilitic, mycotic), systemic lupus erythematosus, ankylosing spondylitis and rarely due to granulomatous disease.

Nevertheless, in many patients, the aetiology of aortic aneurysms is multifactorial, with additional clinical characteristics such as age, hypertension and male gender among others serving as risk factors.

Acute or chronic type A dissections of the aorta is also a cause for valve regurgitation, resulting from commissural detachment due to the proximally propagating dissection. Patients with dissection may also have aortic regurgitation secondary to pre-existing aneurysmal disease.

As one of the most common congenital cardiac anomalies, bicuspid aortic valves (BAV) are found in between 1-2% of the population. BAVs may be anatomically or purely 'bicuspid' (Type 0), that is, consisting of two completely developed cusps, sinuses and commissures. However, most BAVs are functionally bicuspid (Type 1), in that three sinuses exist, with two cusps of different sizes whereby the larger cusp contains a median raphe, representing an obliterated or malformed commissure. This raphe extends from the mid-point of the cusp's free margin to the aortic annulus, inserting at a lower level than the other commissures.

Patients with BAV are at increased risk of developing aortopathy such as aortic dilatation and acute dissection. This may be due to a combination of 1) genetic predisposition, whereby the aortic tissue weakness and fragility responsible for dilatation is a manifestation of a development defect afflicting both the aortic valve and wall and 2) the haemodynamic abnormality caused by a bicuspid valve such as eccentric turbulence is responsible for aortic dilatation. Although there is widespread support for the genetic theory, some debate still exists as to which process exerts the most dominant effect [7].

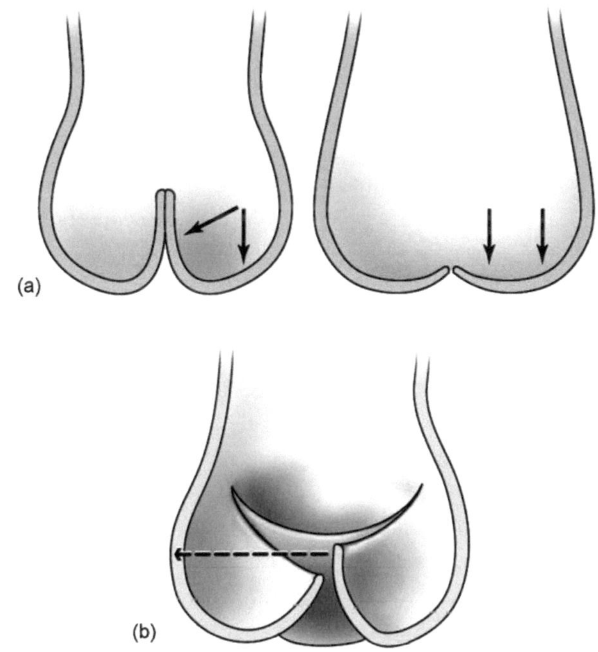

Reprinted from Heart, Lung and Circulation, 2004;13 Suppl 3, Matalanis G, Valve sparing aortic root repairs--an anatomical approach. S13-18., Copyright (2004), with permission from Elsevier

Fig. 5. Leaflet prolapse (a) results in reduction of the area of coaptation between the leaflets and thus the security of the "seal" in diastole. Asymmetrical prolapse (b) will result in aortic regurgitation at a much earlier stage

3.1 Classification of aortic regurgitation

While the Carpentier classification for mitral valve regurgitation has seen widespread application, in recent years, a similar functional classification system for aortic regurgitation has been developed by El Khoury and colleagues [8]. In this system, the aortic valve is viewed as two components, the annulus and valve leaflets, the former consisting of the ventriculo-aortic junction and the sinotubular junction.

The system classifies aortic regurgitation as secondary to I) dilatation of the aortic root structures, II) excessive leaflet motion (ie. prolapse) or III) restriction in leaflet motion such as that in bicuspid, rheumatic and other degenerative processes. One or more of these lesions may be present in to a given case of aortic regurgitation [8].

3.2 Clinical consequences of aortic regurgitation

Untreated symptomatic aortic regurgitation carries a poor prognosis. In patients with New York Heart Association Class III or IV symptoms, 4-year survival is around 30% [9] Symptomatic patients should be offered prompt surgical intervention for aortic regurgitation. Asymptomatic patients should be considered for surgery when left ventricular dimensions increase above the normal range or when ventricular function begins to decline.

In patients with aneurysms of the aortic root, valve-sparing aortic root surgery should be considered when root diameter exceeds 50mm. In those with Marfan's syndrome or a history of aortic dissection, surgery should be considered at 45mm regardless of the prospect of valve preservation.

Conditions when 45mm is a trigger for replacement
1. Marfan's, Loeys-Dietz, etc
2. Bicuspid valve needing an operation alone
3. Strong family history of rupture/dissection
4. Rapid progression of aneursym (>5mm/year)

Table 2. Conditions where aortic dilatation of 45mm is a trigger for replacement

Surgery for replacement of the ascending aorta should be considered when the diameter reaches 50mm.

Surgery may be offered earlier in the presence of a rapidly enlarging aneurysm or co-existing moderate to severe aortic regurgitation. In the case of the latter, earlier surgery before the aneurysm has reached a substantial size may increase the chances of valve preservation by limiting further stretching of valve cusps beyond repair. Aneurysms of the aortic root are the most common indication for surgery

4. Surgical management

4.1 Peri-operative evaluation

Trans-oesophageal echo (TOE) affords an excellent tool for the diagnosis of the mechanism of aortic regurgitation and is essential intra-operatively to assess the quality of the repair. The two dimensional axial and longitudinal views of the aortic root allow measurement of the aortic annulus, STJ, ascending aorta, as well aortic cusp free margin diameters. The plane of coaptation and leaflet prolapse or folding can be easily demonstrated. Colour

doppler allows quantification of the severity of regurgitation and its direction. Eccentricity of the jet can give vital clues of leaflet prolapse or restriction.
Contrast-enhanced computed tomography of the chest is used to assess aneurysm morphology and coronary angiography should be routinely performed to determine the need for concomitant bypass grafting.

4.2 Intra-operative technique

Access to the heart is obtained via median sternotomy. Cardiopulmonary bypass with ascending aorta, femoral or axillary artery cannulation may be required depending on the specifics of concomitant ascending arch pathology.

4.3 Valve sparing aortic root replacement

Valve-sparing aortic root reconstruction involves preservation of the native aortic valve while replacing the ascending aorta. This procedure was initially described by Dr Tirone David [10] and Sir Magdi Yacoub [11]. The two main techniques in widespread practice are aortic valve re-implantation and aortic root remodelling.
Repair of the aortic valve leaflets may be essential for short and long term success of the operation, if there is significant leaflet prolapse or restriction.

4.3.1 Aortic root remodelling

The first technique for correction of aortic root dilatation was described by Sir Magdi Yacoub [11] and subsequently also by Dr Tirone David (David Remodelling procedure). This procedure corrects STJ dilatation and creates neo-aortic sinuses, but does not affect the annular size.
In this technique, the ascending aorta is transected and the aortic root is excised to within 2-3mm of the valve attachment. Subsequently, a Dacron graft sized to the ideal STJ diameter is incised to create 3 evenly spaced tongues. This mimics the aortic sinuses, thus creating a neo-aortic root (Fig. 6 and 7). The apices of the valve commissures are then anastomosed to the corresponding points on the trimmed graft with pledgeted mattress sutures. The proximal sewing line is completed with a running polypropylene suture.
In a modification of the David Remodelling procedure, a separate Teflon "annuloplasty" is added in an attempt to prevent future annular dilatation. This annular plication is not done circumferentially, but over the length of the fibrous LVOT, which is the component most often affected by dilatation.

4.3.2 Aortic valve re-implantation

The re-implantation technique is performed by excising the aortic sinuses and placing a row of braided non-absorbable horizontal mattress sutures evenly around the left ventricular outflow tract below the level of the annulus (Fig. 8). These are passed through the proximal end of the graft which is tied in position as an external annuloplasty. The commissures are firstly secured within the graft ensuring that they are taught and vertically upright (Fig. 9 and 10), then the remnant of the aortic sinus tissue is then re-implanted inside the prosthesis with running polypropylene suture.
In the David re-implantation procedure, a single Dacron graft is used to achieve both annular and STJ plication. The advantages are greater simplicity and haemostasis. The disadvantages are incorporation of the muscular LVOT in the plication process, which if excessive may result in a higher than normal sub-annular gradient.

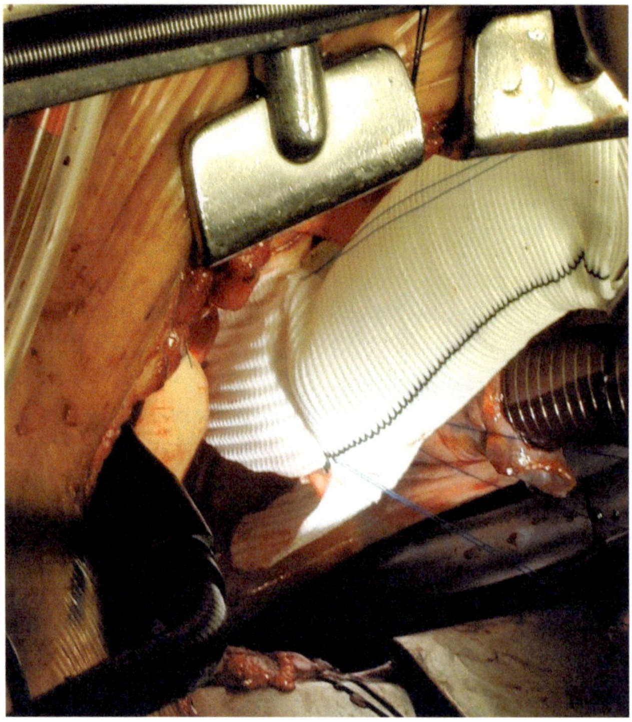

Fig. 6. Insertion of the fashioned graft during the root remodelling procedure

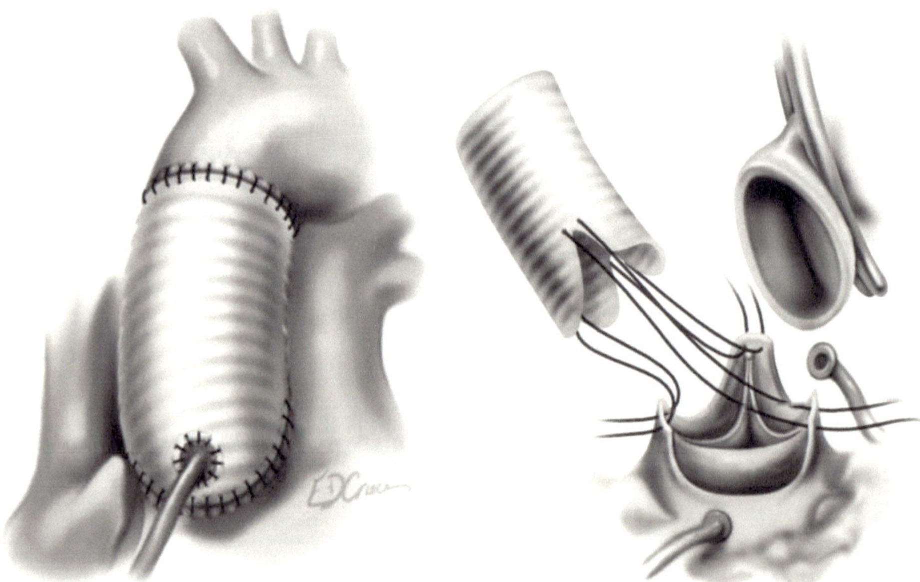

Fig. 7. Final appearance of the aortic root after aortic root remodelling

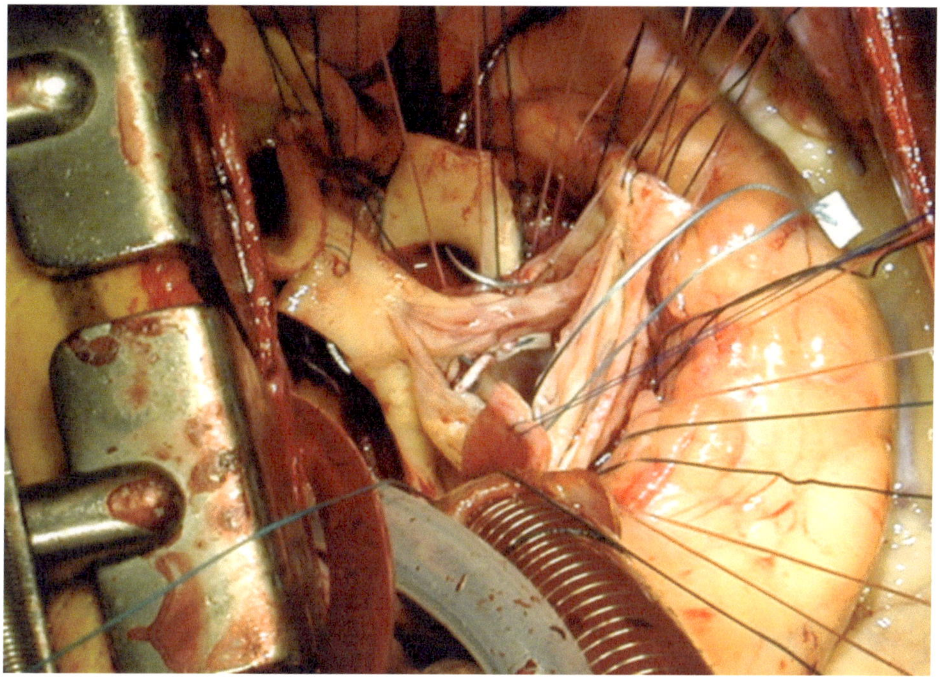

Fig. 8. Placement of horizontal mattress sutures around the left ventricular outflow tract during root re-implantation

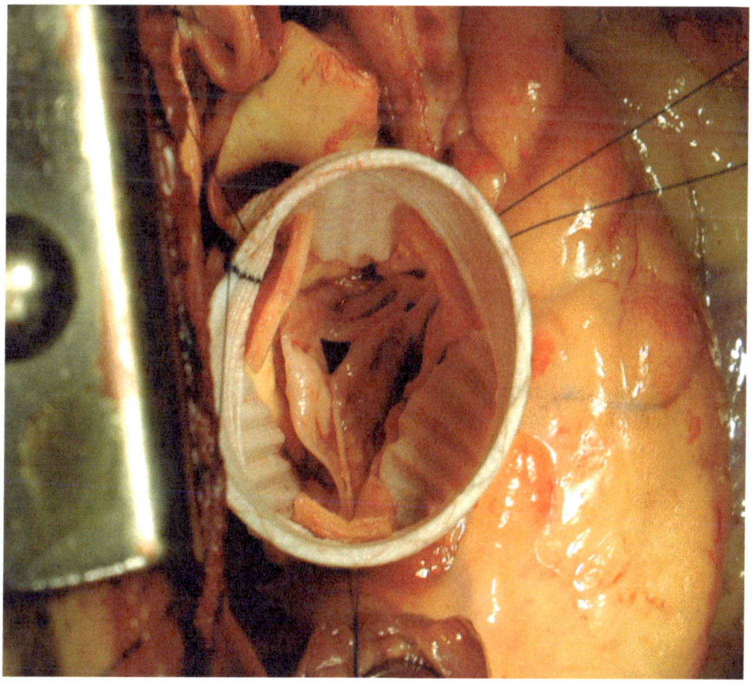

Fig. 9. Re-implantation of the native aortic valve within the vascular graft

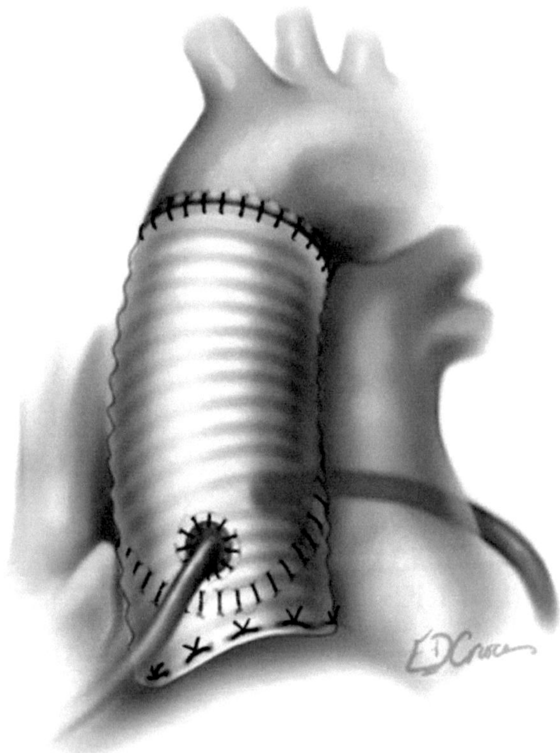

Reprinted from Heart, Lung and Circulation, 2004;13 Suppl 3, Matalanis G, Valve sparing aortic root repairs--an anatomical approach. S13-18., Copyright (2004), with permission from Elsevier

Fig. 10. Final appearance of the reconstructed aortic root following the re-implantation procedure

4.3.3 Recreating the sinuses of Valsalva

When the re-implantation technique was first described by David and Feindel, one perceived disadvantage was the potential physiological disturbance caused by the attachment of a tubular graft to the aortic annulus, thus eliminating the aortic sinuses. Given the role of the sinuses in preventing leafelt stress and strain, there was a concern that their absence would result in abnormal motion of the cusps and contribute toward structural deterioration and late recurrent regurgitation [3].

Subsequently, various modifications were proposed for the creation pseudosinuses to minimise physiological disturbance. The most commonly used technique involves oversizing a tubular graft (diameter which is twice the average height of the cusps) and placing plicating sutures at the level of the annulus and STJ. This acts to "pinch down" the graft, resulting in an outward bulge where the native sinuses would be located [12, 13]. This is sometimes referred to as the "David V" or "Stanford" modification [14].

To minimse the need for technical modifications to the re-implantation procedure, Ruggero De Paulis introduced the Valsava Graft, a Dacron conduit which incorporates the sinuses of Valsalva in the "skirt" portion of the graft [15]. This prosthesis recreates the nomal shape of the aortic sinuses to enable normal valve motion, decrease stress, and potentially increase durability without the need for the manual fashioning of neosinuses.

4.4 Sinotubular junction restoration

In cases where the sinuses of Valsalva and aortic annulus are not dilated, mere reduction of the sinotubular junction to an appropriate diameter will often cure valve incompetence. In such instances the ascending aorta is transected just above the commissures, which are pulled upward and towards each other until satisfactory coaptation of the aortic cusps are achieved. This is the diameter chosen for the graft.

In situations where the aortic cusps are asymmetric, the commissures may need to be spaced in a non-equidistant fashion such that the free margins coapt adequately. The vascular graft is subsequently anastomosed directly to the proximal ascending aorta at the sinotubular junction with a running 4-0 suture.

4.5 Sizing the graft

Much has been said about formulae for choosing the correct diameter of graft. In our institution we prefer placing the three commisural sutures and then elevating them upwards and inward until adequate coaptation of the aortic valve is achieved. A standard prosthetic valve sizer is then used to obtain the diameter of this corrected annulus/STJ and a respective conduit is then chosen.

Care must be made when choosing a conduit size for a re-implantation procedure. After the prosthesis is placed over the annulus, an additional 3-5mm needs to be added to the diameter prior to selection. In our experience, most females have a diameter of 26 to 30mm and males 28 to 32mm. [16]

4.6 Repair of aortic valve prolapse

It is important to note that in late presenting patients with very large aortic roots and severe aortic regurgitation, the leaflets are often overstretched with elongated free margins. Thus, after isolated correction of root dimensions the leaflets will tend to prolapse, even if they did not previously. This is not a contra indication to repair, and can be readily corrected.

Leaflets are assessed for prolapse as determined by a discrepancy in leaflet free margin height relative to its neighbours, and the cusp coaptation height. The latter is considered as indicative of prolapse if the height of coaptation above the level of the annulus is less than half of that of the top of the commissures.

Prolapse can be readily corrected by shortening the free margin back to normal. Minor degrees can be corrected with simple fine plication sutures either at the mid-point of the free margin or at its commissural ends until satisfactory coaptation is achieved (Fig. 11a).

In patients with more extensive degrees of prolapse, or in those with stress fenestrations, a neo-free margin may be constructed with a running polytetrafluoroethylene suture, also known as leaflet "re-suspension", in addition to plication (Fig. 11b).

Patients with connective tissue pathology such as Marfan's syndrome present a unique challenge. Marfan's Syndrome has previously been reported as a predictor of recurrent aortic regurgitation after root replacement. In these patients, the valves are structurally abnormal due to altered fibrillin metabolism, resulting in greater fragility compared to normal cusps [17, 18]. As such, these patients may benefit from additional leaflet reinforcement with running polytetrafluoroethylene sutures in addition to plication, so as to pre-empt further leaflet free margin stretch or tears.

The optimal technique for correction of leaflet prolapse is yet to be established. Previous studies have found recurrence of aortic regurgitation after placing plicating sutures at the commissures, and hence have preferred placing them at the mid point of the free margin

[19]. However, at our centre, we have favored the former technique with encouraging results. It is an attractive approach as the peri-commissural areas are often the most stretched component in prolonged root dilatation and plication here provides support at the most vulnerable site.

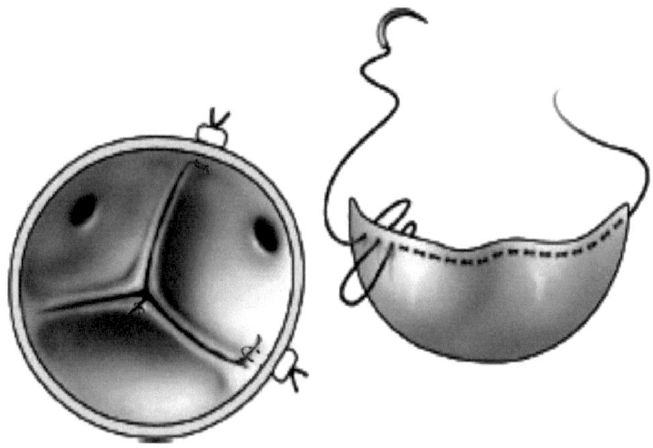

(a) (b)

Reprinted from Heart, Lung and Circulation, 2004;13 Suppl 3, Matalanis G, Valve sparing aortic root repairs--an anatomical approach. S13-18., Copyright (2004), with permission from Elsevier

Fig. 11. Methods of leaflet prolapse correction with (a) plication and (b) leaflet resuspension

4.7 Isolated aortic valve repair

Isolated prolapse of trileaflet aortic valve cusps without co-existent aortic root dilatation is uncommon. However, when encountered, valve repair can be accomplished using the techniques described. Cusp perforation, such as that secondary to endocarditis, can be easily corrected by using autologous pericardium.

4.8 Bicuspid aortic valves

A bicuspid valve's anterior cusp is most commonly prolapsed. Here, repair may be accomplished by placing plicating sutures at the free margin, or by placing a running polytetrafluoroethylene suture as with trileaflet valves. This approach works well for anatomically "pure" bicuspid valves (Type 0).

In functionally bicuspid valves (Type 1), attention must be paid to the raphe. If the raphe has adequate mobility and morphology, it may be shaved and preserved. However if it is severely restricted in movement or heavily calcified, a triangular resection of the raphe may be performed, the leaflet edges primarily reapproximated with running polypropylene sutures. If adequate tissue is not present, autologous or bovine pericardium may be used. Coaptation may be further enhanced with additional free margin plication and resuspension.

Where there is co-existent aortic root dilatation subcommissural triangle plication may be needed to enhance coaptation.

4.9 Completion assessment / Post repair Transeophageal Echo (TOE)

Following completion of the root repair saline testing is performed and leaflets are assessed for competance, symmetry, prolapse or any restriction.

Once pulsatile flow is reastablished, intra-operative trans-oesophageal echocardiography is essential to assess the quality of the operation.
In our institution we do not accept regurgitation >1+ or eccentric jets. The level at which the FM coapts needs to be more than half way between the annulus and STJ, and the amount of coaptation needs to be greater than or equal to 5mm.

5. Outcomes of valve-sparing aortic root replacement and valve repair

Dr Tirone David and colleagues from the Toronto Group recently published their results on 289 patients undergoing valve-sparing aortic root replacement using both the re-implantation (n=228) and remodelling (n=61) techniques [12]. Nine percent of patients underwent surgery for acute type A dissection. Overall, freedom from recurrent regurgitation was high at 86.8% ± 3.8% at 12 years follow-up. Patients undergoing the re-implantation technique experienced greater freedom from recurrent regurgitation compared to those undergoing remodeling (91.0% ± 3.8% versus 82.6% ± 6.2%, p = 0.035), however technique was not an independent predictor of late recurrent regurgitation. In this publication, the Toronto Group also showed that patient survival after undergoing valve-reimplantation was comparable to that of the general population when matched for age and gender.
The largest published series on the re-implantation technique is from Kallenbach and colleagues from Hannover, Germany, who in 2005, published their results of 284 consecutive patients undergoing the re-implantation procedure [20]. The series showed that the re-implantation procedure leads to excellent mid-term and late outcomes with freedom from re-operation due to recurrent aortic regurgitation was 91.1±2.5% at 5 years and 87.1±4.5% at 10 years. Late survival at 10 years was also high at 80.4±5.7% at 10 years.
In recent years, most surgeons have favoured the re-implantation technique, given the reinforcement of the aortic annulus which prevents subsequent dilatation, which is particularly important in patients with connective tissue diseases such as Marfan syndrome. Indeed, the evidence suggests that the re-implantation technique is less likely to result in recurrent regurgitation in the long-term [12, 21].

5.1 Valve-sparing root replacement with concomitant valve repair

Valve-sparing aortic root replacement was principally conceived for patients with morphologically normal valve leaflets where aortic regurgitation was caused solely by a dilated root. They were initially applied to patients with early grades of aortic regurgitation and less severe aortic root dilatation where the leaflets have only been minimally stretched.
However, combining leaflet prolapse correction with aortic valve sparing techniques permits extension of the benefits of valve sparing procedures to patients with advanced aortic regurgitation or aneurysms. In the past decade, there has been growing interest in such an approach.
In David and colleagues' earlier experience, published in 2001 [22], only 11% of patients underwent repair of cusp prolapse. However, almost a decade later, the group's latest report shows that 40% of patients had at least one leaflet free margin plicated while 22% underwent reinforcement of the free margin with a running polytetreafluoroethylene suture [12].
In a seminal publication, the Brussels Group, recently presented their results on 264 patients undergoing elective aortic valve repair for regurgitation occuring in isolation (43%) and in combination with aortic dilatation (57%) [8]. Leaflet repair techniques included free margin plication, resuspension as well as trangular resection with pericardial patch repair, while

combinations of valve-sparing procedures, sinotubular plication, and subcommissural annuloplasty was used to stabilise the annulus. The series is notable in that pre-operatively, 75% of patients had >2+ aortic regurgitation with a mean aortic diameter of 53 ± 9mm, suggesting the presence of long-standing disease whereby leaflets were reasonably stretched, which a decade ago would have been viewed to be a relative contraindication to valve preservation. Despite this, Freedoms from aortic regurgitation greater than 2+ were high at 88± 3% at 5 years and 79± 11% at 8 years, reflecting good durability of repair [8].

In a separate paper, the group reported their results on 111 patients with tri-leaflet valves undergoing repair of cusp prolapse with (n=61) or without (n=50) an associated aortic aneurysm. The re-implantation and sub-commissural annuloplasty techniques were predominantely used to correct aortic root dimensions, while free margin plication and resuspension were performed for cusp repair. At 8 years, freedom from recurrent regurgitation was high at 93±5% and 87±7% for patients with and without aortic aneurysms respectively. The number of cusps repaired and the technique used were not associated with recurrent regurgitation [23].

Performing valve repair alongside valve-sparing root replacement has gained popularity in recent years with several groups finding it to lead to strong mid-term results, with most studies reporting 5 year freedom from recurrent regurgitation rates of 85-95%.

We recently reported our local experience of 61 cases [16] with a relatively aggressive approach towards valve-preservation. Seventy-seven percent of patients had >2+ aortic regurgitation pre-operatively and a total of 69% of patients in the series required aortic valve repair for prolapse (Fig. 12). At mid-term follow-up, 5-year freedom from recurrent regurgitation was encouraging at 88±5.3%.

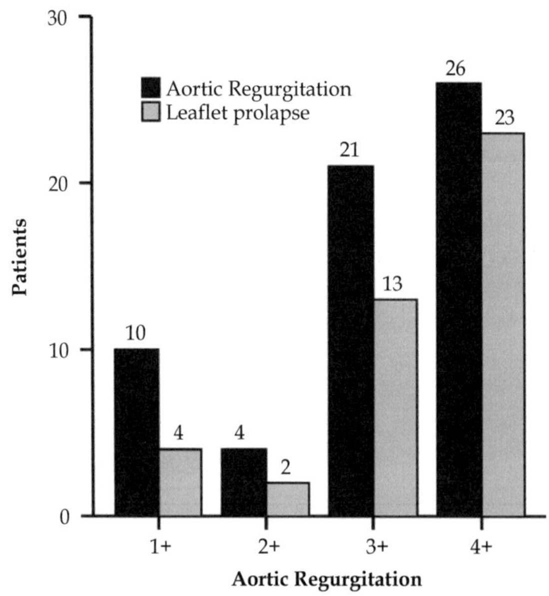

Reprinted from the European Journal of Cardio-Thoracic Surgery, 2010;37:6, Matalanis G, Shi WY, Hayward PAR, Correction of leaflet prolapse extends the spectrum of patients suitable for valve-sparing aortic root replacement.1311-1316., Copyright (2010), with permission from Elsevier

Fig. 12. In our local experience, greater than 2+ regurgitation and leaflet prolapse was present in a significant proportion of patients

A recent report from Luebeck presenting data on 191 remodeling and re-implantation procedures suggested that cusp repair was associated with an increased rate of late recurrent regurgitation. The authors attributed this to a number of factors including the presence of valves unsuitable for repair, fibrotic retraction of the repaired cusps, improper surgical techniques and other tissue properties [24]. Indeed, in our recent published experience, we observed a trend towards greater recurrent regurgitation in patients who had prolapsed leaflets, which did not reach statistical significance [16] (Fig. 13).
We have addressed this by use of more aggressive valve reinforcement with free margin running polytetrafluoroethylene sutures in selected patients with particularly stretched leaflets. Furthermore, in extreme cases, valve-preservation is judiciously avoided with replacement performed instead. In doing so, we hope to minimize the rate of recurrent aortic regurgitation such that it approaches the level seen in patients without leaflet prolapse.

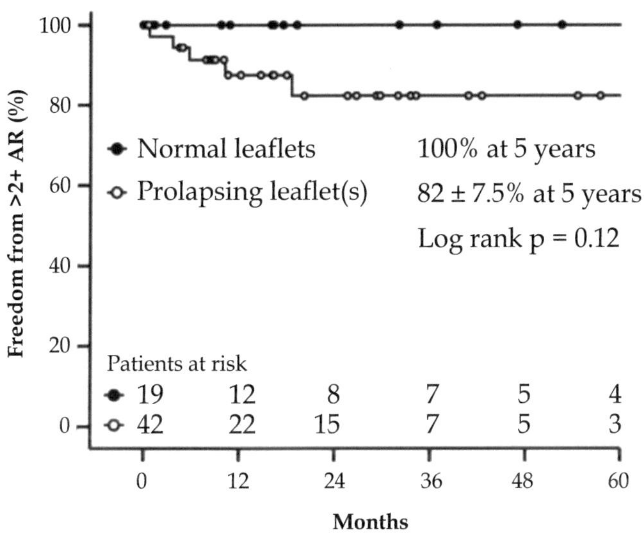

Reprinted from the European Journal of Cardio-Thoracic Surgery, 2010;37:6, Matalanis G, Shi WY, Hayward PAR, Correction of leaflet prolapse extends the spectrum of patients suitable for valve-sparing aortic root replacement.1311-1316., Copyright (2010), with permission from Elsevier

Fig. 13. Our local experience with valve-sparing aortic root replacement with concomitant valve repair

Even if we acknowledge an early marginal reduction in valve durability after very aggressive prolapse correction, it is still an excellent option for many patients, particularly those for whom long term anticoagulation is unacceptable, as seems increasingly common in clinical practice.

5.2 Bicuspid aortic valves

The largest reported series concerning repair of bicuspid aortic valves again comes from the Brussels Group, who recently published their outcomes on 122 consecutive patients undergoing bicuspid repair [25]. Of these, 57% had aortic regurgitation due to aortic dilatation while the remaining exhibited isolated valve insufficiency. Free margin plication and resuspension was performed in the 20% of patients with anatomically bicuspid (Type 0) valves. Those with functionally bicuspid (Type 1) valves, raphe repair was accomplished by either shaving, resection or use of a pericardial patch. At 5 years, freedom from recurrent regurgitation was high at 94±3%. Furthermore, in unadjusted analyses, patients undergoing a root procedure (remodelling or reimplantation) had a greater freedom from recurrent regurgitation compared to those undergoing subcommissural annuloplasty or sinotubular junction plication (95± 5%vs 80±6% at 5 years, p=0.03) [25].

5.3 Impact of the vascular prosthesis

De Paulis and colleagues showed that early valve motion after re-implantation inside the Valsalva prosthesis was similar to those of normal subjects, with graft distensibility being retained at the neosinuses [26]. At late follow-up, the elasticity of the graft's sinuses were also to an extent maintained, with the graft reponding to the changes in pressure between systole and diastole [27]. Further studies may elucidate any haemodynamic or clinical differences between techniques used to create neosinuses. Implantation of the Valsalva prosthesis removes the need to fashion neosinuses from a tube graft, which may prove advantageous by reducing aortic cross clamp times in cases where the aortic pathology extends into the aortic arch requiring complex reconstruction.

6. Conclusions

Evidence thus far shows that preservation and repair of the native aortic valve can be achieved with promising mid-term outcomes. It is rapidly becoming an accepted part of routine clinical practice. We believe that further studies with long-term follow up will reveal the greater potential of valve-sparing aortic root replacement and aortic valve repair.

7. Acknowledgements

The authors wish to acknowledge Ms Beth Croce for her illustrative work.

8. Disclosures

Professor Matalanis, Dr . Shi and Dr. O'Keefe report no conflicts of interest.

9. References

[1] Swanson M, Clark RE. Dimensions and geometric relationships of the human aortic valve as a function of pressure. Circ Res 1974;35:871-882.

[2] Silver MA, Roberts WC. Detailed anatomy of the normally functioning aortic valve in hearts of normal and increased weight. Am J Cardiol 1985;55:454-461.

[3] Kunzelman KS, Grande KJ, David TE, Cochran RP, Verrier ED. Aortic root and valve relationships. Impact on surgical repair. J Thorac Cardiovasc Surg 1994;107:162-170.

[4] Katayama S, Umetani N, Sugiura S, Hisada T. The sinus of valsalva relieves abnormal stress on aortic valve leaflets by facilitating smooth closure. J Thorac Cardiovasc Surg 2008 136:1528-1535.

[5] Bellhouse BJ Bellhouse FH. Mechanism of closure of the aortic valve. Nature 1968;217:86-87.

[6] Robicsek F, Thubrikar MJ. Role of sinus wall compliance in aortic leaflet function. Am J Cardiol 1999;84:944-946.

[7] Girdauskas E, Borger MA, Secknus MA, Girdauskas G, Kuntze T. Is aortopathy in bicuspid aortic valve disease a congenital defect or a result of abnormal hemodynamics? A critical reappraisal of a one-sided argument. Eur J Cardiothorac Surg 2011;doi:10.1016/j.ejcts.2011.01.001.

[8] Boodhwani M, de Kerchove L, Glineur D, Poncelet A, Rubay J, Astarci P, Verhelst R, Noirhomme P, El Khoury G. Repair-oriented classification of aortic insufficiency: Impact on surgical techniques and clinical outcomes. J Thorac Cardiovasc Surg 2009;137:286-294.

[9] Dujardin KS, Enriquez-Sarano M, Schaff HV, Bailey KR, Seward JB, Tajik AJ. Mortality and morbidity of aortic regurgitation in clinical practice. A long-term follow-up study. Circulation 1999;99:1851-1857.

[10] David TE., Feindel CM. An aortic valve-sparing operation for patients with aortic incompetence and aneurysm of the ascending aorta. Journal of Thoracic and Cardiovascular Surgery 1992;103:617-621.

[11] Sarsam MA, Yacoub M. Remodeling of the aortic valve anulus. J Thorac Cardiovasc Surg 1993;105:435-438.

[12] David TE, Maganti M, Armstrong S. Aortic root aneurysm: Principles of repair and long-term follow-up. J Thorac Cardiovasc Surg 2010;140:S14-19.

[13] David TE. The aortic valve-sparing operation. J Thorac Cardiovasc Surg 2011 141:613-615.

[14] Demers P, Miller DC. Simple modification of "T. David-v" Valve-sparing aortic root replacement to create graft pseudosinuses. Ann Thorac Surg 2004 78:1479-1481.

[15] De Paulis R, De Matteis GM, Nardi P, Scaffa R, Buratta MM, Chiariello L. Opening and closing characteristics of the aortic valve after valve-sparing procedures using a new aortic root conduit. Ann Thorac Surg 2001;72:487-494.

[16] Matalanis G, Shi WY, Hayward PA. Correction of leaflet prolapse extends the spectrum of patients suitable for valve-sparing aortic root replacement. Eur J Cardiothorac Surg 2010;37:1311-1316.

[17] Fleischer KJ, Nousari HC, Anhalt GJ, Stone CD, Laschinger JC. Immunohistochemical abnormalities of fibrillin in cardiovascular tissues in marfan's syndrome. Ann Thorac Surg 1997;63:1012–1017.

[18] Missirlis YF, Armeniades CD, Kennedy JH. Mechanical and histological study of aortic valve tissue from a patient with marfan's disease. Atherosclerosis 1976;24:335–338.

[19] Hans-Joachim S, Diana A, Frank L. Correction of leaflet prolapse in valve-preserving aortic replacement: Pushing the limits? Ann Thorac Surg 2002;74:S1762-1764.

[20] Kallenbach K, Karck M, Pak D, Salcher R, Khaladj N Leyh R, Hagl C, Haverich A. Decade of aortic valve sparing reimplantation: Are we pushing the limits too far? Circulation 2005;112:I-253-259.

[21] Liu L, Wang W, Wang X, Tian C, Meng YH, Chang Q. Reimplantation versus remodeling: A meta-analysis. J Card Surg 2011;26:82-87.

[22] David TE, Armstrong S, Joan I, Christopher FM., Ahmad O, Gary W. Results of aortic valve-sparing operations. Journal of Thoracic and Cardiovascular Surgery 2001;122:39-46.

[23] Boodhwani M, de Kerchove L, Watremez C, Glineur D, Vanoverschelde JL, Noirhomme P, El Khoury G. Assessment and repair of aortic valve cusp prolapse: Implications for valve-sparing procedures. J Thorac Cardiovasc Surg 2011;141:917-925.

[24] Hanke T, Charitos EI, Stierle U, Robinson D, Gorski A, Sievers HH, Misfeld M. Factors associated with the development of aortic valve regurgitation over time after two different techniques of valve-sparing aortic root surgery. J Thorac Cardiovasc Surg 2009;137:314-319.

[25] Boodhwani M, de Kerchove L, Glineur D, Rubay J, Vanoverschelde JL, Noirhomme P, El Khoury G. Repair of regurgitant bicuspid aortic valves: A systematic approach. J Thorac Cardiovasc Surg 2010;140:276-284.

[26] De Paulis R, De Matteis GM, Nardi P, Scaffa R, Bassano C, Chiariello, L. Analysis of valve motion after the reimplantation type of valve-sparing procedure (david i) with a new aortic root conduit. Ann Thorac Surg 2002:53-57.

[27] Monti L, Mauri G, Balzarini L, Tarelli G, Brambilla G, Vitali E, Ornaghi D, Citterio E, Settepani F. Compliance of the valsalva graft's pseudosinuses at midterm follow-up with cardiovascular magnetic resonance. Ann Thorac Surg 2011;91:92-96.

6

Aortic Valve Sparing Operations

Bradley G. Leshnower and Edward P. Chen
Division of Cardiothoracic Surgery,
Emory University School of Medicine
USA

1. Introduction

The treatment of aortic root and ascending aortic aneurysms often requires addressing concomitant aortic valve pathology. In the setting of aortic stenosis secondary to cusp degeneration, aortic valve replacement (AVR) is performed. However, when patients present with aortic insufficiency and normal cusp anatomy, a dilemma arises. Historically valve replacement has been performed; however, current options are all associated with their own specific issues. Implantation of a mechanical prosthesis commits the patient to lifelong anticoagulation and the concomitant risks of bleeding and thromboembolism. Use of a bioprosthetic valve eliminates the burden of anticoagulation, but these prostheses suffer from structural valve deterioration and commit the young patient to the potential need for a second or third operation. The optimal solution is to remove all diseased aorta while preserving and restoring the normal aortic cusps to their original geometry to allow for adequate coaptation and valve competency. The term "aortic valve-sparing operations" (AVS) was introduced by David in the 1990's to describe procedures which preserved, rather than replaced the aortic valve cusps during the treatment of aneurysms of the aortic root or ascending aorta with associated aortic insufficiency (1). These are technically demanding procedures which require in-depth knowledge and comprehension of aortic root anatomy and physiology. In this chapter we will review the anatomy and physiology of the aortic root and discuss the various AVS operations which have been used in the treatment of aortic root and ascending aortic aneurysms.

2. Anatomy

The aortic root is a complex structure composed of several components including the aortic annulus, valve cusps, sinus of Valsalva segments, and the sinotubular junction. The aortic annulus is defined by the attachment or hinge point of the cusp and has been described as scalloped or coronet shaped. It is attached to ventricular myocardium in 45% of its circumference and fibrous structures in the remaining 55%. The annulus rises from the nadir of one cusp and peaks at the commissure, the highest point of the annulus and the junction between two adjacent cusps. The area below the commissures is referred to as the subcommissural triangle.

The shape of the aortic cusps is semilunar. The base (hinge point) of the cusp is 1.5 times longer than the length of the free margin (Figure 1). The cusps have three component parts: the hinge point, the body and the coapting surface (free margin). The hinge point has the ability to bend repeatedly without weakening or fracturing due to stress. The body of the cusp has a limited degree of distensibility due to a sliding movement of the different layers that compose the valve. The coapting surface has a specific length which is important in ensuring valve competence under different loading conditions (3). Histopathology studies have revealed that the thick collagenous bundles which comprise the cusps are oriented in an optimal way to transmit stress to the aortic wall (4). Normal aortic valves have three cusps with three corresponding sinus of Valsalva segments. Bicuspid aortic valve is a heritable condition which occurs in 1-2% of the population. These patients have two functional cusps and three sinus segments.

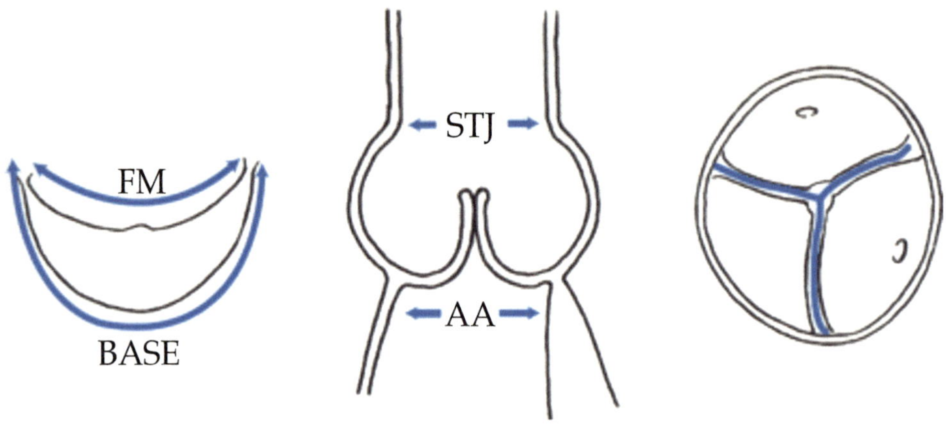

Fig. 1. Geometric relationships of various components of the aortic root. The base of the aortic cusp is 1.5 times longer than its free margin (FM). The diameter of the aortic annulus (AA) is 10 to 15% larger than the diameter of the sinotubular junction (STJ) in children and young adults, but it tends to become equal with aging. Three semilunar cusps seal the aortic orifice. The height of the cusps must be longer than the radius of the aortic annulus. From David TE. Aortic Valve Repair and Aortic Valve-Sparing Operations. In: Cohn LH, ed. *Cardiac Surgery in the Adult.* New York, NY: McGraw Hill:935-948, 2008

Beginning at the aortic annulus, the aorta bulges outward to form three sinuses of Valsalva segments which end at the sinotubular junction (STJ). The shape of the sinus segment is thought to be important in creating vortices which have an effect on both valve opening and closing as well as coronary blood flow (4). In vitro finite element analysis has proven that the shape of the sinus segments plays a vital role in limiting the stress and strain on the cusps (5). The important relationship between the shape of the sinus and its physiologic function has led to the development of prosthetic aortic root grafts with pre-made bulging sinus segments, in attempt to recreate normal aortic root geometry (6).
The sinotubular junction (STJ) is a ridge which lies above the aortic valve commissures and marks the transition from the aortic root to the ascending aorta. The circumference of the sinotubular junction is 15-20% smaller than the aortic annulus in young people, but normalizes to approximately a 1:1 relationship in older age (2). The close relationship of

the STJ and the aortic valve commissures is realized when aneurysmal dilation of the STJ moves the commissures apart and results in loss of leaflet coaptation and aortic insufficiency.
The aortic root is a dynamic structure that expands and contracts throughout the cardiac cycle in a manner which maximizes blood flow through the aortic valve and minimizes stress on the aortic valve cusps. The components of the aortic root complex have a specific geometric relationship with each other to produce optimal hemodynamics. Pathologic alterations in any of the four components can change their interactions and result in valvular dysfunction (4, 7).

3. Pathophysiology

AVS operations were designed for patients with aortic root or ascending aortic aneurysms and competent or regurgitant aortic valve function in the setting of normal cusps. Highly stenotic valves are rarely able to be preserved. The most common cause of aortic insufficiency in North America is annuloaortic ectasia. Young patients develop aortic root aneurysms beginning with dilatation of the sinus segments, followed by annular and STJ dilatation. Elderly patients can develop aortic insufficiency from ascending aortic aneurysms and subsequent dilatation of the STJ. In these patients, the aortic annulus and sinus segments are relatively normal. Marfan syndrome is the most common cause of aortic root aneurysms in young patients. Other connective tissue disorders such as ankylosing spondylitis, Ehlers-Danlos, osteogenesis imperfecta, rheumatoid arthritis, and lupus can cause aortic insufficiency. Aortic dissection is another common indication for an AVS operation. This dissection flap can extend into the aortic root and disconnect one of the aortic valve commissures from the aortic wall causing cusp prolapse and aortic insufficiency (2).

4. Indications

Indications for surgical intervention upon aortic root and ascending aneurysms include the presence of symptoms, aortic size, rapid growth, and the degree of aortic insufficiency. Most patients with aortic aneurysms are asymptomatic. Symptomatic patients complain of chest pain, which is considered a sign of rapid growth, dissection or impending rupture(8). The guidelines for the treatment of asymptomatic patients are drawn from natural history studies which correlated serial aortic measurements and aortic complications (rupture or dissection). It has been demonstrated that the ascending aortic grows at a rate of 1mm/year, and by the time the diameter of ascending aneurysms reaches 6cm, patients have been subjected to a lifetime 34% risk of rupture or dissection (9).
In the largest reported series from the Yale Aortic Institute comparing growth rates and complications, 50% of patients with ascending aortic aneurysms suffered aortic rupture or dissection at a median aortic diameter of 5.9 cm (10). Furthermore, there is a "hinge" point in the data which identifies a significant increase in the probability of rupture or dissection when an aneurysm reaches a size of 6.0cm. Therefore, elective repair of aortic root or ascending aneurysms in trileaflet valves is recommended at a diameter of ≥ 5.5cm or a growth rate of ≥0.5cm/year (8,10). Patients with genetic disorders such as bicuspid aortic valve, Marfan syndrome, Ehlers-Danlos, Turner syndrome, or a familial history of aneurysm

and dissection should undergo elective aortic replacement at a diameter of <5cm depending upon the specific disease (8). These patients have a higher risk of rupture or dissection at smaller aortic diameters. It should be noted that the diameter for aortic intervention can be adjusted for body size based upon published nomograms correlating the aortic rupture/dissection risk to aortic diameter and body surface area (9).

In other situations, the primary indication for surgical intervention is aortic insufficiency and not aneurysmal disease. Current recommendations for aortic valve repair or replacement in the setting of chronic severe aortic insufficiency include: (1) symptoms of congestive heart failure, (2) left ventricular dysfunction with an ejection fraction ≤ 50% at rest, (3) concomitant cardiac or aortic surgery, (4) LV end-diastolic dimension of > 75mm, (5) LV end-systolic dimension of > 55mm and (6) declining exercise tolerance (11). When operating for a valvular indication or aortic dissection, concomitant aortic root or ascending replacement is recommended at aortic diameters ≥4.5cm. In the setting of severe aortic insufficiency and aortic aneurysmal disease, aggressive operative intervention earlier rather than later may enable AVS operation to be performed. Long-standing, severe aortic insufficiency can damage the cusps, causing stress fenestrations or thickening of the free margin which may render the cusps unrepairable and mandate valve replacement.

In addition to the indications listed above, the surgeon must exhibit judgment in patients selected to receive a valve sparing operation. The patient's age and comorbid status must be taken into consideration. Given the excellent durability of bioprosthetic valves, patients with a life expectancy < 15 years should probably undergo aortic valve replacement. The aortic cusps must be carefully inspection both preoperatively on the transesophageal echocardiogram and at the time of surgery once the aorta is transected. Significant calcification of the annulus and cusps are generally considered prohibitive of an AVS operation. Severe free margin thickening has also been demonstrated to limit long term valve durability following AVS operations (7, 12). However stress fenestrations and free margin elongation are not contraindications to a valve sparing procedure, and valve repair techniques are often added to an AVS operation. Due to the extensive reconstruction involved in valve-sparing root replacement, myocardial protection is paramount, as the possibility of a second period of myocardial ischemia exists if the valve repair fails. All of these factors must be considered prior to proceeding with a valve-sparing procedure.

5. Ascending aortic replacement with remodeling of the sinotubular junction

Aortic insufficiency can occur in the setting of either isolated ascending aortic aneurysms or due to aortic root aneurysms. Isolated ascending aortic aneurysms cause aortic insufficiency due to dilation of the STJ which pulls the commissures apart and prevents valve coaptation during diastole (2). If the remainder of the aortic root components are normal, then a reduction of the STJ diameter will restore valve competence. Typically these patients are older and have a large ascending aortic aneurysm and aortic insufficiency. The preoperative echocardiogram will demonstrate loss of STJ definition, minimal dilation of the sinuses and central aortic insufficiency due to lack of cusp coaptation.

During the operation, the aorta is transected approximately 5mm distal to the STJ and the cusps are inspected. Often the cusps are small, there is minimal annular dilatation and the ridge of the STJ is unrecognizable. If the aortic insufficiency has been chronic, there may be pathologic alterations in the cusps. The two most common alterations are elongation of the free margin or stress fenestrations near the commissures. Free margin elongation results in cusp prolapse, which can be corrected with a plication stitch in the center of cusp free margin at the nodule of Arantii. In the case of extensive stress fenestrations, the free margin is reinforced with a double layer 6-0 polytetrafluoroethylene suture. David and colleagues have shown that both of these adjunctive valve repair techniques are durable methods of achieving long-term valve competence with this operation. (1).

Restoring the normal diameter of the STJ is the key to achieving aortic valve competence in this procedure. There are two methods which are used to select the appropriate graft size which will define the neo-sinotubular junction. Once the aorta is transected, traction sutures are placed at the commissures and pulled up until the cusps achieve coaptation. The diameter of an imaginary circle which includes all three commissures is the ideal diameter of the neo-sinotubular junction (13). Next a transparent valve sizer (e.g. Medtronic Freestyle, Medtronic, Minneapolis, MN) is used to determine the annular diameter. The STJ and the annulus should be approximately the same diameter in order to recreate the normal aortic root geometry in this population. Furthermore, the location of the commissures should be marked on the graft and lined up accordingly during construction of the anastomosis in an effort to maintain normal root geometry (Figure 2). Once the graft has been sewn to the aorta, aortic valve competence can be tested by injecting cardioplegia into the graft under pressure. If the left ventricle remains decompressed and there is no distension, then the aortic valve is competent. (1).

David and colleagues reported their outcomes following ascending aortic replacement with reduction of the diameter of the sinotubular junction in 103 patients over a 15 year period. The mean age of these patients was 65 years and all patients had >3+ aortic insufficiency. 9% of patients had bicuspid aortic valves. The mean diameter of the neo-sinotubular junction following ascending replacement was 26mm, and leaflet repair was performed in 40 patients. There were two operative deaths, and 5 and 10 year survival was 80% and 54%. Freedom from moderate or severe aortic insufficiency at 5 and 10 years was 96% and 80%. Two patients in the entire series required reoperation for aortic valve replacement. One patient had severe aortic insufficiency and the other had infective endocarditis. The overall 10 year freedom from aortic valve replacement was 97% (1).

El-Khoury's group also reported their experience with remodeling the STJ for the treatment of supracoronary aortic aneurysms and associated aortic insufficiency. In a smaller series of 55 patients with a mean age of 65, these authors reported an overall survival of 94% and 75% at 5 and 7 years follow-up. 31% of patients had bicuspid aortic valves. Adjunctive cusp repair procedures were performed in 51% of patients and 69% of patients underwent subcommissural annuloplasty. Freedom from recurrent >2+ aortic insufficiency 87% at 5 years, and none of their patients required subsequent aortic valve replacement (14).

The outcomes from these two series provide data that a durable aortic valve sparing operation can be accomplished by remodeling the sinotubular junction with a supracoronary graft and simple leaflet repair techniques in both bicuspid and trileaflet valves. Patient selection and careful examination of the aortic valve cusps with preoperative echocardiography and intraoperative examination is the key to achieving short and long-term success. If the leaflets are severely damaged, the aortic valve should be replaced.

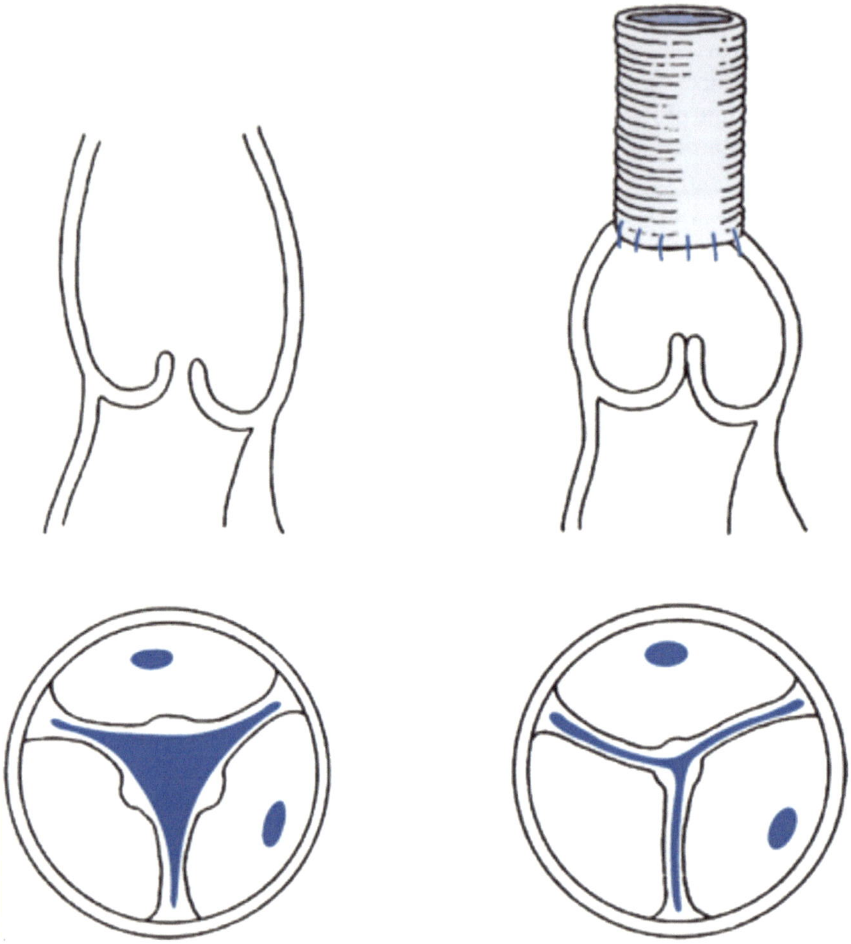

Fig. 2. Sinotubular Junction Remodeling. From David TE. Aortic Valve Repair and Aortic Valve-Sparing Operations. In: Cohn LH, ed. *Cardiac Surgery in the Adult.* New York, NY: McGraw Hill:935-948, 2008

6. Valve sparing aortic root replacement- remodeling technique

Yacoub developed the aortic root remodeling procedure to treat patients with aortic root aneurysms, aortic insufficiency and normal aortic valve cusps. In this population of patients, the pathology is confined to the aortic wall. He reported the first series of valve sparing root replacements for the treatment of 10 patients with aortic root aneurysms and aortic insufficiency in 1993 (15). In this series he described the technique of aortic root remodeling by replacing all diseased aortic root tissue with a tailored Dacron graft. One end of the graft was fashioned to produce three individual tongues which became the neo-aortic sinus segments of the remodeled root (Figure 3). The operative technique is described below.

After initiating cardiopulmonary bypass, the aorta is transected and a careful examination of the aortic valve cusps is performed. If abnormal cusps are discovered and found to be

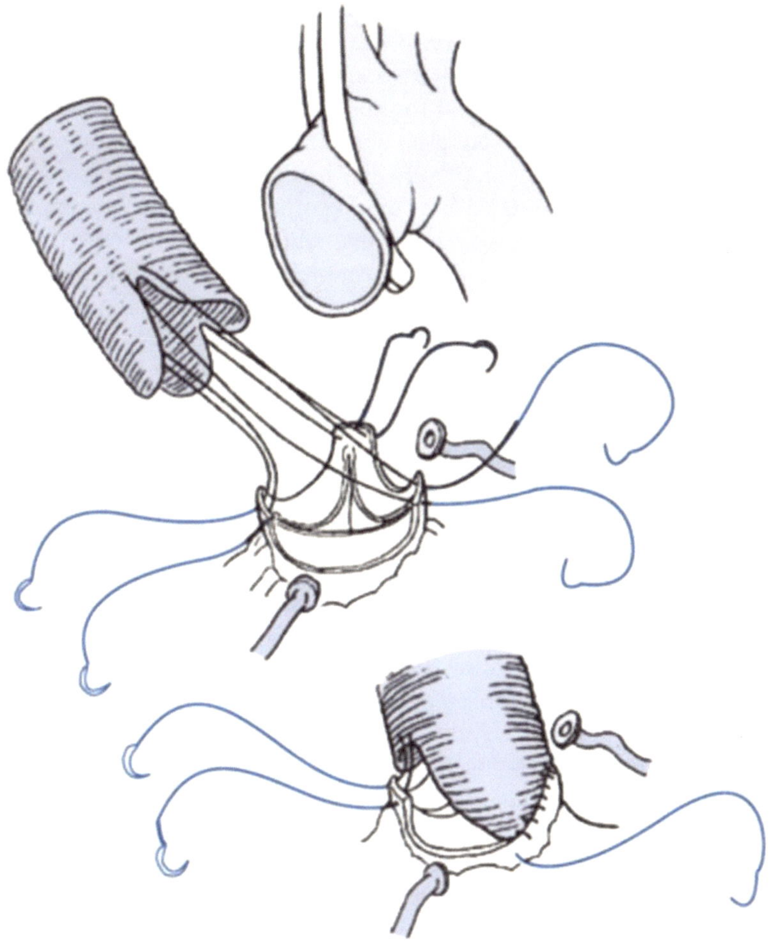

Fig. 3. Aortic Root Remodeling. From David TE. Aortic Valve Repair and Aortic Valve-Sparing Operations. In: Cohn LH, ed. *Cardiac Surgery in the Adult.* New York, NY: McGraw Hill:935-948, 2008

"unsalvageable" despite leaflet repair techniques, then the valve is excised and a conventional Bentall root replacement is performed (16). If the cusps are normal, then the aortic root is dissected out from the surrounding cardiac chambers all the way down to the aortic annulus. The abnormal aneurysmal sinus tissue is excised, leaving a 5mm remnant of aortic wall above the annulus. Traction sutures are placed at the top of each commissure. Additionally, the orifice and proximal portions of the left and right coronary arteries are dissected away form the surrounding structures leaving 5mm circumferentially of sinus tissue to form "coronary buttons". Next, a Dacron graft is sized in a manner similar to the STJ remodeling procedure previously described. The traction sutures above each commissure are pulled up until the cusps achieve coaptation. The graft diameter is the diameter of an imaginary circle which includes all three commissures. A transparent valve sizer (e.g. Medtronic Freestyle) can be used to help determine the optimal graft diameter. The positions of the commissures are marked on the graft. The graft is then tailored with three longitudinal cuts at the positions of the commissures with the ends rounded to create neo-aortic sinuses which are the width of the intercommissural distance. It is important to make the heights of the three neo-sinuses (two in the case of bicuspid valve) approximately the same size as the diameter of the graft to properly recreate normal aortic root geometry. Once the neo-sinus segments of the root graft are created, the commissural posts are sutured outside the graft above the neo-sinus (Figure 3). Then the remnant aortic wall tissue above the annulus is sutured to the graft with a running stitch. Once this is complete, holes are made inside the root graft with an ophthalmic cautery and the coronary buttons are reimplanted. At this point the leaflets are inspected again, and any leaflet repairs are performed at this time. The ideal level of coaptation is 5-6mm above the level of the nadir of the aortic annulus, and the optimal length of the coaptation zone is 4mm. Before proceeding with the remainder of the planned procedure, valve competency is re-tested by injecting cardioplegia into the graft under pressure. If the left ventricle remains decompressed and there is no distension, then the aortic valve is competent. (2, 17)

Yacoub reported the long term results of his remodeling procedure in 158 patients over an 18 year period. All patients had aortic root aneurysms, and 31% were performed in the setting of acute Type A aortic dissection. 43% of these patients had Marfan syndrome. 49% of patients had preoperative moderate aortic insufficiency and 18% had severe aortic insufficiency. The elective aneurysm group had a 1 and 10 year survival of 97% and 82%, while the acute dissection cohort had survival rates of 73% and 53%. Post-operative echocardiography revealed that 64% of patients had trivial or no aortic insufficiency, 33% had mild to moderate aortic insufficiency, and only 3% had severe aortic insufficiency. Freedom from reoperation was 99% and 89% at 1 and 10 years (18).

David modified Yacoub's remodeling technique for patients with annuloaortic ectasia or Marfan syndrome by adding an annuloplasty to the fibrous portion of the aortic annulus in an attempt to prevent future annular dilatation (19). This was accomplished by passing multiple horizontal sutures from inside to out on the fibrous aspect of the left ventricular outflow tract underneath the annulus. These sutures are then passed through a narrow strip of Dacron or Teflon felt and tied down to reduce the diameter of the aortic annulus (Figure 4). David recently reported his 12 year follow-up data from 61 patients who underwent his modified remodeling procedure. 42% of these patients had Marfan syndrome and 12% were performed in the setting of acute Type A dissection. 34% of patients had preoperative moderate aortic insufficiency, and 21% had severe aortic insufficiency. There was 1 operative death and survival rates were 97% and 83% at 1 and 12 years. At 12 years, freedom from moderate or severe aortic insufficiency was 83%, and freedom from reoperation upon the aortic valve was 90% (17). Other groups have also reported durable long-term valve function following root remodeling including patients with bicuspid valves (20, 21).

The root remodeling has been adopted by many surgeons and has produced excellent long term results with durable aortic valve function. However, due to its lack of an annuloplasty, many surgeons prefer the reimplantation technique, especially in patients with annular dilatation or connective tissue disorders.

7. Valve sparing aortic root replacement-reimplantation technique

In 1989, David performed the first valve sparing root replacement using the reimplantation technique. The patient was a young woman with Marfan syndrome and a 5.4cm aortic root

aneurysm who had elected to get an aortic valve homograft so that she could eventually have children. Instead, David reimplanted her native valve into a cylindrical Dacron tube graft (22). Since the original operation, this pioneering procedure has undergone several modifications and has been adopted by surgeons worldwide as their primary AVS operation. The technical aspects of the most recent iteration of the David V reimplantation procedure are described in the following paragraphs.
Once the decision is made to proceed with valve-sparing root replacement, the root is circumferentially dissected down to the nadir of the aortic annulus. All abnormal sinus tissue is excised, leaving a 5mm rim of aortic tissue above the annulus. Coronary buttons are also fashioned, and 4-0 pledgeted polypropolene sutures are placed from inside to out just above the top of each commissure.

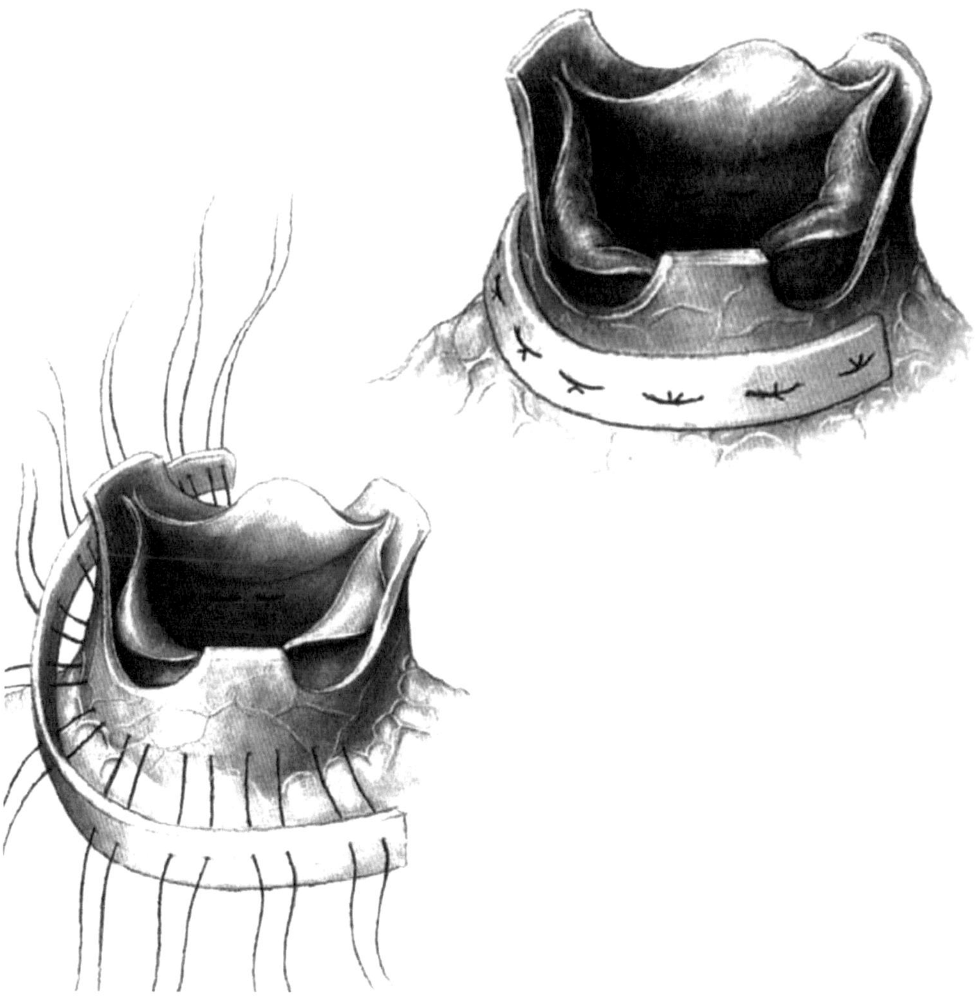

Fig. 4. Aortic Root Remodeling with Annuloplasty. From David TE. Remodeling of the Aortic Root and Preservation of the Native Aortic Valve. *Operative Techniques in Cardiac & Thoracic Surgery*. 1996; 1:44-56

In the reimplantation procedure, correct graft size selection is paramount to achieving a successful result. In the David V procedure, the diameter of the graft = 2(2/3 average cusp height) + 8mm. This is a slight modification of the original David-Feindel formula, as it enlarges the graft by 2mm to create neo-sinus segments (23,24) A ruler is used to measure the height of the cusp from the hinge point at the nadir of the annulus to the free margin edge at the nodule of Arantius. This formula is based upon the anatomic relationships of the normal human aortic root. Cusp height (as opposed to the annulus, STJ, or sinus) is used as the measured distance upon which graft size is based because it is the only relatively fixed measurement in the aortic root complex. In large series, most grafts range from 30-36mm in diameter (24).

Sizing the graft in this fashion allows for a graft larger than the ideal STJ and annulus, which can be plicated down at the top and bottom to create neo-sinus segments. A transparent valve sizer is used to measure the annulus. If annular dilatation is present, a valve sizer smaller than the anuulus is selected and the graft sizer is placed through the bottom of the graft. A series of interrupted pleating stitches approximately 4mm above the end of the graft plicates the annular end of the graft down to the diameter of the valve sizer. The positions of the commissures are also marked on the graft, and a small triangle is cut out at the position of the left/right commissure.

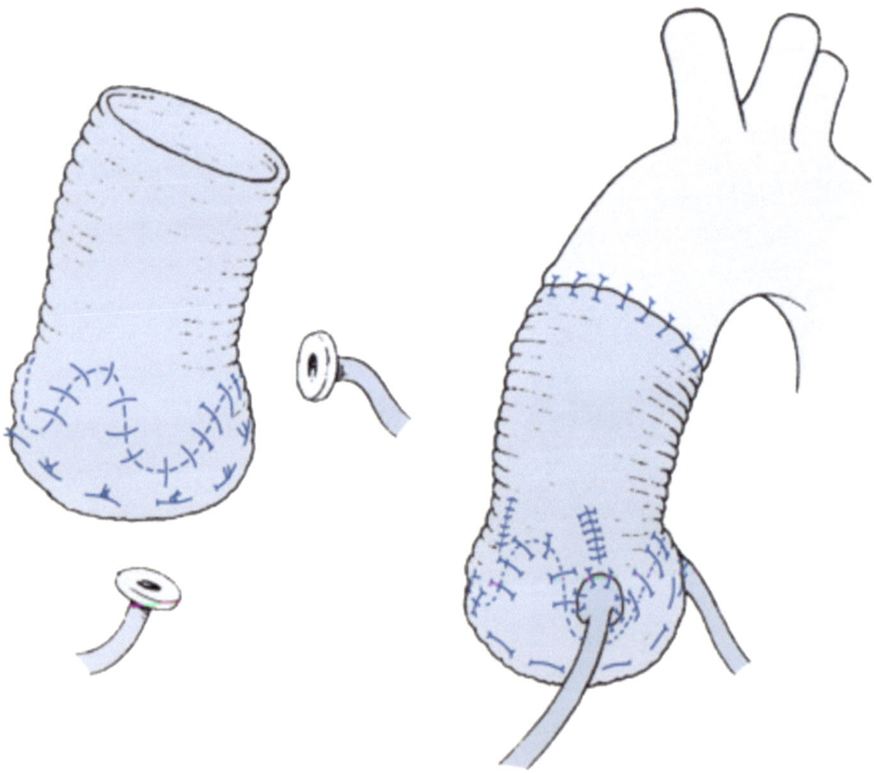

Fig. 5. David V Reimplantation Procedure. From David TE. Aortic Valve Repair and Aortic Valve-Sparing Operations. In: Cohn LH, ed. *Cardiac Surgery in the Adult.* New York, NY: McGraw Hill:935-948, 2008

Multiple (9-12) 2-0 or 3-0 horizontal pledgeted mattress stitches are placed circumferentially from inside to out of the left ventricular outflow tract at the level of 2mm below the nadir of the annulus in a horizontal plane. These stitches go through the fibrous portion of the outflow tract and the muscular interventricular septum and are passed through the tailored end of the Dacron graft. If the aortic annulus is not dilated, these sutures are spaced symmetrically. In the case of annular dilatation, the sutures which are placed in the area of the subcommissural triangles of the non-coronary cusp should be placed closer together, as this is where annular dilatation occurs. Next the commissural stitches are brought through the inside of the graft and the graft is seated around the outside of the annulus. The sutures are tied to secure the graft to the outside of the annulus, but not too tightly, which would pursestring the graft (2).

The graft is cut to about 5-7 cm in height and the commissural sutures are pulled up vertically and the cusps are assessed for the position of optimal coaptation. Once the ideal position of each commissure is recognized, the sutures on each commissure are passed through the root graft. This resuspends the valve inside the graft, and the cusps and commissures are inspected carefully for proper alignment and coaptation. Optimal position results in coaptation of all cusps at the same level approximately 5-6mm above the nadir of the annulus and a 4mm coaptation zone. The sutures of the commissures are tied outside the graft. Next, the annulus is secured to the graft by a 4-0 running polypropylene stitch by passing the needle from inside to out on the graft 1mm above the annulus and outside to in on the graft. Multiple sutures are used to secure the scalloped aortic annulus to the graft. Once this is complete, holes are made in the appropriate positions and the coronary artery buttons are reimplanted. Pleating stitches are again placed between each commissure to create bulges in the graft which form the neo-sinuses. Each 3mm of plication reduces the diameter of the neo-sinotubular junction by 1mm. Pressurized cardioplegia is injected into the graft to test for valve competence and hemostasis. Any necessary cusp repair procedures are performed at this time. When valve competence is satisfactory, the graft is sutured to the distal aorta.

In 2010, David reported his long-term results of 228 patients who underwent valve-sparing root replacement with the reimplantation technique. This series represented his entire experience with the reimplantation procedure including modifications of his own technique. 34% of patients had Marfan syndrome, 10% had bicuspid valves, and 8% of patients were operated on in the setting of acute Type A dissection. 24% of patients had moderate aortic insufficiency preoperatively, and 27% had severe aortic insufficiency. There were 4 operative deaths and survival at 1 and 12 years was 97% and 83%. 6 patients developed postoperative moderate aortic insufficiency and 2 patients developed severe aortic insufficiency. Freedom from moderate or severe aortic insufficiency at 4 and 12 years was 98% and 91 %. Two patients required reoperation on the aortic valve resulting in a freedom from reoperation at 4 and 12 years of 99% and 97% (17).

The importance and reproducibility of David's reimplantation technique is underscored by its adoption by surgeons worldwide who perform reimplantation procedures. In 2005 the Hannover group reported their 11 year experience with the reimplantation technique in 284 patients. 19% of patients had Marfan syndrome, 6% had bicuspid aortic valves and 19% of patients were operated on in the setting of acute Type A dissection. Elective operative mortality was 1.3%, and overall operative mortality was 3.1%. At 10 years follow-up, survival was 80%, and freedom from reoperation due to aortic valve dysfunction was 87%. In their analysis, the authors discovered that Marfan syndrome was an independent risk factor for requiring reoperation on the aortic valve (25).

The contribution of the shape of the sinus segments to minimizing stress and strain on the cusps and has led to the creation of the Valsalva graft, a graft with premade spherical sinus segments (6) (Vascutek, Renfrewshire, Scotland). In 2010, DePaulis reported a multi-center study from 8 Italian surgeons reporting the long-term results of performing the reimplantation technique with the Valsalva graft in 278 patients. 15% of patients had Marfan syndrome, 11% had bicuspid aortic valves, and 5% of patients underwent valve-sparing procedures in the setting of an acute Type A dissection. 49% of patients had preoperative moderate-severe aortic insufficiency. Operative mortality was 1.8%. At 10 year follow-up, survival was 95% and freedom from significant aortic insufficiency was 88%. 17 patients underwent subsequent AVR for a 10 year freedom from reoperation of on the aortic valve of 91%. The results of this multi-center study highlights the reproducibility of the David V procedure. Although many surgeons prefer to tailor their own graft, the use of a standardized, commercially available graft which has proven excellent long-term valve durability has both simplified and standardized the procedure (26).

8. Remodeling vs reimplantation

Valve-sparing root replacement has evolved from Yacoub's original remodeling procedure to the current David V reimplantation procedure. These two operations have sparked many debates over which is the optimal procedure to restore the natural anatomy and physiology of the aortic valve.

It has been argued that the remodeling procedure is superior to the reimplantation procedure in recreating native aortic root physiology because remodeling maintains the independent mobility of the individual sinus segments. Sinus segment mobility is crucial to facilitating changes in aortic root distensibility throughout the cardiac cycle. Root expansion and contraction throughout systole and diastole is thought to maximize blood flow through the valve apparatus while minimizing stress and strain on the leaflets. Based upon echocardiography data evaluating valve opening and closing characteristics, patients who received a remodeling procedure displayed more physiologic leaflet movements throughout the cardiac cycle compared to patients who underwent a reimplantation procedure inside a straight tube graft (27). Remodeling also preserves the dynamic properties of the annulus which becomes rigid when it is confined by a Dacron graft in the reimplantation technique.

The main arguments for the superiority of the reimplantation procedure is that the remodeling procedure fails to stabilize the annulus, which is important in preventing future annular dilatation, especially in patients with annuloaortic ectasia, Marfan syndrome or other connective tissue disorders. David provided data to support this theory by comparing the results of the remodeling and reimplantation procedures in his own personal series of valve-sparing root replacements in Marfan patients. Using echocardiographic measurements of the different components of the reconstructed aortic root, David showed that patients undergoing the remodeling procedure had progressive dilatation of the aortic annulus and neo-sinus segment over a 13 year period. The annular dilatation occurred even in patients who received an annuloplasty as an adjunctive part of their remodeling procedure. Annular and sinus dimensions were unchanged in patients who received a reimplantation procedure. This translated into more stability in aortic valve function in the reimplantation cohort with regards to progression of aortic insufficiency over time. David hypothesized that the reason for the progression of dilatation in the remodeling cohort, even in the presence of an annuloplasty is that either the small amount of remnant connective tissue between the annuloplasty line and the remodeling suture line dilated, or the annuloplasty sutures cut through the abnormal fibrous tissue of the LVOT (28). David abandoned the use of the remodeling procedure in favor of reimplantation for patients with Marfan syndrome in 1998.

It has been recognized by multiple surgeons who perform both procedures that the remodeling procedure is a simpler, faster procedure as it requires one less suture line and requires less dissection and mobilization of the root (29, 30). The David V is a considerably more complex procedure, but it allows the surgeon the flexibility to adjust all of the components of the aortic root complex in order to achieve normal physiologic function. Despite its complexity, it has gained worldwide adoption and is the procedure of choice by the majority of surgeons who perform valve-sparing root replacements. Furthermore, many surgeons have published modifications of the David V technique with excellent results (31, 32, 33, 34).

Both the remodeling and the reimplantation procedures have demonstrated excellent long-term aortic valve durability. The two operations should be viewed as complementary rather than competing procedures. Most surgeons recommend that patients with annuloaortic ectasia, Marfan syndrome and other connective tissue disorders are best served by a reimplantation procedure. The remodeling procedure should be reserved for older patients with a normal aortic annulus (($\leq$25mm woman, $\leq$27mm man) (17, 34)

9. Conclusions

The treatment of patients with aortic root and ascending aortic aneurysms has been evolving over the past three decades. The majority of patients are still currently receiving Bentall procedure with a mechanical or bioprosthetic valved conduit. However, the number of surgeons performing AVS operations is increasing, and the indications are expanding. More surgeons are beginning to perform these procedures on patients with bicuspid valves, severe aortic insufficiency, and in the setting of acute Type A dissection. Again, patient selection and cusp examination are paramount to achieving success, but the addition of cusp repair techniques to the AVS operation has enabled an increasing number of patients to retain their native valves. The long-term data has proven that these operations can be performed with low morbidity and mortality, and provide durable aortic valve function. When feasible, AVS operations are the optimal treatment for patients with aortic disease and normal leaflets, as they avoid the burden of lifelong anticoagulation and significantly reduce their risk of endocarditis or requiring a subsequent operation for structural valve deterioration.

10. References

[1] David TE, Feindel CM, Armstrong S, Maganti M. Replacement of the ascending aorta with reduction of the diameter of the sinotubular junction to treat aortic insufficiency in patients with ascending aortic aneurysm. *J Thorac Cardiovasc Surg.* 2007;133:414-8.

[2] David TE. Aortic Valve Repair and Aortic Valve-Sparing Operations. In: Cohn LH, ed. *Cardiac Surgery in the Adult*. New York, NY: McGraw Hill:935-948, 2008.

[3] Yacoub MH. Valve-Conserving Operation for Aortic Root Aneurysm or Dissection. *Operative Techniques in Cardiac & Thoracic Surgery* 1996;1:57-67.

[4] Yacoub MH, Kilner PJ, Birks EJ, Misfeld M. The aortic outflow and Root: A Tale of Dynamism and Crosstalk. *Ann Thorac Surg*. 1999;68:S37-43.

[5] Katayama S, Umetani N, Suquira S, Hisada T. The sinus of Valsalva relieves abnormal stress on aortic valve leaflets by facilitating smooth closure. *J Thorac Cardiovasc Surg*. 2008; 136(6):1528-35.

[6] De Paulis R, De Matteis GM, Nardi P, Scaffa R, Colella DF, Chiarello L. A new aortic Dacron conduit for surgical treatment of aortic root pathology. *Ital Heart J*. 2000;1:457-63.

[7] Gleason TG. Current Persepctive on Aortic Valve Repair and Valve-Sparing Aortic Root Replacement. *Semin Thorac Cardiovasc Surg*. 2006;18:154-164.

[8] Hiratzka LF, Bakris GL, Beckman JA et al. 2010 ACCF / AHA / AATS / ACR / ASA / SCA / SCAI / SIR / STS / SVM Guidelines for the Diagnosis and Management of Patients with Thoracic Aortic Disease: A Report of the American College of Cardiology Foundation/American Heart Association Task Force on Practice Guidelines, American Association for Thoracic Surgery, Amercian College of Radiology, American Stroke Association, Society of Cardiovascular Anesthesiologists, Society for Cardiovascular Angiography and Interventions, Society of Interventional Radiology, Society of Thoracic Surgeons, and Society for Vascular Medicine. *Circulation* 2010;121:e266-e369.

[9] Elefteriades JA. Indications for aortic replacement. *J Thorac and Cardiovasc Surg*. 2010;140(6):S5-S9.

[10] Coady MA, Rizzo JA, Hammond GL et al. Surgical intervention criteria for thoracic aortic aneurysms: A study of growth rates and complications. *Ann Thorac Surg*. 67:1922-1926, 1999.

[11] Bonow RO, Carabello BA, Chatterjee K, De Leon AC Jr. et al. 2008 Focused Update Incorporated Into the ACC/AHA 2006 Guidelines for the Management of Patients With Valvular Heart Disease. *J Am Coll Cardiol*. 2008;52:e1-142.

[12] Casselman FP, Gillinov AM, Akhrass R, Kasirajan V et al. Intermediate-term durability of bicuspid aortic valve repair for prolapsing leaflet.*Eur J Cardiothorac Surg*. 1999; 15:302-308.

[13] Morishita K, Abe T, Fukada J, Sato H, Shiiku C. A surgical method for selecting appropriate size of graft in aortic root remodeling. *Ann Thorac Surg*. 1998;65: 1795-6.

[14] Boodhwani M, De Kerchove L, Glineur D, Rubay J et al. Aortic valve repair with ascending aortic aneurysms: associated lesions and adjunctive techniques. *Eur J Cardiothorac Surg*. 2011 Jan 12 epub.

[15] Sarsam MA, Yacoub M. Remodeling of the aortic valve annulus. *J Thorac Cardiovasc Surg*. 1993;105:435-438.

[16] Bentall H, De Bono A. A technique for complete replacement of the ascending aorta. *Thorax*. 1968; 23:338-339.

[17] David TE, Maganti M, Armstrong S. Aortic root aneurysm: Principles of repair and long-term follow-up. *J Thorac Cardiovasc Surg*. 2010; 140:S14-19.

[18] Yacoub MH, Gehle P, Chandrasekaran V, et al. Late results of a valve-preserving operation in patients with aneurysms of the ascending aorta and root. *J Thorac Cardiovasc Surg.* 1998; 115:1080-1090.
[19] David TE. Remodeling of the Aortic Root and Preservation of the Native Aortic Valve. *Operative Techniques in Cardiac & Thoracic Surgery.* 1996; 1:44-56.
[20] Aicher D, Langer F, Lausberg H, Bierbach B, Schafers HJ. Aortic root remodeling: ten-year experience with 274 patients. *J Thorac Cardiovasc Surg.* 2007;134(4):909-15.
[21] Erasmi AW, Sievers HH, Bechtel JF, Hanke T et al. Remodeling or reimplantation for valve-sparing aortic root surgery? *Ann Thorac Surg.* 2007; 83(2):S752-76.
[22] David TE. The aortic valve-sparing operation. *J Thorac Cardiovasc Surg.* 2011;141:613-5.
[23] David TE, Feindel CM. An aortic valve-sparing operation for patients with aortic incompetence and aneurysm of the ascending aorta. *J Thorac Cardiovasc Surg.* 1992;103:617-22.
[24] David TE. Sizing and tailoring the Dacron graft for reimplantation of the aortic valve. *J Thorac Cardiovasc Surg.* 2005;130:243-4.
[25] Kallenbach K, Karck M, Pak D, Salcher R et al. Decade of Aortic Valve Sparing Reimplantation: Are We Pushing the Limits Too Far? Circulation 2005;112[S1]:I-253-259.
[26] De Paulis R, Scaffa R, Nardella S, Maselli D et al. Use of the Valsalva graft and long-term follow-up. *J Thorac Cardiovasc Surg.* 2010;140:S23-7.
[27] Leyh RG, Schmidtke C, Sievers HH, Yacoub MH. Opening and Closing Characteristics of the Aortic Valve After Different Types of Valve-Preserving Surgery. *Circulation* 1999;100:2153-2160.
[28] De Oliveira NC, David TE, Ivanov J, Armstrong S et al. Results of surgery for aortic root aneurysm in patients with Marfan syndrome. *J Thorac Cardiovasc Surg.* 2003;125:789-96.
[29] Miller DC. Valve-sparing aortic root replacement in patients with the Marfan syndrome. *J Thorac Cardiovasc Surg.* 2003;125:773-8.
[30] David TE, Armstrong S, Maganti M , Colman J, Bradley TJ. Long-term results of aortic valve-sparing operations in patients with Marfan syndrome. *J Thorac Cardiovasc Surg.* 2009;138:859-64.
[31] Gleason TG. New graft formulation and modification of the David reimplantation technique. *J Thorac Cardiovasc Surg.* 2005;130:601-3.
[32] Patel ND, Williams JA, Barreiro CJ, Bethea BT, et al. Valve-Sparing Aortic Root Replacement: Early Experience with the De Paulis Valsalva Graft in 51 Patients. *Ann Thorac Surg.* 2006;82:548-53.
[33] Kerendi F, Guyton RA, Vega JD, Kilgo PD, Chen EP. Early results of valve-sparing aortic root replacement in high-risk clinical scenarios. *Ann Thorac Surg.* 89(2):471-8.
[34] Svensson LG, Cooper M, Batizy LH, Nowicki ER. Simplified david reimplantation with reduction of annular size and creation of artificial sinuses. *Ann Thorac Surg.* 2010;89(5):1443-7.
[35] Hanke T, Charitos EI, Stierle U, Robinson D et al. Factors associated with the development of aortic valve regurgitation over time after two different techniques of valve-sparing aortic root surgery. *J Thorac Cardivasc Surg.* 2009;137:314-9.

[36] Cameron DE, Alejo DE, Patel ND, Nwakanma LU, et al. Aortic root replacement in 372 Marfan patients: evolution of operative repair over 30 years. *Ann Thorac Surg.* 2009;87(5):1344-9.

Part 4

Aortic Valve Allograft

7

Clinical Outcome of Aortic Root Replacement With Cryopreserved Aortic Valve Allografts

Aya Saito [1,2] and Noboru Motomura [1,2]
[1]Department of Cardiothoracic Surgery, the University of Tokyo
[2]University of Tokyo Tissue Bank
Japan

1. Introduction

Cryopreserved heart and vascular allografts are major prostheses of choice in cardiac surgery today, used in variety of treatment situations. Right and left ventricular outflow tract reconstruction in congenital heart diseases, cases of infective endocarditis, mitral valve plasty, and aortic aneurysm of infective etiology are the major indications for allograft use. Saphenous vein grafts with small-sized valves have also been reported to be beneficial in particular cases in reconstructing the right ventricular flow to the pulmonary artery for neonates and infants, since these valved vein grafts offer good performance in preserving right ventricular function in small children, thus leading to better clinical outcomes [Murakami, 2002; Tam, 2001].

It has been over 40 years since the first heart valve allograft was performed by Dr. Ross for a case of congenital heart defect [Ross and Somerville, 1966]. Since then, heart valve allografts have entered into clinical use steadily, starting with the use of fresh grafts. Emerging techniques of cryopreservation, including programmed freezing methods and innovation of cryoprotective agents, have enabled long-term graft storage without the loss of morphological and biological benefits, and banking systems have made elective use possible. Tissue Banking system was introduced into Japan in 1997, and gradually became established as the method of choice mainly for congenital heart defects and infective cardiovascular diseases. The University of Tokyo Tissue Bank (UTTB) houses one of the biggest banks in Japan where related clinical investigations and scientific research is also conducted.

In this chapter we describe the allograft processing, the characteristics, and the clinical results of cryopreserved aortic valve allograft that were shipped from UTTB.

2. Tissue processing

2.1 Procurement

The tissues are usually collected in the operating theatre under sterile conditions, in the same manner as in an ordinary surgical procedure. Informed consent is obtained from the donor family in advance by the tissue bank donor coordinators. The procurement team consists of 4-6 surgeons, including cardiovascular surgeons for heart valve procurement and liver transplantation surgeons for venous graft procurement. A small piece of each allograft or adjacent connective tissue is sent for a culture test to rule out any contamination with microorganisms. A blood specimen of the donor is also obtained in advance or during the procurement for serological study. Following a median sternotomy, the whole heart is excised and the heart valves and superior caval vein are dissected on a side table in the theatre. The descending thoracic aorta, inferior caval vein, and portal vein system, and veins from the lower extremities are also retrieved accordingly. Care is taken to process the tissues obtained from the thoracic cavity, the abdominal cavity, and the femoral region separately to avoid cross-contamination. The dissected tissues are immersed in disinfection medium: RPMI 1640 medium + l-glutamate (GIBCO, Invitrogen Corp., Grand Island, NY, USA) containing cefmetazole (240 µg/ml), lincomycin (120 µg/ml), and vancomycin (50 µg/ml), and polymyxin B (1000 µg/ml). Tissues from the thoracic cavity, abdominal cavity, and lower extremities are separately incubated in this antibiotic solution for 24 to 48 hours at 4°C. Up to December 2000, amphotericin B (5 µg/ml) was added to the disinfection medium at the University of Tokyo Tissue Bank, since at the time the trachea was also recovered from the donor, which was considered to be contaminated with yeast.

2.2 Trimming

After immersion in the antibiotic solution, tissues are trimmed to an appropriate size and shape in a laminar flow cabinet (Figure 1 a,b). A surgeon performs the tissue dissection dressed in a sterile disposable operating theatre gown. Tissues are packed in double-sterile bags (Figures 2a to 2d). Samples for microbiological testing are also taken from each graft at this time. Sediments obtained from filtration of the disinfection solution are also sent for microbiological testing. The tissues that are positive for microbes at trimming are excluded from clinical use.

2.3 Cryopreservation

The tissues are cryopreserved in RPMI 1640 containing 10% dimethyl sulfoxide (Me_2SO) in a final volume of 100 ml, including the tissue graft. The doubly packed tissues are cooled at a rate of -1°C/min down to -40°C, and then at a rate of -5°C/min to -80°C, using a programmable freezer (Profreeze, Nippon Freezer Co., Ltd, Tokyo, Japan). The grafts are then stored in vapor-phase liquid nitrogen at -180°C until used. Ketheesan et al demonstrated that a freezing rate of -1°C/min best maintained the viability of cells [Ketheesan et al, 1996], and this is the standard method of cryopreservation regimen today. As for the duration of graft storage, we keep the grafts for a maximum of 5 years, because of possible damage to the packages.

2.4 Thawing and clinical use

Grafts are rapidly thawed in a 37°C sterile saline bath and rinsed by sequential dilution using 1000 ml lactate Ringer solution (Lactec G®) to completely remove Me_2SO, because Me_2SO can cause tissue damage at normal body temperature. A small piece of thawed tissue is submitted for microbiological and pathological tests for the final check of quality control of the graft.

3. Characteristics of the heart valve allografts

3.1 Immunogenicity

In the past 40 years heart valve allografting, cryopreservation techniques (programmed freezing methods, innovation of cryoprotective agent, etc.) have improved significantly, and

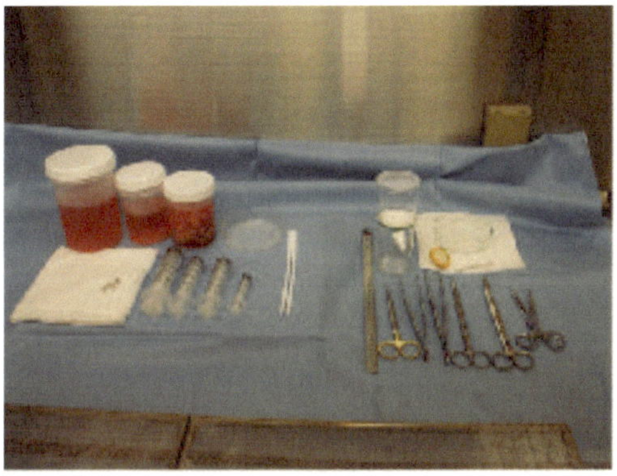

(a)

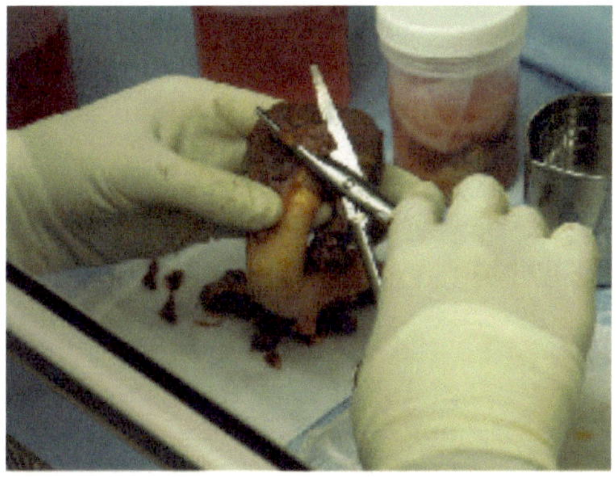

(b)

Fig. 1. (a) Tissues trimming is performed in a laminar flow chart; (b) Muscle skirt is trimed to 4mm thick and 20mm long

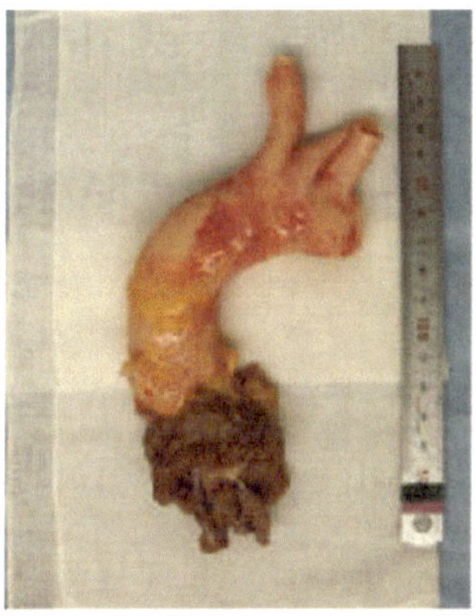

(a)

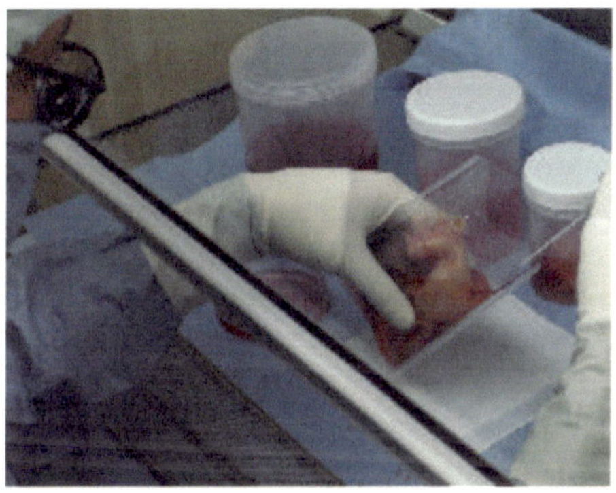

(b)

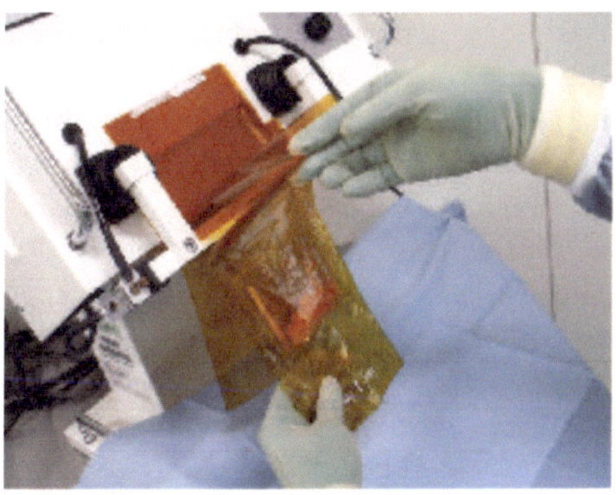

(c)

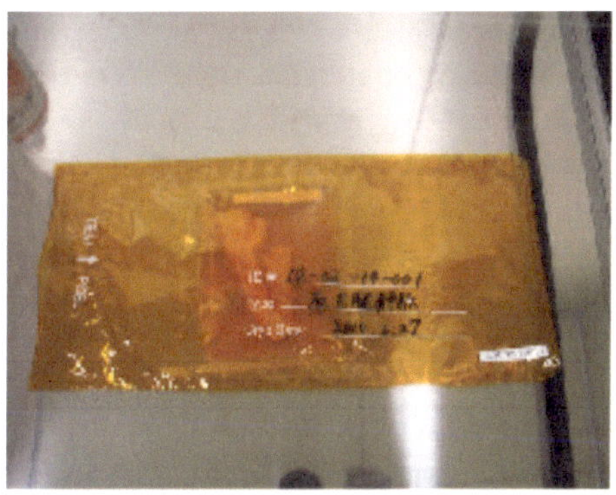

(d)

Fig. 2. (a) Allograft after trimming; (b) The graft is immersed in medium containing cryoprotectant (first package); (c) First and second packages are sealed tight with a heat sealer; (d) Final view of the package progress in techniques and establishment of tissue banking systems have enabled long-term graft storage. With more frequent use of allografts, questions related to the extent of the allografts' antigenicity and the influence of the cryopreservation method on immunogenicity of the allografts has become a matter of discussion [Hoekstra et al., 1996].

Results of clinical investigations and animal experimentation have shown that both fresh and cryopreserved valve allografts have a certain, albeit, low degree of immunogenicity. Such studies date back back to the 1990s and continue up to the present. Fischlein et.al. reported that allograft valves caused immunological reaction after implantation by monitoring the circulation mononuclear cell in the recipients' peripheral blood; the immunological reaction was reversible without immunosuppressive treatment [Fischlein, 1995]. The authors concluded that aortic valve allografts were able to induce an immune response in the recipient that was related to early graft destruction and failure. In further studies using a rat transplantation model, it appeared that cryopreservation diminished but did not eliminate the immunogenicity of the allograft [Oei, 2001]. O'Brien et al presented data showing a donor-specific immune response after aortic valve allografting in the rat [Zhao, 1994], also confirmed in a clinical study [Hogan et al, 1996]. Graft rejection was also observed in infant cases receiving heart valve allografts [Rajani et al, 1998]. In several studies, mixed lymphocyte reaction (MLR) results showed recipient alloreactivity in rats [Rajani et al, 1998; Ketheesan et al, 1996; Oei et al, 2001; Saito et al, 2006]. The impact of cryopreservation manipulation on the alteration in the graft's allogenicity is still under investigation, and it is worth noting that two previous studies [Ketheesan et al, 1996; Oei et al, 2001] have concluded that cryopreservation decreases the immunogenicity of allografts. However, our analyses have shown that there was no difference in immunogenicity before and after cryopreservation [Saito et al, 2006]. This discrepancy in the results may arise from the difference in the conduits used (valved conduits vs non-valved aortic grafts), or the experimental methodology, or may be related to the method of measurement, i.e., whether antigen non-specific T cell response induced by concanavalin A stimulation was used [Ketheesan et al, 1996; Oei et al, 2001], or antigen-specific T cell response to donor antigen was employed using a third alloantigen [Saito et al, 2006].

Histological investigation was the major method of estimating the allogenicity of the cryopreserved allografts compared with fresh grafts [Legare et al, 2000; Moustapha et al, 1997; O'Brien et al, 1987; Oei et al, 2002], and our experimental results also added some data on the alteration of allogenicity in cryopreserved tissues from a molecular perspective [Saito et al, 2006]. Consistent with the results of T cell responses, our investigation of graft revealed that cryopreservation did not modify the graft's immunogenicity. Real-time PCR studies showed that the gene expression of TNFα, IFNγ, and iNOS (as a downstream effector of IFNγ pathway) in response to cryopreservation. In other words, cryopreservation did not modify graft allogenicity. Consistent with our results, Solanes et al recently reported that the cryopreservation method maintained immunogenicity of porcine arterial allografts [Solanes et al, 2005].

Cellular viability of grafts is important in that it preserves the long term viability of grafts [O'Brien et al, 1987], and numerous studies have addressed the status of endothelial cell viability in cryopreserved heart valves and vascular allografts [Oei et al, 2002]. The importance of preserving endothelial cell viability after cryopreservation is a matter of controversy, since there are two opposite interpretations; one being that graft endothelial cell viability is decreased after cryopreservation and also after transplantation because of depletion of donor cellular population [Armiger,1995; Mitchell et al, 1995; Neves et al, 1997;

Niwaya et al, 1995; O'Brien et al,1987; Redwood and Tennant, 2001], and the other that graft cell viability is maintained to a certain degree even after cryopreservation, from morphological, metabolic, and chromosomal perspectives [Fischlein et al, 1995; Lang et al, 1994; Oei et al, 2001]. Duration of warm ischemic time (i.e., the period from cardiac arrest of the donor and retrieval of the heart valve tissues to insertion in medium with antibiotic cocktail at 4°C), differences in the graft preparation method, and the antibiotic treatment regimen, may influence the outcome. In our animal experiments [Saito et al, 2006], eNOS gene expression level was measured in fresh and cryopreserved aortic allografts, which were processed in the same manner, including warm ischemic time and antibiotic treatment for a precise comparison. Levels of eNOS gene expression were similar in fresh and cryopreserved grafts, suggesting that endothelial cell viability is well-preserved at the molecular level after cryopreservation at the molecular level. Endothelial cells are also recognized as MHC class II antigen-presenting cells and may induce T-cell mediated immune responses after allotransplantation [Fischlein et al, 1995; Le Bas-Bernardet et al, 2004; Mitchell and Lichtman, 2004; Ono et al, 1998].

3.2 Resistance against infection

Invasive infective endocarditis of the aortic root is a critical and challenging post-operative complication that needs to be treated, especially when it forms an abscess at the juxtavalvular structure that can perforate to other neighboring cardiac structures. Short-term mortality rates due to this complication are reported to be 5% to 39% [Anguera et al, 2006; Cabell et al, 2005; Chu, 2004; Hasbun, 2003; Motomura et al, 2002; Kilian et al, 2010; Perrotta et al, 2010]. Gram positive cocci such as *Staphylococcus aureus* are frequently isolated, and among these *Methicillin-resistant Staphylococcus aureus* (MRSA) bacteremia is associated with significantly higher mortality rates than other infections. Surgical treatment at the appropriate time is crucial, including complete resection of the infected area and substitution of the defect with valvular prostheses. The choice of valve prosthesis is a key issues for a better prognosis. As regards the choice of substitutes, a heart valve allograft is considered superior to the other prosthesis like mechanical valves and bioprosthetic valves. Since the 1990s, several retrospective studies have shown that possible superiority of the valve allograft use for severe infective endocarditis and prosthetic valve endocarditis cases from the clinical results [Grinda et al, 2005; Haydock et al, 1992; Leyh et al, 2004; Sabik et al, 2002; Vogt et al, 1997; Yankah et al, 2005] ; however, there is no final consensus of an allografts' potential of antimicrobial capacity due to the absence of randomized controlled studies and scientific evidence supporting this mechanism [Eichinger et al, 2002; Rowe et al, 1999], and the presence of opposing opinions [El-Hamamsy et al, 2010; Klieverik et al, 2009]. Further information was contributed in 2008 by our group to strongly support the allografts' property to overcome infection from a scientific point of view; the key substance conferring the antibacterial property was found to be indoleamine 2,3-dioxygenase (IDO) [Narui et al, 2009; Saito et al, 2008].

IDO is a IFN-γ induced, rate-limiting enzyme of the L-tryptophan (Trp) -L-kynurenine (Kyn) pathway [Mellor and Munn, 2004; Munn et al, 1998]. IDO is an important factor in induction of immunological tolerance by suppressing T cell proliferation through Trp degradation, and by producing toxic Trp metabolites that have anti-bacterial properties [Bauer et al, 2005; Bozza 2005; Silva 2002]. A possible mechanism linking antimicrobial activity and possible immune tolerance of allografts is the contribution of IDO. Our study was based on an aortic transplantation model using inbred rats. Aortic allografts, isografts, and control grafts were analyzed to determine the extent of IFNγ, TNFα, and IDO gene expression by quantitative RT-PCR. Also, Trp metabolite production in the graft was measured by liquid chromatography/tandem mass spectrometry analysis. The bacteriostatic effect of each graft and Trp metabolite production was determined by a MRSA proliferation assay. These experiments showed significant gene expression of IFNγ, TNFα, and IDO in the allografts but not in the isografts and MRSA growth was suppressed when incubated with allografts but not with isografts (Figure 3A). Among Trp metabolites, the bacteriostatic effect against MRSA was remarkable with 3-hydroxykynurenine (3-HK) (Figure 3B), and 3-HK was actually isolated from allografts but not from the isografts. It may be concluded that the allograft anti-infection property arises as a consequence of the biological reaction following allotransplantation, which is not expected to occur with

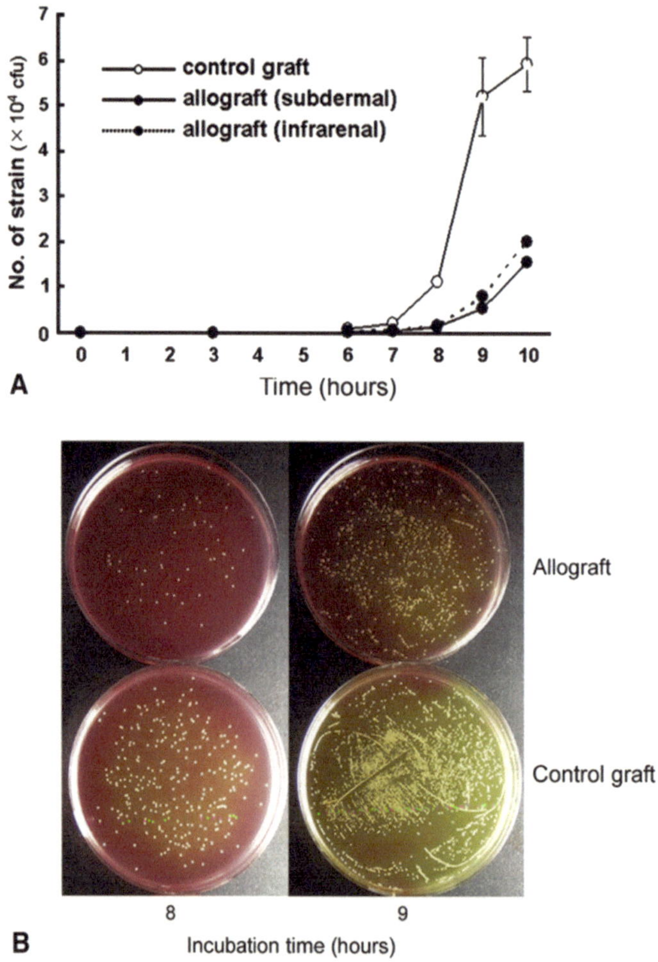

Fig. 3. A) Antimicrobial activity of the allografts against MRSA growth in vitro. MRSA proliferated remarkably when cultured with control grafts, whereas allografts showed MRSA growth suppression. B) MRSA proliferation was visualized on the mannitol salt agar. (Saito et al., 2008)

artificial biomaterial or mechanical prosthesis. Because of this, the allograft heart valve will still be a prime material of choice in surgical procedures related to infective endocarditis.

3.3 Allograft calcification

Although durability of allografts is generally as good as that of bioprosthetic valves, they tend to fail sooner in young recipients, especially neonates and infants than in adults, because of progressive calcification and degeneration [Baskett et al, 1996; O'Brien et al, 2001]. The precise mechanism regarding allograft calcification especially in the younger patients is still not fully understood; however, some studies have been reported [Mennander et al, 1991; Religa et al, 2003; Shioi et al, 2002; Tintut et al, 2000].

Factors related to calcium metabolism in the young (e.g., hyperphosphatemia) are thought to be a possible mechanism promoting allograft calcification. Graft calcification in young rats was inhibited by restriction of dietary inorganic phosphate (Pi) or by blocking of Pi transport via the sodium-phosphate cotransporter by phosphonoformic acid (unpublished data).

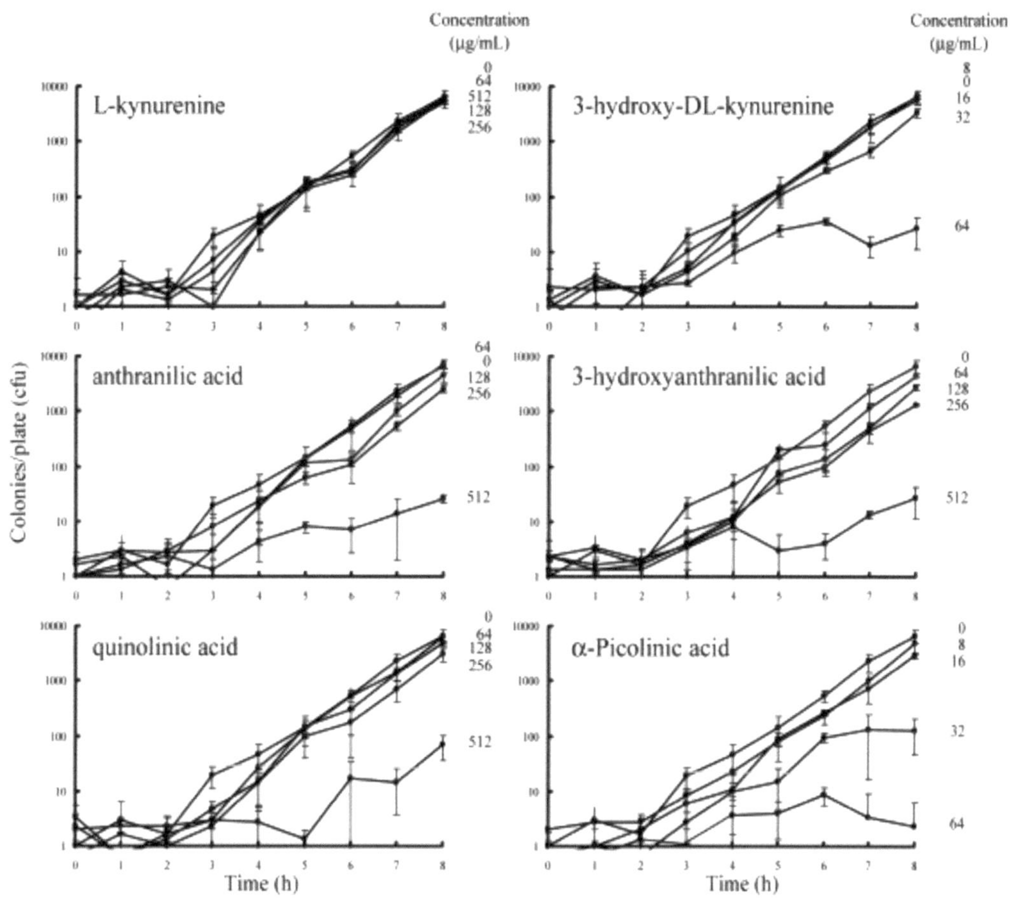

Fig. 4. MRSA Growth Curves with or without Tryptophan Metabolites at Various Concetrations (Narui et al., 2009)

4. Clinical experience from UTTB case series

Heart valve allografts have proven to be useful in the management of aortic valve and aortic root pathology. It has been more than 40 years since an aortic valve allograft was first inserted. Although they are not the only device available for valve replacement, they provide superior clinical outcome compared with the other types of devices such as prosthetic valves (mechanical and bioprosthetic valves) when they are used for infective endocarditis. The purpose of this section is to present the clinical performance of cryopreserved aortic valve allografts, which were provided by the University of Tokyo Tissue Bank (UTTB).

4.1 Patients and methods

Between December 1998 and September 2010, 60 aortic valve allografts were provided from UTTB for aortic root reconstruction. All the patients' characteristics were evaluated preoperatively (age, gender, indication for allograft transplantation and aortic allografts') profiles, and short- and long-term outcomes were analyzed. Recipients and the allografts were matched by size; blood-type or gender match were not mandatory. Follow-up data including the survival, performance status, graft function, and cause of deaths or graft loss were collected by follow-up with the surgeons in charge at 1, 3, 6, and 12 months after the surgery, followed by yearly updates.

The end points of the analysis of graft survival were repeat graft replacement for any reason, reoperation on the graft, or death of the patient with the graft in place. Long-term survival, freedom from recurrence of infection, reoperation, and cardiac death were assessed by Kaplan-Meier method using statistical analysis computer software, SAS ver. 5 (SAS Institute Inc., Cary NC, USA). Patients who survived more than 30 days after the procedure were included in the calculation for long-term analysis.

4.2 Results

A total of 60 patients received allograft transplantation during the observation period. Follow-up ranged from 2 days to 144.6 months (mean, 35.5 months). Mean age at time of operation was 52+/-16 years (range, 9 months - 74 years), and the majority of the patients were between 40 and 70 years of age. Most of the patients (48, 80%) were male. The majority of patients were diagnosed with active infective endocarditis (56/60, 93.3%) including 42 prosthetic valve endocarditis (29 mechanical prostheses, 10 bioprosthetes, 2 homografts, and 1 autograft), and 14 cases of native valve endocarditis. Forty-five cases (75%) presented with advanced infection with aortic annular abscess formation or extensive destruction of the aortic root structure. Microorganisms were isolated from 43 cases by preoperative blood culture, most of them being *Staphylococcus.spp.* or *Streptococcus spp.*, and MRSA was isolated from 6 of the 43 cases (14.0%). All the cases received antibiotic regimen prior to the surgery, however, urgent decision making was required to decide on surgery in most cases because of their hemodynamic instability and arrhythmia resulting from sudden onset of valvular disorders (in most cases, acute regurgitation), large amounts of vegetation on the valve leaflets, and progression of prosthetic valve dehiscence from the annulus. Four cases received allografts for non-infective reason; 2 cases for aortic root pseudoaneurysm after aortic root replacement, 1 for prosthetic valve dehiscence from the annulus because of Behcet's disease, and 1 for congenital aortic stenosis after balloon valvuloplasty. Fifty-four cases (90%) were the repeat surgery of the aortic root. Almost all cases were considered very high risk for surgical intervention (Figure 5 a,b).

Surgical techniques especially for proximal anastomosis at the aortic root have changed overtime; circumferential interrupted proximal suture technique in early days, intermittent continuous suture anastomoses with 6 to 8 stitches in the next era, and interrupted suture at the posterior anastomosis line and intermittent continuous suture in the anterior side of the proximal anastomosis line recently. The method of coronary artery reconstruction was carried out by direct reimplantation of the coronary buttons or interposition between the coronary ostium and allograft wall using the aortic arch branches of the allografts especially in repeat cases (Figure 5c) [Ohtsuka et al, 2001]. Coronary artery bypass grafting was added, if necessary. Short-term outcome showed a 30-day operative mortality of 11.7% (7/60), and the causes of death were uncontrolled infection in 3 cases, low output syndrome in 2 cases, multisystem organ failure (MOF) in 1 case, and bleeding in 1 case. Long-term results showed that the 1-year, 5-year, and 10-year survival rates were 88%, 61% and 53%, respectively (Figure 6a). Freedom from recurrent infection was 94%, 91%, and 91%, respectively (Figure 6c), and freedom from reoperation rates were 92%, 69%, and 55%,

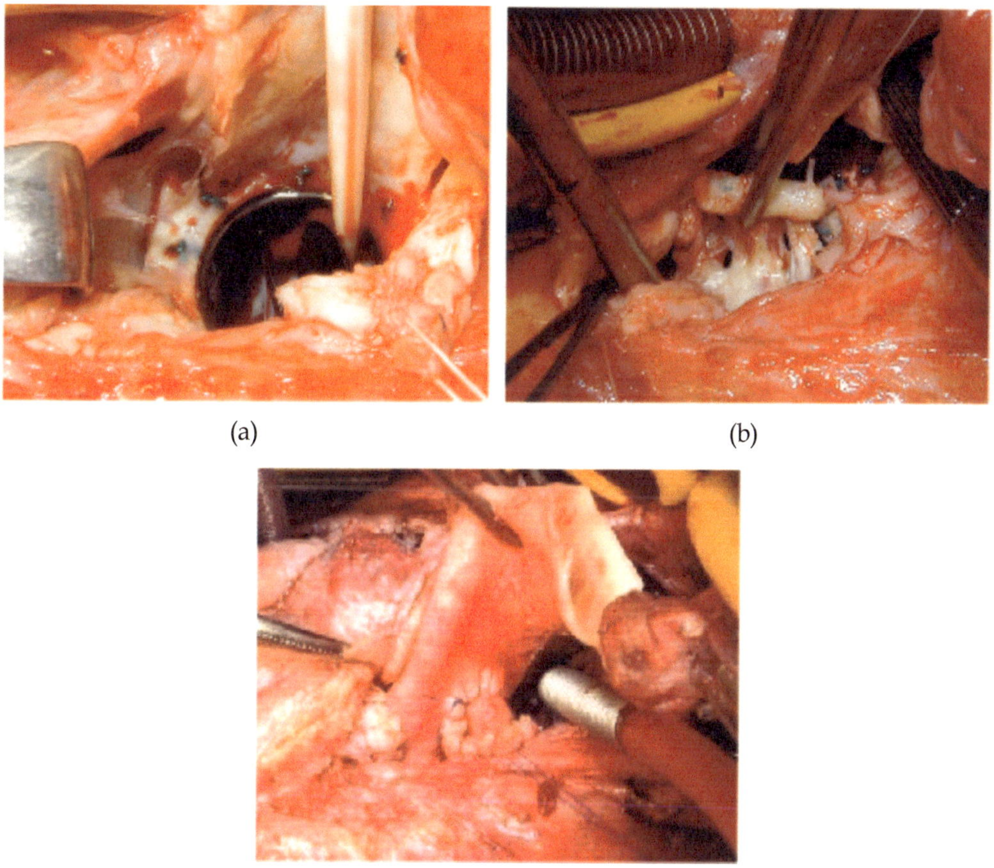

(a) (b) (c)

Fig. 5. (a) Annular abscess at the aortic root; (b) Prosthetic valve is detatched from the annulus due to the infection; (c) Reconstruction of the aortic root with coronary artery reconstruction using a piece of arterial allograft respectively (Figure 6d). The longest surviving graft has lasted 144.6 months. The causes of allograft loss were: uncontrolled infection in 4 cases, heart failure arising from aortic insufficiency in 3 cases, bleeding in 1 case, and MOF in 1 case. The other 6 cases were lost due to non-cardiac reasons. The major indications for reoperation were pseudoaneurysm at the anastomosis sites (either proximal or distal anastomosis line), allograft aortic valve insufficiency due to perforation of the non-coronary cusp [Saito et al, 2003], and bleeding at the proximal anastomosis.

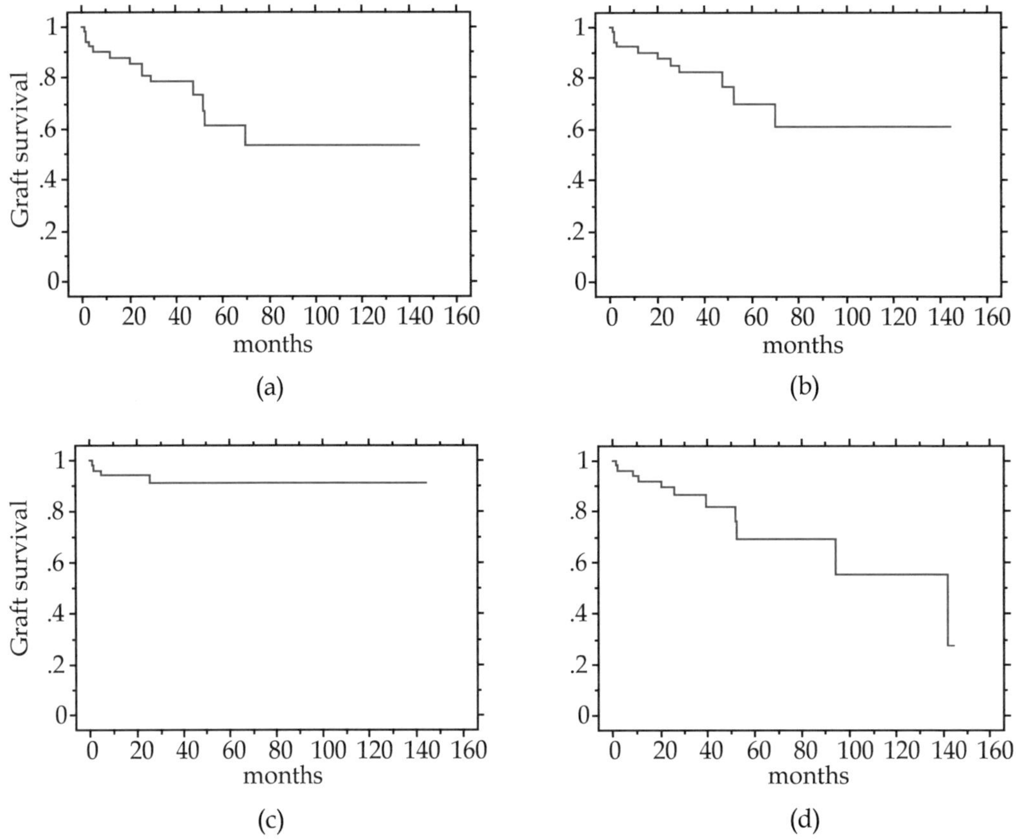

Fig. 6. (a) Cumulative survival after aortic root replacement with allograft (conditional survival); (b) Freedom from cardiac death; (c) Freedom from recurrence of infection; (d) Freedom from reoperation

5. Conclusions

The aortic root replacement with heart valve allograft was carried out successfully in patients with extensive infective lesions around the aortic root for whom the estimated operative mortality was very high. The allografts' nature of anti-infection property was thought to be beneficial in those critical infective disease, and long-term prognosis was satisfactory once the infection was controlled by surgery. Pseudoaneurysm formation at the anastomosis line appeared to be the major issue to overcome in order to improve the operative outcome.

6. References

Anguera, Miro, San Roman, de Alarcon, Anguita, Almirante, Evangelista, Cabell, Vilacosta, Ripoll, Munoz, Navas, Gonzalez-Juanatey, Sarria, Garcia-Bolao, Farinas, Rufi, Miralles, Pare, Fowler, Mestres, de Lazzari, Guma, del Rio, Corey.2006.Periannular complications in infective endocarditis involving prosthetic aortic valves. *Am J Cardiol*, 98.9.1261-1268

Armiger. 1995. Viability studies of human valves prepared for use as allografts. *Ann Thorac Surg*, 60.2 Suppl. S118-120; discussion S120-111

Baskett, Ross, Nanton, Murphy. 1996. Factors in the early failure of cryopreserved homograft pulmonary valves in children: preserved immunogenicity? *J Thorac Cardiovasc Surg*, 112.5.1170-1178; discussion 1178-1179

Bauer, Jiga, Chuang, Randazzo, Opelz, Terness. 2005. Studying the immunosuppressive role of indoleamine 2,3-dioxygenase: tryptophan metabolites suppress rat allogeneic T-cell responses in vitro and in vivo. *Transpl Int*, 18.1.95-100

Bozza, Fallarino, Pitzurra, Zelante, Montagnoli, Bellocchio, Mosci, Vacca, Puccetti, Romani. 2005. A crucial role for tryptophan catabolism at the host/Candida albicans interface. *J Immunol*, 174.5.2910-2918

Cabell, Abrutyn, Fowler, Hoen, Miro, Corey, Olaison, Pappas, Anstrom, Stafford, Eykyn, Habib, Mestres, Wang. 2005. Use of surgery in patients with native valve infective endocarditis: results from the International Collaboration on Endocarditis Merged Database. *Am Heart J*, 150.5.1092-1098

Chu, Cabell, Benjamin, Kuniholm, Fowler, Engemann, Sexton, Corey, Wang. 2004. Early predictors of in-hospital death in infective endocarditis. *Circulation*, 109.14.1745-1749

Eichinger, Goppel, Mendler, Mattes, Lankes, Botzenhardt, Bauernschmitt, Lange. 2002. In-vivo bacterial adherence to intracardiac prosthetic materials: a new experimental model. *J Heart Valve Dis*, 11.3.438-446

El-Hamamsy, Eryigit, Stevens, Sarang, George, Clark, Melina, Takkenberg, Yacoub.Long-term outcomes after autograft versus homograft aortic root replacement in adults with aortic valve disease: a randomised controlled trial. *Lancet*, 376.9740.524-531

Fischlein, Schutz, Haushofer, Frey, Uhlig, Detter, Reichart. 1995. Immunologic reaction and viability of cryopreserved homografts. *Ann Thorac Surg*, 60.2 Suppl.S122-125; discussion S125-126

Grinda, Mainardi, D'Attellis, Bricourt, Berrebi, Fabiani, Deloche. 2005. Cryopreserved aortic viable homograft for active aortic endocarditis. *Ann Thorac Surg*, 79.3.767-771

Hasbun, Vikram, Barakat, Buenconsejo, Quagliarello. 2003. Complicated left-sided native valve endocarditis in adults: risk classification for mortality. *Jama*, 289.15.1933-1940

Haydock, Barratt-Boyes, Macedo, Kirklin, Blackstone. 1992. Aortic valve replacement for active infectious endocarditis in 108 patients. A comparison of freehand allograft valves with mechanical prostheses and bioprostheses. *J Thorac Cardiovasc Surg*, 103.1.130-139

Hoekstra, Knoop, Vaessen, Wassenaar, Jutte, Bos, Bogers, Weimar. 1996. Donor-specific cellular immune response against human cardiac valve allografts. *J Thorac Cardiovasc Surg*, 112.2.281-286

Hogan, Duplock, Green, Smith, Gall, Frazer, O'Brien. 1996. Human aortic valve allografts elicit a donor-specific immune response. *J Thorac Cardiovasc Surg*, 112.5.1260-1266; discussion 1266-1267

Ketheesan, Kearney, Ingham. 1996. The effect of cryopreservation on the immunogenicity of allogeneic cardiac valves. *Cryobiology*, 33.1.41-53

Kilian, Fries, Kowert, Vogt, Kreuzer, Reichart.Homograft implantation for aortic valve replacement since 15 years: results and follow-up. *Heart Surg Forum*, 13.4.E238-242

Klieverik, Yacoub, Edwards, Bekkers, Roos-Hesselink, Kappetein, Takkenberg, Bogers. 2009. Surgical treatment of active native aortic valve endocarditis with allografts and mechanical prostheses. *Ann Thorac Surg*, 88.6.1814-1821

Lang, Giordano, Cardon-Cardo, Summers, Staiano-Coico, Hajjar. 1994. Biochemical and cellular characterization of cardiac valve tissue after cryopreservation or antibiotic preservation. *J Thorac Cardiovasc Surg*, 108.1.63-67

Le Bas-Bernardet, Coupel, Chauveau, Soulillou, Charreau. 2004. Vascular endothelial cells evade apoptosis triggered by human leukocyte antigen-DR ligation mediated by allospecific antibodies. *Transplantation*, 78.12.1729-1739

Legare, Lee, Ross. 2000. Cryopreservation of rat aortic valves results in increased structural failure. *Circulation*, 102.19 Suppl 3.III75-78

Leyh, Knobloch, Hagl, Ruhparwar, Fischer, Kofidis, Haverich.2004.Replacement of the aortic root for acute prosthetic valve endocarditis: prosthetic composite versus aortic allograft root replacement.*J Thorac Cardiovasc Surg*,127.5.1416-1420

Mellor, Munn. 2004. IDO expression by dendritic cells: tolerance and tryptophan catabolism. *Nat Rev Immunol*, 4.10.762-774

Mennander, Tiisala, Halttunen, Yilmaz, Paavonen, Hayry. 1991. Chronic rejection in rat aortic allografts. An experimental model for transplant arteriosclerosis. *Arterioscler Thromb*, 11.3.671-680

Mitchell, Jonas, Schoen. 1995. Structure-function correlations in cryopreserved allograft cardiac valves. *Ann Thorac Surg*, 60.2 Suppl.S108-112; discussion S113

Mitchell, Lichtman. 2004. The link between IFN-gamma and allograft arteriopathy: is the answer NO? *J Clin Invest*, 114.6.762-764

Motomura, Takamoto, Murakawa, Yoneda, Shibusawa, Maeda, Suematsu, Murakami, Nakajima, Kotsuka. 2002. Short-term result of aortic valve replacement with cryopreserved homograft valve in the University of Tokyo Tissue Bank. *Artif Organs*, 26.5.449-452

Moustapha, Ross, Bittira, Van-Velzen, McAlister, Lannon, Lee. 1997. Aortic valve grafts in the rat: evidence for rejection. *J Thorac Cardiovasc Surg*, 114.6.891-902

Munn, Zhou, Attwood, Bondarev, Conway, Marshall, Brown, Mellor. 1998. Prevention of allogeneic fetal rejection by tryptophan catabolism. *Science*, 281.5380.1191-1193

Murakami, Takamoto, Takaoka, Kobayashi, Maeda, Takayama, Motomura, Murakawa, Ono. 2002. Saphenous vein homograft containing a valve as a right ventricle-pulmonary artery conduit in the modified Norwood operation. *J Thorac Cardiovasc Surg*, 124.5.1041-1042

Narui, Noguchi, Saito, Kakimi, Motomura, Kubo, Takamoto, Sasatsu. 2009. Anti-infectious activity of tryptophan metabolites in the L-tryptophan-L-kynurenine pathway. *Biol Pharm Bull*, 32.1.41-44

Neves, Gulbenkian, Ramos, Martins, Caldas, Mascarenhas, Guerreiro, Matoso-Ferreira, Santos, Monteiro, Melo. 1997. Mechanisms underlying degeneration of cryopreserved vascular homografts. *J Thorac Cardiovasc Surg*, 113.6.1014-1021

Niwaya, Sakaguchi, Kawachi, Kitamura. 1995. Effect of warm ischemia and cryopreservation on cell viability of human allograft valves. *Ann Thorac Surg*, 60.2 Suppl.S114-117

O'Brien, Harrocks, Stafford, Gardner, Pohlner, Tesar, Stephens. 2001. The homograft aortic valve: a 29-year, 99.3% follow up of 1,022 valve replacements. *J Heart Valve Dis*, 10.3.334-344; discussion 335

O'Brien, Stafford, Gardner, Pohlner, McGiffin. 1987. A comparison of aortic valve replacement with viable cryopreserved and fresh allograft valves, with a note on chromosomal studies. *J Thorac Cardiovasc Surg*, 94.6.812-823

Oei, Stegmann, Vaessen, Marquet, Weimar, Bogers. 2001. Immunological aspects of fresh and cryopreserved aortic valve transplantation in rats. *Ann Thorac Surg*, 71.5 Suppl.S379-384

Oei, Stegmann, van der Ham, Zondervan, Vaessen, Baan, Weimar, Bogers. 2002. The presence of immune stimulatory cells in fresh and cryopreserved donor aortic and pulmonary valve allografts. *J Heart Valve Dis*, 11.3.315-324; discussion 325

Ohtsuka, Takamoto, Ono, Motomura. 2001. Aortic root replacement and coronary interposition using a cryopreserved allograft and its branch. *Eur J Cardiothorac Surg*, 20.3.631-632

Ono, Nakajima, Lee, Hirata, Kobayashi, Kawauchi, Kotsuka, Takamoto, Furuse. 1998. Influence of cryopreservation on human vascular endothelial cell immunogenicity. *Transplant Proc*, 30.7.3915-3916

Perrotta, Aljassim, Jeppsson, Bech-Hanssen, Svensson.Survival and quality of life after aortic root replacement with homografts in acute endocarditis.*Ann Thorac Surg*,90.6.1862-1867

Rajani, Mee, Ratliff. 1998. Evidence for rejection of homograft cardiac valves in infants. *J Thorac Cardiovasc Surg*, 115.1.111-117

Redwood, Tennant. 2001. Cellular survival in rat vein-to-artery grafts. Extensive depletion of donor cells. *Cell Tissue Res*, 306.2.251-256

Religa, Bojakowski, Gaciong, Thyberg, Hedin. 2003. Arteriosclerosis in rat aortic allografts: dynamics of cell growth, apoptosis and expression of extracellular matrix proteins. *Mol Cell Biochem*, 249.1-2.75-83

Ross, Somerville. 1966. Correction of pulmonary atresia with a homograft aortic valve. *Lancet*, 2.7479.1446-1447

Rowe, Impellizzeri, Vaynblat, Lawson, Kim, Sierra, Homel, Acinapura, Cunningham, Burack. 1999. Studies in thoracic aortic graft infections: the development of a porcine model and a comparison of collagen-impregnated dacron grafts and cryopreserved allografts. *J Thorac Cardiovasc Surg*, 118.5.857-865

Sabik, Lytle, Blackstone, Marullo, Pettersson, Cosgrove. 2002. Aortic root replacement with cryopreserved allograft for prosthetic valve endocarditis. *Ann Thorac Surg*, 74.3.650-659; discussion 659

Saito, Motomura, Kakimi, Narui, Noguchi, Sasatsu, Kubo, Koezuka, Takai, Ueha, Takamoto. 2008. Vascular allografts are resistant to methicillin-resistant Staphylococcus aureus through indoleamine 2,3-dioxygenase in a murine model. *J Thorac Cardiovasc Surg*, 136.1.159-167

Saito, Motomura, Kakimi, Ono, Takai, Sumida, Takamoto. 2006. Cryopreservation does not alter the allogenicity and development of vasculopathy in post-transplant rat aortas. *Cryobiology*, 52.2.251-260

Saito, Ohtsuka, Motomura, Kotsuka, Takamoto, Takazawa. 2003. Early valvular obliteration of cryopreserved aortic valve allograft. *Jpn J Thorac Cardiovasc Surg*, 51.8.384-386

Shioi, Katagi, Okuno, Mori, Jono, Koyama, Nishizawa. 2002. Induction of bone-type alkaline phosphatase in human vascular smooth muscle cells: roles of tumor necrosis factor-alpha and oncostatin M derived from macrophages. *Circ Res*, 91.1.9-16

Silva, Rodrigues, Santoro, Reis, Alvarez-Leite, Gazzinelli. 2002. Expression of indoleamine 2,3-dioxygenase, tryptophan degradation, and kynurenine formation during in vivo infection with Toxoplasma gondii: induction by endogenous gamma interferon and requirement of interferon regulatory factor 1. *Infect Immun*, 70.2.859-868

Solanes, Rigol, Khabiri, Castella, Ramirez, Roque, Agusti, Roig, Perez-Villa, Segales, Pomar, Engel, Massaguer, Martorell, Rodriguez, Sanz, Heras. 2005. Effects of cryopreservation on the immunogenicity of porcine arterial allografts in early stages of transplant vasculopathy. *Cryobiology*, 51.2.130-141

Tam, Murphy, Parks, Raviele, Vincent, Strieper, Cuadrado.2001.Saphenous vein homograft: a superior conduit for the systemic arterial shunt in the Norwood operation. *Ann Thorac Surg*, 71.5.1537-1540

Tintut, Patel, Parhami, Demer.2000.Tumor necrosis factor-alpha promotes in vitro calcification of vascular cells via the cAMP pathway. *Circulation*, 102.21.2636-2642

Vogt, von Segesser, Jenni, Niederhauser, Genoni, Kunzli, Schneider, Turina.1997.Emergency surgery for acute infective aortic valve endocarditis: performance of cryopreserved homografts and mode of failure. *Eur J Cardiothorac Surg*, 11.1.53-61

Yankah, Pasic, Klose, Siniawski, Weng, Hetzer.2005.Homograft reconstruction of the aortic root for endocarditis with periannular abscess: a 17-year study. *Eur J Cardiothorac Surg*, 28.1.69-75

Zhao, Green, Frazer, Hogan, O'Brien.1994.Donor-specific immune response after aortic valve allografting in the rat. *Ann Thorac Surg*, 57.5.1158-1163

Part 5

Outcome Assessment

Forecasting of the Possible Outcome of Prosthetics of the Aortal Valve on Preoperational Anatomo-Functional Hemodynamics and According to Heart Indicators

F. F. Turaev[1], A. M. Karaskov[2] and S. I. Zheleznev[2]
[1]*V.Vakhidov Republican Specialized Center for Surgery, Tashkent,*
[2]*E.N.Meshalkin Novosibirsk State Research Institute of Circulation Pathology, Novosibirsk,*
[1]*Uzbekistan*
[2]*Russia*

1. Introduction

Prosthetics of the aortal valve is recommended as a standard surgical procedure for the majority of patients with defects of the aortal valve, who need surgical treatment [1]. Being the most simple technically possible to make nowadays, prosthetics of the aortal valve makes 13 % from all operations in case of acquired valve defects [2,3]. The 5-year survival rate without operation makes 50-80 % whereas surgical treatment leads to recovery and survival rate increase even at a serious clinical course of aortal defect [4,5,6]. At present stage of cardiosurgery development there are some methods of estimation of risk of operation [7,8,9]. However indicators under which it would be possible to estimate the forecast of AV prosthetics in the postoperative period are quite poor [10,11]. Available scales of risk estimation sometimes limit an exact prediction of risk or overrate the risk at patients who undergo valve surgery with or without coronary shunting [12,13,14,15]. The estimation of preoperative indicators which characterize the postoperative forecast can be useful for preoperative stratification of risk.
The aim of the research was to estimate the influence of initial anatomic-functional and hemodynamic indicators when forecasting the nearest results at patients after prosthetics of the aortal valve.

2. Material and methods

To estimate the influence of initial anatomic-functional indicators on the results of AV prosthetics 394 patients who underwent isolated AV prosthetics in 2001-2007 have been examined. Out of 394 people there are 311men and 83women at the age of 10 – 78, middle age is 36,9 ± 1,3 years. In Functional ClassI on New York Heart Association there were 14 (3,6 %) patients, in class II - 42 (10,7 %), in class III - 296 (75,0 %), in class IV - 42 (10,7%). Patients have been divided according to hemodynamic implication of defect into two groups: I group patients with an aortal stenosis and combined aortal defect with prevalence of stenosis (AS) - 165 (41,9 %) patients and II group with aortal insufficiency and combined aortal defect with prevalence of insufficiency (AI) - 229 (58,1 %) patients. The reasons of aortal defect (AD) were: rheumatic disease in 74,8 % of cases, an infectious endocarditis (IE) - 16,3 %, congenital defect AV - 8,5 %, an atherosclerotic degeneration and a calcification - 0,4 %. All patients took chest X-ray, ECG, EchoCG, laboratory examination. Patients condition at baseline was a landmark to determine all totality of defect pathogenetic disorders, and evaluation of the factors affecting the separate components of complete clinical picture creation permitted to consider specially the causes, conditions and consequences of systemic positions.

Calculations were performed with the help of «STATISTICA for Windows», v.6.0 and original programs developed in "Excel - 2000" in "Visual Basic for Application" integrated computer language. Group data was divided into numeral and classification ones; additional tables for deviations (abs. and %) of variables from baseline levels were calculated. Difference of significance was evaluated by χ^2criterion and 2x2 tables – by adjusted Fisher test.

Distribution parameters were evaluated by formulas as follows:

$$M = \frac{1}{N}\sum_{i=1}^{n} Xi; \qquad S = \sqrt{\frac{1}{N-1}\sum_{i=1}^{n}(Xi - M)2}; \qquad m = M\frac{S}{\sqrt{N}}$$

Consistency of numerical data with normal distribution law was assessed with help of Kolmogorov test. If the numerical data did not correspond to normal distribution law, non-parametric statistical methods were used - Wilcoxon rank test. Power and direction of correlation between the signs were determined by Pearson correlation coefficient **(r)** and by Spearmanrank correlation, if distribution of the baseline data was deviant. The values of these tests range from -1 to +1. The extreme values are observed in signs associated with linear functional relation. The significance of selected correlation coefficient is assessed by statistics value: r* $\sqrt{n-2}$ / $\sqrt{1-r2}$ =ta,f(1). The expression (1) permits to determine *a*, possibility of correlation coefficient difference from zero depending on *r* and sample size *n*. This, in turn, allows comparing the correlation of the same signs in the different sample sizes by possibility. Correlation power was assessed by a value of the correlation coefficient: strong, if $r \geq 0.7$, moderate, if r = 0.3-0.7, weak, if$r<0.3$. The differences between compared values were significant if $p<0.5$, it is consistent with criteria accepted in medical and biological researches.

Prognosis model is based on the regression analysis. Regression analysis was directed to the test of significance of one (dependent) variable Y from set of other ones, so called independent variables Xj = {X1, X2, … Xp}. The values of the prognostic parameter are defined according to the result of determination of the risk factors based on analysis of the clinical materials. The purpose of linear regression analysis in this study was to predict the values of the resulted variable Y according to the known values of physical parameters, EchoCG parameters and various additional features related to surgery specificity. The index of favorable surgery outcome was calculated as an arithmetic mean of risk factors.

As a result of these calculations, the model was developed. Based on this model the program was created in "Excel–2000»-« The Program of forecasting of probability of a favorable outcome of surgical treatment of aortal valve defects » (CERTIFICATE SPD RUzbDGU 01377) which helps to calculate a percentage of favorable surgery outcome and dynamics of LV ejection fraction after surgery with prognostic significance of 75-90%.

3. Results

As a result of the performed analysis the variables put into factor groups (F) affecting the surgery prognosis were determined: F1 - blood supply disturbance (HF, NYHA FC), F2 - physical parameters (gender, age*, weight*, height*, body surface area*, Ketle index*, CTI*), F3 - hemodynamic parameters (SBP*, DBP*, MBP*, BSV, HR*, BMV*, TPR*, SPR, HI*, LV stroke work*), F4 - heart parameters (EDD*, ESD*, EDV*, ESV*, SV*, EF*, FS*, RF*, SVE*, RV*, LA*, RA*, PA*), F5 - myocardial parameters (IVS*, LVPW*, LVMM*, sPLVWT and dPLVWT*, 2HD*), F6 -valve morphology (calcification degree on AV, regurgitation degree on AV, MV, and TV), F7- - valve parameters (FA and ascending aorta diameter*, AV gradients*, AO* surface, MO* surface, MV gradients*, Emv, Amv, E/A mv). Indexed parameters, reverse values and second degree were considered in «*» variables, it has been leading to increase in prognosis efficacy (see Table 1).
During research it has been defined, that for patients with isolated AV prosthetics greater influence on the operation forecast was made by factors heart characteristics, the central hemodynamics, indicators of valves, anthopometrical data and myocardium indicators (Fig. 1)

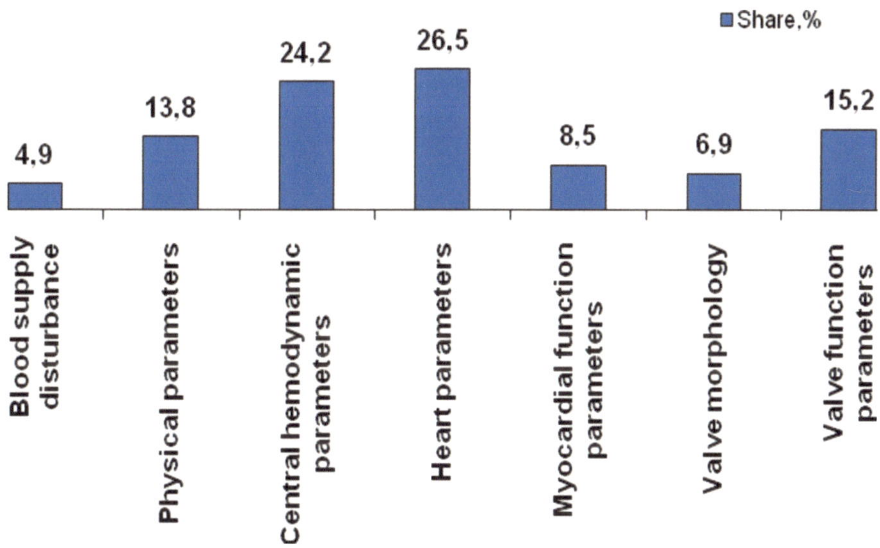

Fig. 1. Share of influence of factors on the forecast

№	Variable	Unit	defenition	Variable nomenclature
			I Blood supply disturbance (F 1)	
1	HF		I, IIA, IIB, III	Heart failure
2	FC		I , II, III, IV	Functional class
			II Physical parameters (F 2)	
1	Gender		1 - man, 2 – woman	Patient gender
2	Age*	years		Age
3	Weighr*	kg		Weight
4	Height*	cm		Height

№	Variable	Unit	defenition	Variable nomenclature
5	BSA*	m^2	BSA= 0.007184 * Weight^0.423 * Height^0.725	Body surface area
6	Ketle index*	U	Ketle index = 10000* Weight / Height^2	Ketle index (body weight index)
7	CTI*	%		Cardiothoracic index
			III Central hemodynamic parameters (F 3)	
1	SBP*	mmHg		Systolic blood pressure
2	DBP*	mmHg		Diastolic blood pressure
3	MBP*	mmHg	MBP = DBP+[(SBP - DBP)/3]	Mean blood pressure
4	PBP*	mmHg	SBP-DBP	Pulse blood pressure
5	BSV		BSV = 90,97 + 0,54 * PBP - 0,57 * DBP - 0,61*Age	Blood stroke volume by Starr (39)
6	HR*	beat per minute		Heart rate
7	CO*	l/min	CO= SV * HR / 1000	Cardiac output (blood supply)
8	TPR*	dyne*cm-5	TPR = 79,92*MBP/CO	Total peripheral resistance (59)
9	RPR		RPR = TPR / BSA	Relative peripheral resistance (110)
10	HI*	U	HI =CO / BSA	Heart index (109)
11	Asw*	U	Asw(LV) = SV*1,055* (MBP-5)*0,0136	LV stroke work (153)
12	LVMW	U	LVMW = 0,0136 * 1,055 *CO * (MBP-5)	LV minute work (157)
13	LVWI		LVWI = 0,0136 * 1,055 * HI * (MBP-5)	LV work index (160)
14	LVWSI		LVWSI = 0,0136 * 1,055 * SI * (MBP-5)	LV work stroke index (161)
15	HFi		HFi= SBP* HR / LVMM	Heart functioning index
			IV Heart parameters (F4)	
1	EDD*	cm		End-diastolic dimension
2	ESD*	cm		End-systolicdimension
3	EDV*	cm^3	EDV= 7 * EDD^3 / (2.4 + EDD)	End-diastolic volume
4	ESV*	cm^3	ESV = 7 * ESD^3 / (2.4 + ESD)	End-systolic volume
5	SV*	cm^3	SV = EDV - ESV	Stroke volume
6	SI*	u	SI = SV / BSA	Stroke index (108)
7	LVEF*	%	LVEF = 100*(EDV-ESV)/EDV	Ejection fraction
8	LVFS*	%	LVSF = 100*(EDD-ESD)/EDD	Fractional shortening
9	RF	%	RF = ESV / EDV * 100	Residual fraction (55)
10	SVE*	%	SVE = EDV / ESV *100	Systolic ventricular ejection (56)

№	Variable	Unit	defenition	Variable nomenclature
11	TC*		TC = (EDV-ESV)/ (EDD-ESD)*1/ESV	Ventricular wall tensility coefficient (57)
12	RV*	cm		Right ventricle
13	LA*	cm		Left atrium
14	RA*	cm		Right atrium
15	PA*	cm		Pulmonary artery
16	PAP	mmHg		Pulmonary artery pressure
17	PA FAD	mm		PA fibrous annulus diameter
V Myocardial function parameters (F5)				
1	dIVST*	cm		Diastolic interventricular septum thickness
2	dPLVWT*	cm		Diastolic posterior LV wall thickness
3	LVMM*	g	LVMM = 1,04 * ((EDD+VST+ PLVWT)^3 - EDD^3)-13,6	LV myocardial mass
4	rsPLVWT *	U.	rsPLVWT = dPLVWT / EDD	Relative systolic posterior LV wall thickness
5	rdPLVWT *	U.	rdPLVWT = dPLVWT / ESD	Relative diastolic posterior LV wall thickness
6	2HD*	U.	2HD = (dIVST + dPLVWT)/EDD	Relative double thickness
VI Valve morphology (F 6)				
1	AVca	score	1,2,3,4	AV calcification, degree
2	AVreg	score	1,2,3,4	AV regurgitation, degree
3	MVreg	score	1,2,3,4	MV regurgitation, degree
4	TVreg	score	1,2,3,4	TV regurgitation, degree
VII Valve function parameters (F 7)				
1	ARD*	cm		Aortic root diameter
2	AAD *	cm		Ascending aorta diameter
3	AVppg*	mmHg		AV peak pressure gradient
4	AVmpg*	mmHg		AV mean pressure gradient
5	AVsfs	m/s		AV systolic flow speed
6	AO s*	cm^2		Aortic orifice surface area
7	E mv			MV E peak
8	A mv			MV A peak
9	E/A mv	U.	E/A mv = E mv / A mv	E/A ratio
10	MO s*	cm^2		Mitral orifice surface area
11	MV ppg	mmHg		MV peak pressure gradient
12	MV mpg	mmHg		MV mean pressure gradient

Table 1. Risk factors and variables and their components

During the correlation analysis of relation of factors with the operation forecast the following patterns have been revealed.
The moderate force of correlation of blood supply disturbance indicators **(F1)** (r=0,683) with the operation forecast has been revealed. It is accounted for the fact that among the operated patients there were more patients at a serious stage of HF and FC, age-specific patients with the long rheumatic anamnesis complicated with a current aortal defect and acute IE. Thus the bigger dependence of the operation forecast on circulatory unefficiency indicators was in the group of patients with AI (r=0,707), than in the group of patients with AS(r=0,580). The less was HF (r =-0,346) and FC degree on NYHA (r =-0,606), the more favorable there was an operation forecast (Fig. 2).

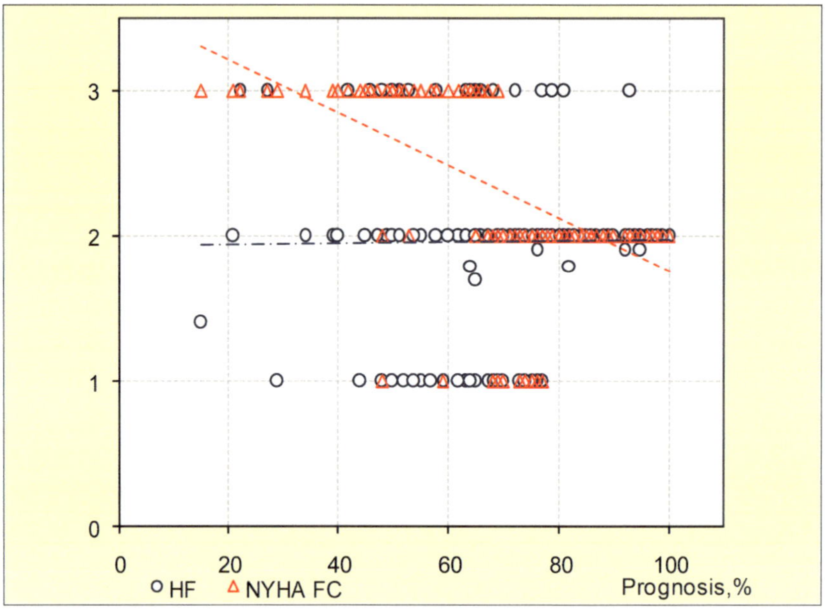

Fig. 2. Influence of degree HF and FC NYHA on the operation forecast

The analysis of the influence of physical parameters indicators **(F2)** has shown, that the younger the patient was (r =-0,626) and the less Ketle index (r =-0,324) and CTI (r =-0,584) were, at appropriate height (r=0,385) (that testifies the constitutional maturity of the patient), the more accurate the operation forecast was. Whereas the indicator of body surface had very weak correlation (r =-0,011), that is bound up with the absence of patients with «prosthesis-patient mismatch» in the surveyed group. In hemodynamic groups the correlation was discernible. Dependence of the operation forecast on CTI was shown at patients with AI (r =-0,567) more than at patients with AS (r =-0,298). The great values of indicator CTI shown by radiological signs of a LV arch protrusion on the left side contour and an aortic arch on the right side contour of a heart shade arise and testify the evidence of aortal defect thatis observed at patients who suffer from AV insufficiency. In both groups the patients of the young-age group had more accurate operation forecast. However the influence of an indicator of the body surface area with the forecast was observed more at patients with AS (r=0,363), than at patients with AI (r =-0,184). If to estimate influence of age on peak AV mpg in both groups then the value was higher in the senior age group (AI r = 0,470;

AS r = 0,612). The loss of aorta elasticity at the expense of sclerotic processes, which occur after a number of years, leads to increase of AV mpg value.

The analysis of influence of hemodynamic parameters indicators **(F3)** has shown, that hemodynamic indicators had moderate correlation with the operation forecast (r=0,424). The patients with the big stroke output of blood circulation had the best operation forecast, which means indemnification and adequate regulation of the central hemodynamic. Thus the influence of indicators (F3) on the operation forecast was more in group of patients with AI (r=0,232), than in a subgroup with AS (r=0,124).

The analysis of influence of heart parameters **(F4)** on the operation forecast has shown that the linear and LV volume indicators have direct correlation with SV and LV EF indicators. The patients with LV sufficient volume indicators at smaller changes on a small circle of blood circulation had more accurate operation forecast (Fig. 3).

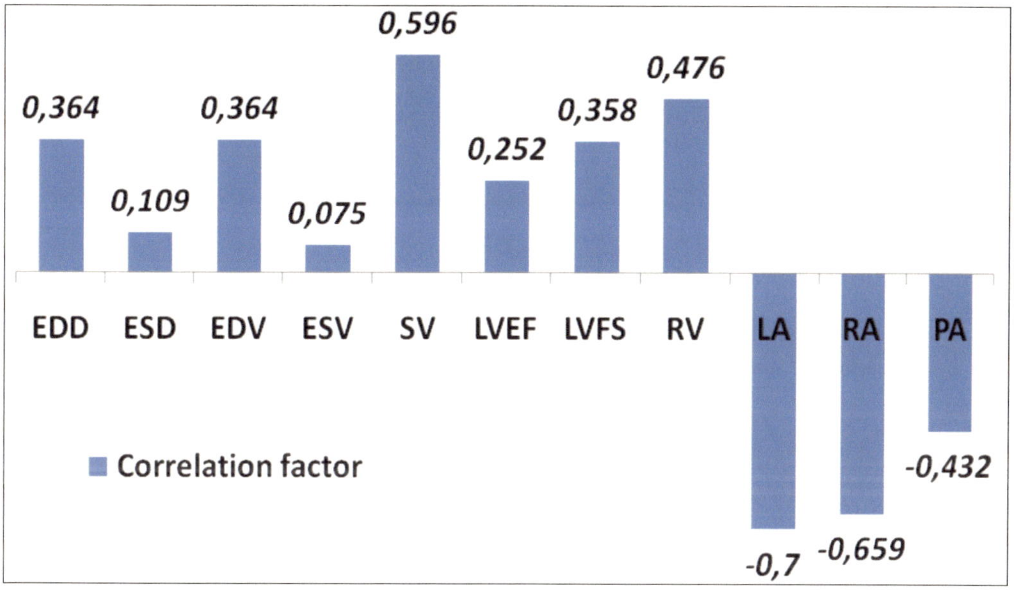

Fig. 3. Correlation of an indicator with an operation outcome

One of the important indicators was the indicator of SV size. The more the SV size was, the more accurate an operation forecast in groups was. SV= (EDV LV - ESV LV) size mostly depends on ESV size, which characterizes the force of cardiac muscle reduction, completeness of LV release. The ESV increase reflects cardiac muscle insufficiency and promotes EDV augmentation in the subsequent cycles. The ESV increase, thus, is one of mechanisms of compensatory reaction realizations at a heart failure, in the form of involvement of Franc-Starling mechanism. Therefore at a stage of preoperative treatment for an adequate estimation of the operation forecast it is necessary to estimate dynamics of the systolic LV size. Reduction of the given indicator during preoperative preparation of patients with the complicated current aortal defect will testify sufficient safety of retractive function and reserve possibilities of a myocardium. The fraction of LV emission influenced the operation forecast in group of patients with AI (r=0,402) more, than in a subgroup with AS (r=0,284), whereas the indicator of fraction of shorting had almost identical influence on the forecast (r=0,406 and r=0,387 accordingly).

Almost all indicators of myocardial function parameters **(F5)** had average return correlation close to a strong one (r <-0,603) (Fig. 4).

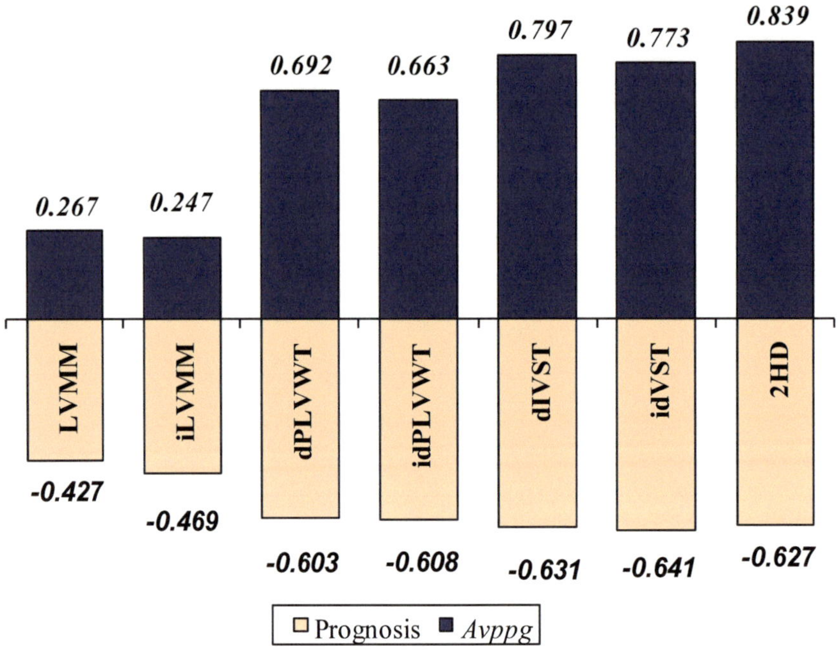

Fig. 4. Correlation of an indicator with the forecast and a systolic gradient of pressure

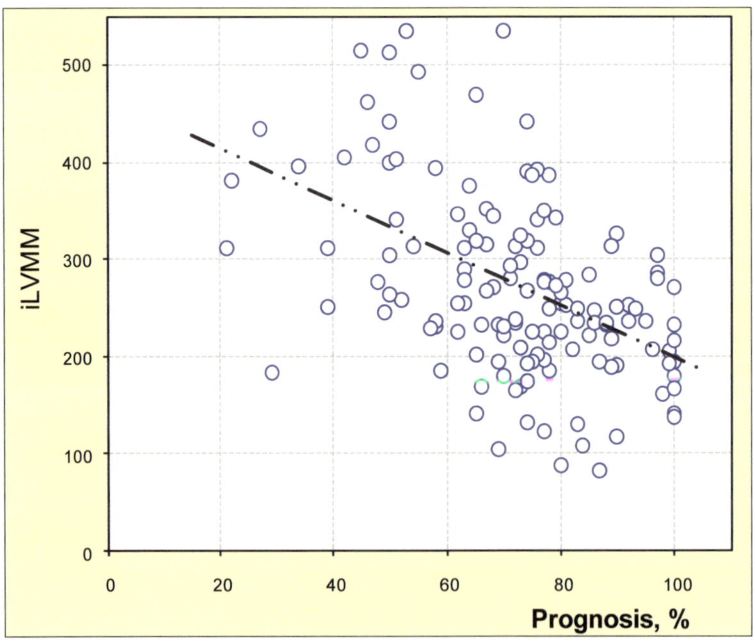

Fig. 5. Influence of an index of myocardium mass on the operation forecast

It has been revealed, that the expressed hypertrophy carries negative influence on the operation forecast. The low the degree of a hypertrophy of LV walls, IVST and myocardium masses is, the better the operation forecast (Fig. 5). Great values of peak AVmpg (r> 0,663) play a great role at expressed LV hypertrophy.

Correlation of indicators of myocardial function parameters **(F5)** on the forecast in hemo dynamic groups has shown an identical direction of force of relation, with prevalence of size of correlation factor for group of patients with AS. In case of identical influence of value of LV myocardium mass on the operation forecast in hemodynamic groups (r =-0,407), the degree of hypertrophy IVST (r =-0,459) had more influence on the AS patients' operation forecast, than hypertrophy PLVWT (r =-0,281) did. Whereas the forecast patients with AI have been influenced more by degree of hypertrophy PLVWT (r =-0,323), than hypertrophies IVST (r =-0,131). Evidence of IVST hypertrophy is bad prognostic sign, both at a stenos is of the aortal valve, and at its insufficiency. It is necessary to use surgical treatment of aortal defect at early stages of defect implication, before the expressed myocardium hypertrophy has development.

In spite of the fact that all patients had been executed with AV prosthetics, valve morphology variables **(F6)** (a calcification exponent (r =-0,563), regurgitation degree on AV (r = 0,639), changes on MV (r =-0,298) and TV (r =-0,631)) had high degree of correlation. The expressed calcification and the related to it inflammatory process sometimes with transiting on ARD aortas and surrounding tissues, as a rule, found in patients with AS, leads to the loss of elastic properties and a destruction of elements of an aorta root, making the basic stages of operation more complicated to perform. At times after prosthesis implantation there is a high gradient on a prosthesis which reduces the possibilities of the return LV remodeling and retrogression of myocardium mass. In cases of AV insufficiency (patients with AI), enlarged ARD aortas and the sufficient sizes of LV cavity allow quickly in the conditions of good visibility to implant a larger prosthesis, even bigger than a settled one and to achieve the least transprosthetic gradient of pressure which promotes improvement of the current post-operative period.

Acknowledgement to it was the estimation of the influence of valve function parameters **(F7)** indicators which has shown, that the more the diameter of a root of an aorta is (r = 0,309) and low indicators of initial AV mpg (r =-0,649) are, the more accurate the operation forecast is. So the analysis of group of patients with AS has shown, that the operation forecast among patients with diameter of a fibrous ring more than 2,4 sm, which allowed to implant a prosthesis of adequate diameter without technical complexities, was more accurate. Whereas, in group with AI the operation forecast was more accurate among patients with no more than 3,5cm ARD diameter. Dilatation aorta ARD and expansion of an ascending aorta makes surgeons think about necessity of aortas binding or replacement of ascending department which leads to operation time extension and risk increase. The influence of a systolic gradient of pressure on the forecast has shown, that the higher its reference value is, the worse the operation forecast. If transprosthetic gradient of pressure does not exceed more than 30-40 mmHg in the postoperative period of prosthesis implantation, it allows achieving a favorable outcome of operation in more than 80 % of cases (Fig. 6).

4. Discussion

Revealing of the indicators, which reference values can define the percent of a favorable outcome of operation, prognosticate possible complications, as well as an estimation of

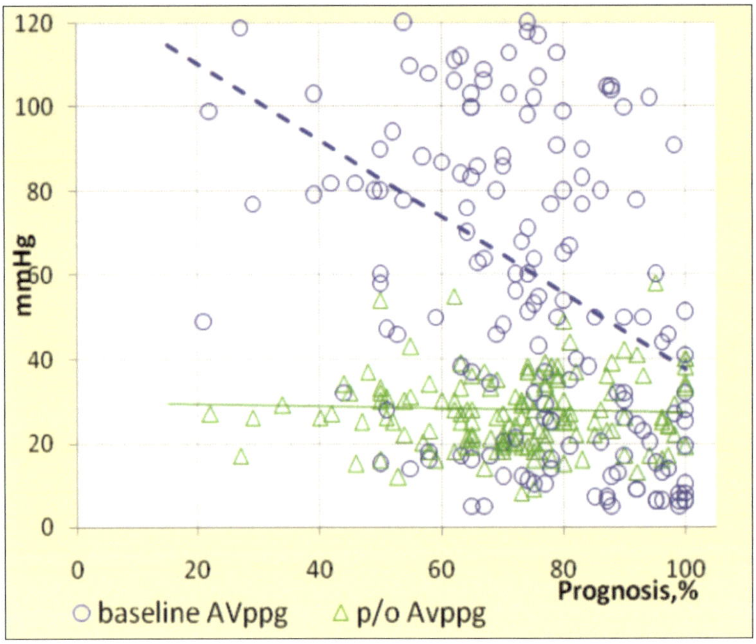

Fig. 6. Influence of a systolic gradient of pressure on the operation forecast

condition gravity in the preoperative period of patients to be operated is one of actual directions of modern cardio surgery. There are scales of risk estimation which sometimes limit an exact prediction of risk or which overrate the risk among patients who undergo valve surgery with or without coronary shunting [9,12,13,14,15].There are intro-operative factors worsening the operation forecast: age, female gender, fraction of LV emission, HF, FC on NYHA, chronic obstructive diseases of lungs, a diabetes, chronic renal insufficiency [3,4].There is convincing data, which say the risk of an early lethality increases if there is immediate surgery among patients of the senior age group and patients with an a trial clottage [5]. These indicators allow estimating results of a wide number of operations on heart. However the analysis and the account of indicators according to which it would be possible to estimate the forecast of operation of AV prosthetics in the postoperative period, taking into account initial data and specificity of operation are poor enough [10,11]. In our research 68 initial anatomic-functional indicators have been the subject of the correlation analysis. The carried analysis has allowed to group indicators in 7 basic groups of factors (F) and to define their influence on the operation forecast: the factor of disturbance of blood circulation (F1) - 4,9 %; the factor of anthropometrical indicators (F2) - 13,8 %; the factor of indicators of the central hemodynamic (F3)-24,2 %; the factor of anatomo-functional indicators of heart (F4)-26,5 %; the factor of indicators of myocardium LV (F5)-8,5 %; the factor of morphology of valves (F6)-6,9%, the factor of valves indicators (F7)-15,2 %. The correlation analysis has shown, that patients with less signs of heart failure (r =-0,346), being in a smaller functional class, have more favorable the operation forecast. Thus these indicators for the operation forecast for patients with AI (r=0,707) was more important, than for group with AS (r=0,580).Patients of a smaller age group (r =-0,626), with smaller Ketle index (r =-0,324),having smaller value of a cardiothoracic index (r =-0,584) had better operation forecast. Thus dependence on the forecast of operation from CTI was more among patients with AI (r =-0,567).Whereas the influence of an indicator of body surface area on the operation forecast was shown more among patients with AS (r=0,363). Influence of indicators characterising a functional condition of the central hemodynamics had moderate correlation with the operation forecast (r=0,424). One of significantly influencing the operation forecast is anatomo-functional indicators in both hemodynamic groups was SV (r=0,596). The ejection fraction of LV influenced the operation forecast in group of patients with AI (r=0,402) more, than in group with AS (r=0,284). The most significant influence was exerted by the indicators characterizing the degree of a myocardium hypertrophies(r=0,839), testifying that the operation forecast is mainly influenced by the condition of initial myocardium. IVST hypertrophy expression (r =-0,407) is a bad prognostic sign, both in case of stenosis of the aortal valve, and at its insufficiency. Calcification expression AV (r =-0,563), regurgitation degree on AV (r = 0,639), changes in MV (r =-0,298) and TV (r =-0,631), expression of an initial systolic gradient of pressure (r =-0,649) negatively affect the operation forecast. As a result of the carried out research there is the prognostic model with calculation of14 various indicators, with prediction reliability of 75-90 % on the basis of which «the Program of forecasting of probability of a favorable outcome of surgical treatment of defects of the aortal valve» in medium "Excel - 2000" has been made and tested. This model is also devoted to forecasting of the surgical treatment results. Type of the realizing COMPUTER - personal computer Intel Celeron (2500 GHz), the programming language - "Visual Basic for Application", a kind and the version of operational system - Microsoft Excel - 2003 in a package «Microsoft Office 2003».

5. Conclusions

Thus, the carried out analysis of influence of initial anatomic-functional indicators on forecasting of results of the aortal valve prosthetics of has shown, that patients with an aortal stenosis and the prevalence of a stenosis are more serious group of defect with less favorable operation forecast, than patients with aortal insufficiency or prevalence of insufficiency. The reason of it is the expressed hypertrophy of LV and IVST having pathological character, with rasping morphological changes in AV in the form of calcification, with transition to FC aortas, the high indicators of a systolic gradient of pressure, with a forwardness of disturbances on a small circle of a blood circulation. Diameter of FC aortas of 2,3-3,5 sm is defined as the optimal size when AV prosthetics will give the best operation forecast as it will allow to implant the adequate prosthesis in both hemodynamic groups. With a smaller size of diameter of an aorta fibrous ring it is necessary to survey adequacy of the effective area of an implanted prosthesis. Value of a transprosthetic gradient of pressure less than 35-40 mm Hg after operation is considered to be optimum indicators which leads to positive results of prosthetics of the aortal valve.

6. References

[1] Braunwald E. Aortic valve replacement: an update at the turn of the millennium. Eur Heart J 2000; 21:1032-1033.

[2] Cohen G, David TE, Ivanov J, Armstrong S, Feindel CM. The impact of age, coronary artery disease, and cardiac comorbidity on late survival after bioprosthetic aortic valve replacement. J Thorac Cardiovasc Surg 1999; 117:273-284. <http://intl-ejcts.ctsnetjournals.org/cgi/ijlink?linkType=ABST&journalCode=jtcs&resid=117/2/273>

[3] Sedrakyan A, Hebert P, Vaccarino V, Paltiel AD, Elefteriades JA, Mattera J, Lin Z, Roumanis SA, Krumholz HM. Quality of life after aortic valve replacement with tissue and mechanical implants. J Thorac Cardiovasc Surg 2004; 128:266-272.

[4] Kvidal P, Bergstrom R, Malm T, Stahle E. Long-term follow-up of morbidity and mortality after aortic valve replacement with a mechanical valve prosthesis. Eur Heart J 2000; 21:1099-1111.

[5] Kvidal P, Bergstrom R, Horte LG, Stahle E. Observed and relative survival after aortic valve replacement. J Am Coll Cardiol 2000; 35:747-756. <http://intl-ejcts.ctsnetjournals.org/cgi/ijlink?linkType=ABST&journalCode=jacc&resid=35/3/747>

[6] Waszyrowski T, Kasprzak JD, Krzeminska-Pakula M, Dziatkowiak A, Zaslonka J. Early and long-term outcome of aortic valve replacement with homograft versus mechanical prosthesis-8-year follow-up study. Clin Cardiol 1997; 20:843-848.

[7] Bolshev L.N., Смирнов N.V.table of mathematical statistics. - M: the Science, 1983.

[8] Nashef SA, Roques F, Michel P, Gauducheau E, Lemeshow S, Salamon R. European system for cardiac operative risk evaluation (EuroSCORE). Eur J Cardiothorac Surg 1999; 16:9-13.

[9] Parsonnet V, Dean D, Bernstein AD. A method of uniform stratification of risk for evaluating the results of surgery in acquired adult heart disease. Circulation 1989; 79 (Suppl. I):I3-I12.

[10] Hannan EL, Racz MJ, Jones RH, Gold JP, Ryan TJ, Hafner JP, Isom OW. Predictors of mortality for patients undergoing cardiac valve replacements in New York State. Ann Thorac Surg 2000; 70:1212-1218.

[11] He GW, Acuff TE, Ryan WH, Douthit MB, Bowman RT, He YH, Mack MJ. Aortic valve replacement: determinants of operative mortality. Ann Thorac Surg 1994; 57:1140-1146.

[12] Bhatti F, Grayson AD, Grotte G, Fabri BM, Au J, Jones MT, Bridgewater B. The logistic EuroSCORE in cardiac surgery: how well does it predict operative risk?. Heart 2006; 92 (12):1817-1820.

[13] Collart F, Feier H, Kerbaul F, Mouly-Bandini A, Riberi A, Mesana TG, Metras D. Valvular surgery in octogenarians: operative risks factors, evaluation of Euroscore and long term results. Eur J Cardiothorac Surg 2005; 27:276-280.

[14] Gogbashian A, Sedrakyan A, Treasure T. EuroSCORE: a systematic review of international performance. Eur J Cardiothorac Surg. 2004; 25:695-700.

[15] Karthik S, Srinivasan AK, Grayson AD, Jackson M, Sharpe DA, Keenan DJ, Bridgewater B, Fabri BM. Limitations of additive EuroSCORE for measuring risk stratified mortality in combined coronary and valve surgery. Eur J Cardiothorac Surg 2004; 26:318-322

9

Aortic Valve Surgery and Reduced Ventricular Function

Dominik Wiedemann, Nikolaos Bonaros and Alfred Kocher
Dep. of Cardiac Surgery, Vienna Med. Univ. & Univ. Clinic of Cardiac Surgery, Innsbruck Med. Univ.
Austria

1. Introduction

Aortic valve disease is a fatal disease with but a single cure. Removal of the mechanical obstruction in aortic stenosis (surgery or TAVI) and replacement of an incompetent valve (so far only surgery) are the only treatment options.

While aortic valve replacement in patients with isolated valve disease and normal pump-function of the heart has become a routine procedure and is performed with excellent results all over the world, it can be a rather challenging procedure in severely ill patients with heart failure and comorbidities. Patients with low ejection fraction are one of the most challenging patient groups in cardiac surgery.

According to the guidelines for the management of patients with valvular heart disease as recommended by all major heart associations including the European Society of Cardiology, American College of Cardiology, American Heart a ventricular function reduced to below 50% ejection fraction is considered a class I, level of evidence B and C indication respectively for aortic valve surgery. (ACC/AHA 2006 Guidelines for the
Management of Patients With Valvular Heart Disease, Bonow et al., 2006) Despite this fact there is a high number of patients presenting with severely reduced ventricular function for aortic valve surgery.

In aortic insufficiency 70% have a function reduced to below 50% and around 10% present with a significantly reduced function of less than 30% EF. In case of aortic stenosis the numbers are a less dramatic but still more than 40 % of patients referred for valve surgery have an ejection fraction below 50%.

This is due to the fact that aortic valve disease can go unnoticed for a very long time resulting in heart failure at time of presentation. Another fact is that at least some patients are treated conservatively for a too long period of time until their EF deteriorates.

Apart from that, due to the demographic development there is an increasing number of patients with aortic valve disease and advanced age resulting in a high number of elderly patients with more comorbidities and reduced ejection fraction.

2. Impaired ventricular function

In the scientific literature there are various definitions with different thresholds describing impaired ventricular function in patients undergoing aortic valve surgery. Ali and co-workers

define reduced left ventricular ejection fraction as <60%, which is in fact an unusual cut off level. (Ali et al., 2006)
Sharony et al. included patients with an ejection fraction < 40% in their study on aortic valve replacement in patients with impaired ventricular function. (Sharony et al., 2003) Mihaljevic T. et al. used a more complex system including 5 subgroups according to cardiac pump-function. Impairment of LV function was graded qualitatively as follows: EF 50% or greater, none; EF 40% to 49%, mild EF 35-39% moderate; EF 26%-34% moderately severe, and EF 25% or less, severe. They demonstrated the prognostic value of this grading system in previous studies. (Mihaljevic T. et al., 2008) For the sake of clearness of this book chapter we include scientific studies with a cut off level of less than 40% and cite the exact values as described in the respective publications.

3. Pathogenesis

Indications for aortic valve replacement are either aortic stenosis, or aortic insufficiency or combined lesions. It is important to distinguish between the indications for aortic valve due to the fact that aortic insufficiency is a risk factor in itself for worse outcome following surgery beyond the impact of reduced left ventricular function.
(Chaliki et al., 2002; Sionis et al., 2010)
34% of all the patients with valve pathologies referred to cardiac surgery are patients with aortic stenosis but only 10% are admitted with aortic insufficiency. (Vahanian et al. 2007 ESC, VHD Guidelines, 2007) Around 10% of the patients with aortic stenosis have combined lesions, but stenosis is the clinically predominant pathology in these cases and therefore these lesions are included into the statistics of aortic stenosis.

3.1 Aortic regurgitation (AR)

The literature regarding aortic valve replacement in patients with aortic insufficiency and impaired ejection fraction is extremely limited with very few patients studied.
Aortic insufficiency as compared to aortic stenosis turns out to be a significant predictor of both mortality and morbidity after aortic valve replacement. Chaliki et al. investigated 450 patients with aortic insufficiency. Only about 10% (n=43) of those patients had a severely impaired left ventricular function (<35%). A major finding of the study is that these patients constitute a high risk group even after successful surgery. The operative mortality rate in this group was excessive with 14% as compared to patients with moderately impaired and normal ejection fraction, with 6.7% and 3.7% mortality rates respectively. This difference becomes even more pronounced in the long term follow-up: At 10 years after surgery only 41% of the patients with low ejection fraction survived as opposed to 56% and 70% in patients with moderately impaired EF and normal EF respectively. Of note, aortic valve replacement for aortic insufficiency does not lead to any significant improvement in pump-function regardless of the preoperative ejection fraction. (Chaliki et al. 2002) (table 1)
In view of the high risk of AVR in patients with heart failure, surgery should ideally be performed before such a severe decrease in EF occurs. However, patients do remain asymptomatic for a long time even if the ejection fraction is already reduced. The decision to recommend operative intervention to asymptomatic patients with chronic, severe aortic regurgitation is very difficult because aortic valve replacement continues to entail immediate risk, and biologic and mechanical valves still have problems resulting in significant mortality and morbidity. (Scognamiglio, et al., 2005) On the other hand for patients who

have AR and already have severe LV dysfunction, an important issue to consider is whether AVR represents too high a risk and conservative treatment is preferable.

	LoEF EF <35% (n=43)			MedEF EF 35%–50% (n=134)			NI EF EF ≥50% (n=273)		
	Preop	Postop	Change	Preop	Postop	Change	Preop	Postop	Change
EF, %	29±6	34±14*	4.9±13.8†	43±6	47±12‡	4±11.9§	58±7	56±10‡	−2.3±10.9
LVD, mm	74±8.3	63±10‡	−10.3±10.4‖	70±8.3	57±9.2¶	−14.4±9.5‖	65±8.7	53±7.4¶	−13.1±8.4
LVS, mm	61±8	51±13‡	−8.5±12.3‖	53±7	41±10¶	−12.4±9.6†	42±8	35±7.9¶	−8.3±7.9
LVD/WT	6.8±1.4	5.1±1.5‡	−1.2±1.1‖	6.7±1.5	4.8±1.1¶	−1.9±1.3‖	6.1±1.4	4.6±1¶	−1.6±1.5
LVS/WT	4.4±1.2	3.2±1.2‡	−1.3±1.2#	3.4±0.7	2.4±0.6¶	−1.1±0.8†	2.5±0.6	2±0.6¶	−0.6±0.7
SWST, $10^5 \cdot dyne \cdot s^{-1}$	159±49	105±49.3‡	−53.7±52.8#	122±34	74.2±25.7¶	−47.6±36.5†	82±30	61±24¶	−27±32

Data presented are mean±SD. Abbreviations as in Table 1.
Postoperative values compared with preoperative values: *$P<0.06$; ‡$P<0.05$; ¶$P<0.001$.
Compared with NI EF group: ‖P=NS; #$P<0.05$; †$P<0.01$; §$P<0.0001$

reprint from Chaliki HP, et al. 2002 with permission of Circulation

Table 1. Comparision of pre- and postoperative echocardiographic values (Chaliki et al. 2002)

Natural history studies have focused mainly on asymptomatic patients with normal function. In a recent study patients were stratified according to their ejection fraction and it was demonstrated that those with markedly lower EF had a higher rate of congestive heart failure than patients who had moderately reduced or normal EF before AVR.

The outcome of conservatively treated patients with even mild LV dysfunction is poor. Indeed, patients with either EF 55% or LV systolic dimension 25 mm/m², even if asymptomatic at presentation, have excessive long-term mortality rates if treated conservatively. Although patients with severe LV dysfunction could not be analyzed specifically, the uniform risk increase with decreasing EF under conservative treatment suggests that such patients are at very high risk if not operated on and that an aggressive approach is justified.

Sionis et al. even evaluated if it is beneficial to offer these patients cardiac transplantation instead of performing aortic valve replacement. But they conclude from their data of only 27 patients that while the mortality of patients with aortic valve insufficiency and impaired ventricular function undergoing aortic valve replacement is high, it is not excessively high justifying listing for transplantation. Additionally a lot of these patients do not develop heart failure and therefore still benefit from AVR. (Sionis et al., 2010)

Conversely, although patients with a markedly low EF and severe AR are at high risk, their medium-term outcome is not uniformly ominous. The usual operative mortality rate reported for AVR ranges from 1% to 7%. Chaliki et al. show excessive operative mortality rates among patients with markedly low EF, but it is not overwhelming. A majority of patients remain free of heart failure 10 years after AVR. Therefore, a notable period of event-free survival can be achieved in most patients after correction of AR despite their very low preoperative EF. The functional status of most patients improves after surgery, irrespective of preoperative EF. Thus, a markedly low EF (<35%) is not, in our judgment, a contraindication to AVR. (Chaliki 2002)

In light of the fact that patients with aortic insufficiency and reduced ejection fraction do not benefit from aortic valve replacement regarding pump function it would be necessary to re-evaluate the guidelines for aortic valve replacement in those patients, since currently AVR in asymptomatic patients is only recommended when EF declines down to <50% or end-diastolic diameter increases >70 mm or end-systolic diameter increases > 50mm (or >25 mm/m^2 body surface area)

However it is difficult to schedule patients with aortic insufficiency and normal EF for surgery because often these patients remain asymptomatic until the pump-function is markedly reduced. When EF is significantly impaired the outcome of surgery is worse but on the other hand the mortality rate of asymptomatic AR patients is rather low and surgery does not improve quality of life. So it remains a matter of debate if the time point of surgery has to be delayed in a later stage if the surgical outcome becomes worse or if surgery should be performed as soon as possible even in asymptomatic patients as long as left ventricular function is still normal

Scognamiglio et al. showed that patients with AR and reduced LVEF can benefit from an unloading therapy with Nifedipine, so that the need for surgery can be delayed by prolonging the asymptomatic period while preserving LVEF (Scognamiglio 2005)

From the data from the literature we conclude that patients with AI and impaired EF should be considered at high risk, carefully evaluated and if suitable scheduled for surgical intervention as soon as possible.

3.2 Aortic stenosis (AS)

In developed countries, aortic stenosis is the most prevalent of all valvular heart diseases. It is primarily a manifestation in patients with advanced age. The disorder is becoming more frequent as the average age of the population is increasing. Symptomatic severe AS is a lethal disease if left untreated. (Figure 1, Figure 2, Carabello, 2009)

Aortic valvular abnormalities are quite frequent in old patients. In the Cardiovascular Health Study, in which 5201 men and women older than 65 years were examined, 26% of

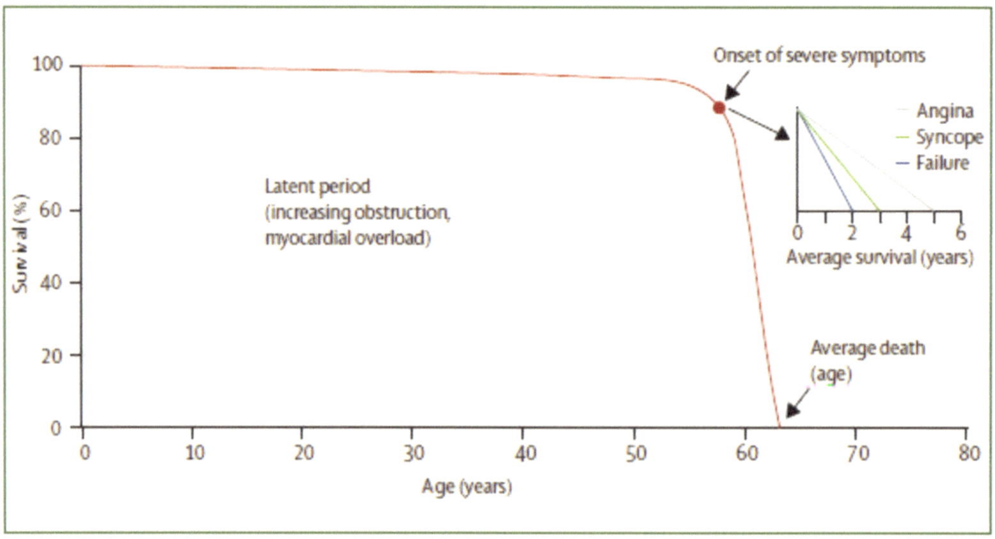

Reprinted with permission of the Lancet

Fig. 1. Survival of patients with aortic stenosis over time. After a long latent asymptotic period. during witch time survival is nearly normal, survival declines precipitously once symptoms develop. Adapted with permission from Ross and colleagues (Carabello et al. 2009)

study participants had aortic sclerosis (a thickening of the valve or calcification without significant obstruction). A slight predominance of the disorder was noted in men. 2% of all patients had frank aortic stenosis.

A clear increase in prevalence of sclerosis was seen with age: 20% in patients aged 65–75 years, 35% in those aged 75–85 years, and 48% in patients older than 85 years. For the same age-groups, 1.3%, 2.4%, and 4% had frank aortic stenosis.

The only effective therapy is the mechanical relief of the obstruction. (Carabello, 2009) with operative replacement of the valve or transcatheter aortic valve implantation (TAVI) as treatment options. Therefore it is one of the clearest decisions for a doctor to recommend valve replacement for aortic stenosis. Balloon valvuloplasty plays an important role in the pediatric population but a very limited role in adults because its efficacy is low while complication rates are high (>10%).

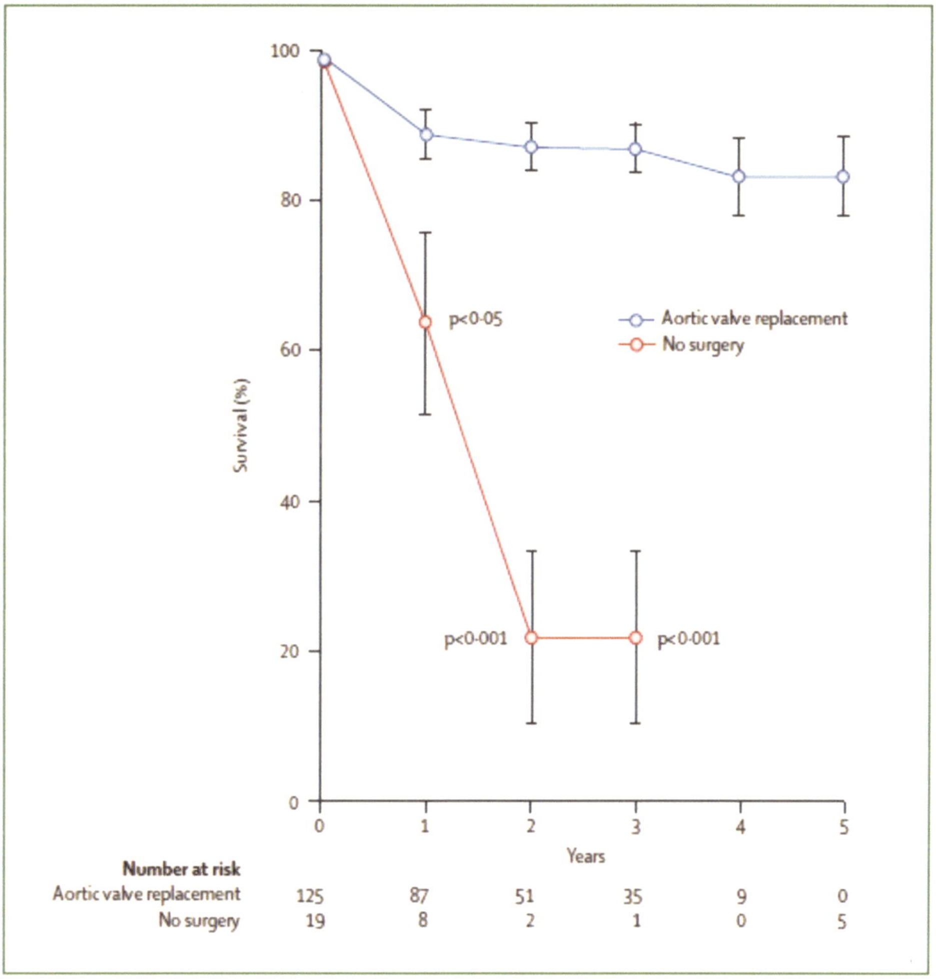

Reprinted with permission of the Lancet

Fig. 2. Mean survival of patients with symptoms of aortic stenosis. (Carabello et al. 2009)

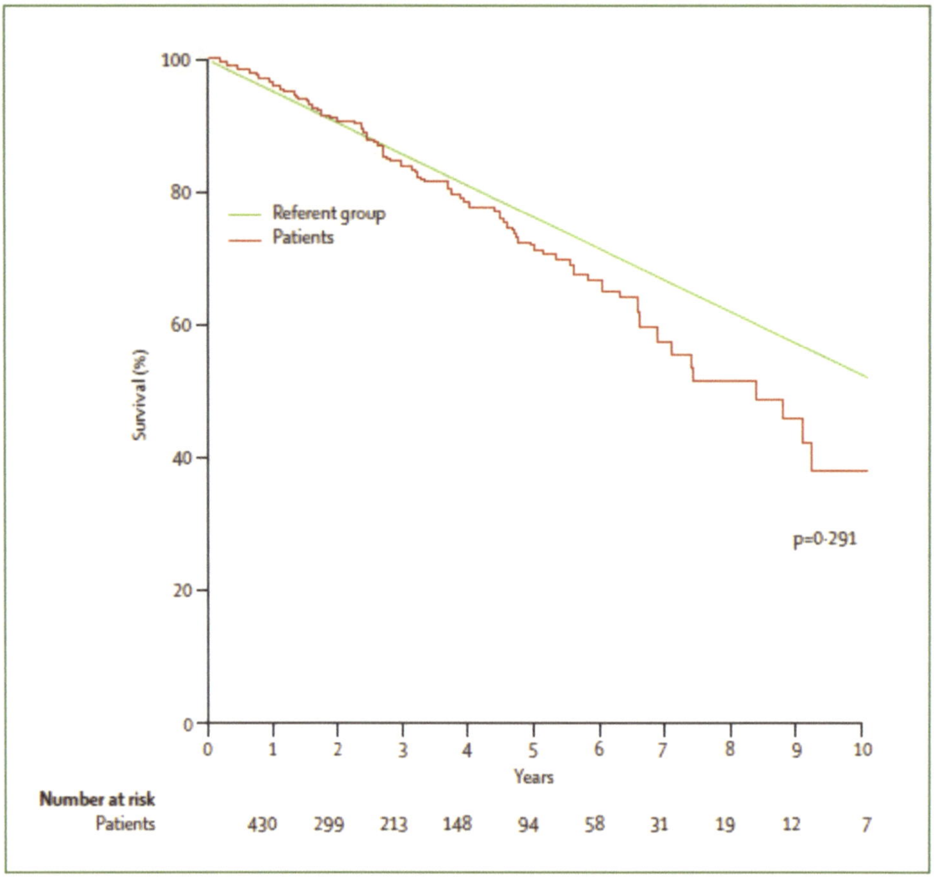

Reprinted with permission of the Lancet

Fig. 3. Survival of asymptomatic patients with severe aortic stenosis versus age-matched US population. (Carabello et al. 2009)

In asymptomatic patients with aortic stenosis survival is comparable to an aged matched population (figure 3). Therefore there is no point in treating asymptomatic patients. As soon as those patients develop symptoms, survival is markedly reduced (Grossi et al. 2008) However one of the problems are asymptomatic patients with severe stenosis and reduced ejection fraction at time of surgery. It is recommended to perform aortic valve replacement in patients with asymptomatic severe aortic stenosis and an ejection fraction <50 (class of recommendation I) however the level of evidence is only C. (Vahanian 2007 ESC Guidelines) According to the paper by Hannan E. and colleagues, as soon as the aortic valve is replaced in these patients risk adjusted survival returns to level that is not statistically different to the survival of people from the general population who are age and sex matched to this group. As with aortic regurgitation reduced ejection fraction emerges as one of the most significant risk factors of early and late mortality (Figure 4, Hannan et al. 2009).

Michaljevic and coworkers showed that among other risk factors like older age, greater degree of aortic stenosis, greater LV mass index, smaller standardized prosthesis-patient size, in addition LV dysfunction and advanced symptoms influence the long term survival of patients undergoing aortic valve replacement (Figure 5, Mihaljevic et al. 2008)

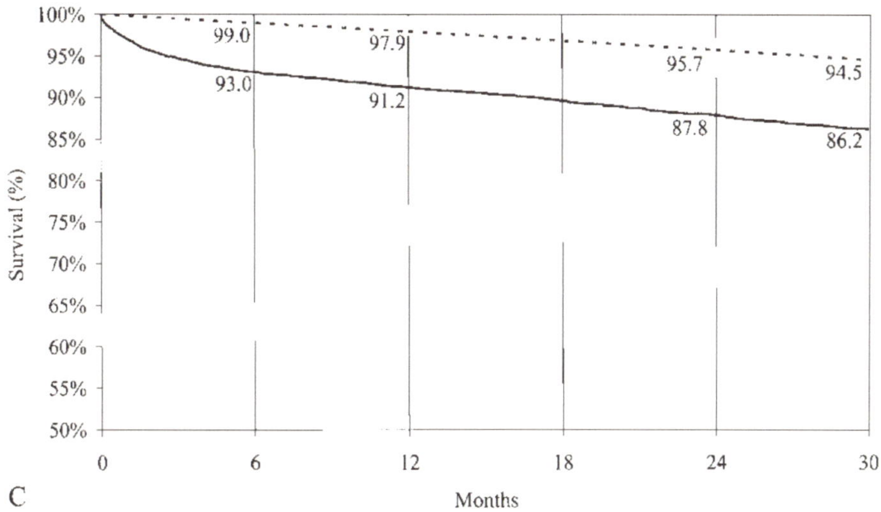

Reprinted with permission of the Journal of Thoracic and cardiovascular surgery

Fig. 4. Hannan and coworkers investigated the survival after aortic valve replacement with concomitant CABG according to cardiac riskfactors. The Dashed line is the survival of age- and sex-matched population. Solid and dash-dotted lines represent survival for aortic valve re- placement patients with and without concomi- tant coronary artery bypass grafting, respectively. (Hannan et al. 2009)

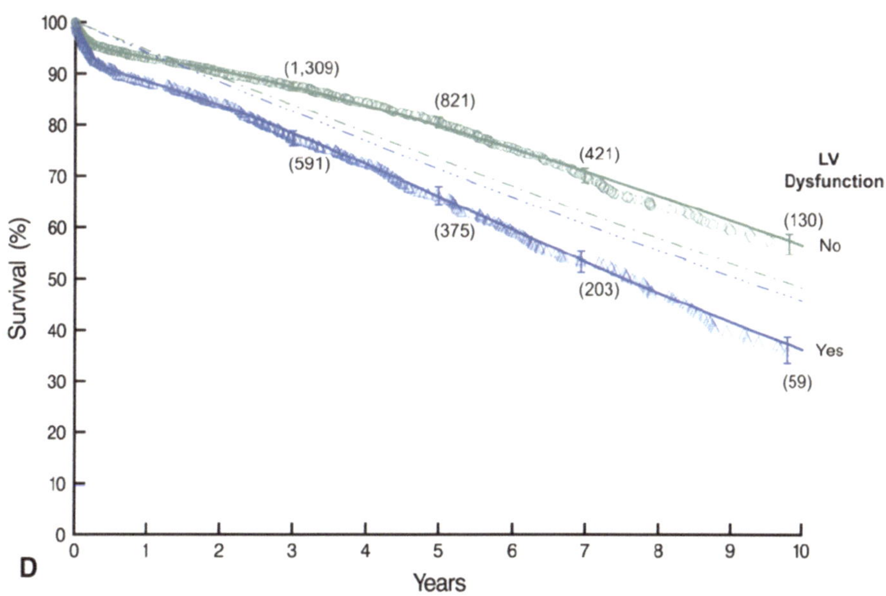

Reprinted with permission of the Journal of Thoracic and cardiovascular surgery

Fig. 5. Long term (> 1 year) survival of patients undergoing AVR with and without ventricular dysfunction (EF<40%) (Mihaljevic et al. 2008)

Since AS is a disease of elderly patients the outcome depends on comorbidities and concomitant surgical procedures (CABG). Onset of dyspnoea and other symptoms of heart failure presage the worst outlook for the patient with aortic stenosis. Whereas concentric hypertrophy helps to maintain systolic performance, increased wall thickness impairs diastolic function. The percentage of patients with low ejection fraction in the surgical population of AS ranges from 10-15%

As in aortic insufficiency, valve replacement for stenosis has become a routine procedure and again patients with reduced ejection fraction represent a challenge for the cardiac surgeon. Low ejection fraction has been identified as a significant risk factor for both reduced early and late mortality after AVR.

3.2.1 Low gradient low flow aortic stenosis

Low gradient low flow AS is defined as aortic stenosis with an effective aortic area <1cm2, LVEF <40% and a mean transaortic pressure gradient of < 30 mmHg. Assessment is usually performed by dobutamine stress testing. This is neccessary to confirm that the reduced effective orifice area is in fact severe rather than an effect of low flow on a mild or moderately stenosed valve (2) Contractile reserve on dobutamine stress testing is defined by an increase in the systolic velocity integral or stroke volume by at least 20% during dobutamine infusion. Aortic valve replacement is recommended by the AHA for patients with low gradient low flow aortic stenosis with contractile reserve (Class1: level of evidence C) (Monin, et al. 2003)

Especially patients without contractile reserve represent a high risk group (figure 6). Monin and colleagues showed that patients with contractile reserve have better prognosis than those without contractile reserve. Both groups of patients have much better life expectancies when the diseased valve is replaced in comparison to medical treatment only. (figure 6)

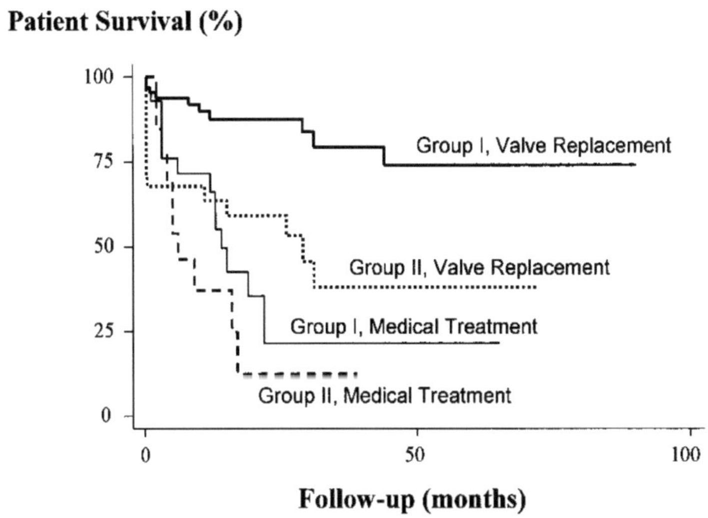

Reprint with permission of Circulation

Fig. 6. Monin et al. showed that patients without contractile reserve (group II) perform worse than those with contractile reserve (group I). Nevertheless for both groups valve replacement has much better results than medical treatment alone

A more recent paper by Clavel et. al. used a slightly different definition with an aortic valve area of <1.2 cm2 and <40% ejection fraction however a mean gradient of <40 mmHg. (Clavel, et al. 2008) This multicenter study showed that patients with low flow low gradient AS are a high risk population with an operative mortality of 18% and 3-year survival rates of only 57%.

In a best evidence topic of Subramanian et al. performed a meta analysis of the current literature on severe aortic stenosis but poor left ventricular function with no contractile reserve. To discuss whether it is ever worth contemplating aortic valve replacement in this setting. Out of the 251 papers screened for this analysis 14 presented the best evidence to answer this question.

The conclusion of the study was that patients with severe aortic stenosis and a contractile reserve of <20% improvement in stroke volume on dobutamine stress testing have a very poor prognosis of only 10-20% at two years. Heart transplant would offer the best chance of survival to those eligible but for those not eligible, a surgical option should not be discounted for selected patients. The American Heart Association guidelines state that prognosis is very poor for either medical or surgical treatment, but the European Society of Cardiology guidelines state that surgery can be performed in these patients but should take into account the clinical condition of the patient. The operative mortality is around 30% and the French Multicentre study on low gradient aortic stenosis has shown that if the patient survives there is likely to be an improvement in symptoms and ejection fraction. Thus, absence of contractile reserve on stress testing does not exclude myocardial recovery after surgery, although it is a strong predictor for operative mortality. (Subramanian et al; 2008)

4. Strategies for improved outcome

As stated above poor left ventricular function is a negative prognostic factor after aortic valve Replacement regardless the type of the aortic valve disease. Therefore it is important to find objective prognostic variables to identify patients who benefit the most from a surgical intervention and to exclude patients with an excessively high operative risk.

Several studies have reported various approaches to improve postoperative outcome in theses patients.

4.1 B-Type natriuretic peptide as a predictor of heart failure following aortic valve surgery

Biomarkers, especially pro-BNP have been associated with heart failure and poor ventricular function.

Pro-BNP might be an objective prognostic variable for outcome after surgical aortic valve replacement. (Nozohoor et al. 2009)

NT pro-BNP levels have been to be elevated in patients with aortic valve stenosis. And has already been suggested to monitor the progression of the disease non-invasively as well as to time surgery for aortic stenosis optimally. Further more pro-BNP correlates with endsystolic wallstress in patients with aortic stenosis.

At our department it has become standard of care to administer a 24 hour infusion course of levosimendan 3 days prior to surgery in patients with low EF and high proBNP levels, in order to precondition patients for surgery (data not yet published). In our experience pro-BNP decrease more than 50% on average due to this treatment.

Järvelä et al. investigated the impact of levosimendan in aortic valve surgery. A total of 24 patients were included in this study, 12 per arm however only with a moderate reduction in pump-function (treatment group 48%, control 54%). Levosimendan was started at induction of anaesthesia and continued over 24 hours. While induction of anesthesia led to reduction of EF in both groups, ejection fraction slowly recovered almost to preoperative levels in the control group. In contrast to that the ejection fraction of patients receiving levosimendan even improved in comparison to the preoperative levels. (Figure 7). (Järvelä et al. 2008)
Eventhough the preoperative ejection fraction was only moderately reduced. The application of levosimendan led to an improvement of EF. This seems rather promising especially when having in mind, that patients with severely reduced EF don not improve in ventricular function after aortic valve replacement without any concomitant treatment.

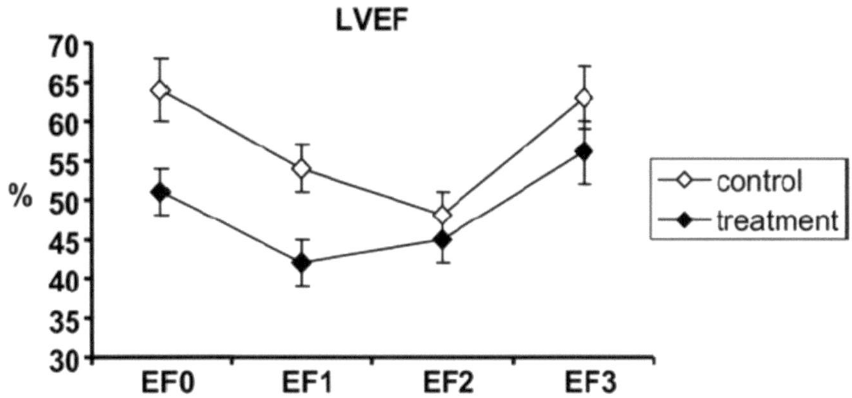

Reprinted with permission of Circulation

Fig. 7. Effects of levosimendan on cardiac performance and recovery in aortic valve surgery (Järvelä et al. 2008)

4.2 Statins

Statins have become a blockbuster drug primarily for artherosclerotic diseases, but they have pleotropic effects. This triggered the interest on potential beneficial effects of these drugs for other indications like aortic aneurysms and calcific valvular heart disease.
Considerations regarding statin-therapy for valvular heart diseases are on the one hand slower progression of calcification in patients with aortic stenosis and on the other hand there are studies showing that statin therapy improves the outcome after aortic valve replacement.
Hyperlipidemia has been suggested as a risk factor for stenosis of the aortic valve, but lipid lowering studies have had conflicting results. There are studies suggesting statin-therapy for every patient with aortic stenosis. (Fedoruk et al. 2008) However Rossebo et al. showed that statin-therapy did not reduce the composite outcome of combined aortic-valve events and ischemic events in AS patients. Statin-therapy resulted in reduced incidence of ischemic cardiovascular events but not events related to aortic-valve stenosis. (Rossebo et al. 2008) Nevertheless the overall outcome of patients with statin-therapy in this study was superior to those without statin-therapy, this might be due to the fact that a high percentage of AS patient have concomitant ischemic cardiovascular diseases. Therefore we would suggest statin-therapy as standard of care for every patient with aortic stenosis.

4.3 Prosthesis patient mismatch

Prosthesis patient mismatch (PPM) occurs when the effective orifice area (EOA) of a prosthetic valve is too small relative to the patient's body size. It is graded as moderate if the ratio of effective orifice area (EOA) in cm square to body surface area in m square is <0.85 cm2/m2 and severe if it is <0.65 cm2/m2. PPM has been a controversial topic ever since valves have been implanted. (Mascherbauer, 2008; Yap CH 2007))
Urso et al. concluded in their best evidence topic that there is no strong evidence that moderate patient-prosthesis mismatch (PPM) (indexed IEOA0.85 and >0.65 cm^2/m^2) is an independent risk factor for 30-day or mid-term overall mortality for adult patients undergoing AVR. An exception could be represented by patients with poor ejection fraction, a condition that can make moderate mismatch a predictor of overall mortality after AVR. On the other hand, severe mismatch is a predictor of overall 30-day or mid-term mortality for patients undergoing AVR independently from the presence of poor ejection fraction. In conclusion, our review suggests that the condition of severe PPM should be always avoided, while the presence of moderate mismatch could be tolerated in patients with normal ejection fraction without any impact on overall survival. (Urso 2009)
Ruel an colleagues concluded that prosthesis–patient mismatch at an indexed effective orifice area of 0.85 cm^2/m^2 or less after aortic valve replacement primarily affects patients with impaired preoperative left ventricular function and results in decreased survival, lower freedom from heart failure, and incomplete left ventricular mass regression. Patients with impaired left ventricular function represent a critical population in whom prosthesis–patient mismatch should be avoided at the time of aortic valve replacement. (Ruel 2005)
There are various ways for reduction of PPM including aortic root enlargement, use of a supra-annular or high performance prosthesis, and the use of a stentless bioprosthesis, aortic homograft, or pulmonary autograft. (Hashimoto 2006)

4.4 The awake patient in cardiac surgeons

Since heart valve surgery in high-risk patients is associated with considerable morbidity and mortality epidural anaesthesia without mechanical ventilation has been proposed to reduce invasiveness. Bottio et al. showed that heart valve surgery utilising cardiopulmonary bypass is feasible and can be safe using epidural anaesthesia. By maintaining autonomic ventilation, a low mid-term morbidity and mortality was observed in patients in whom there was an unacceptable operative risk. (Bottio 2007)
Nevertheless we feel that this is only a niche for cardiac surgical adventurers and only an important step in as far that proof of concept has been demonstrated, however not a method we would recommend to any of our patients.

4.5 Future perspectives

4.5.1 Transcatheter aortic valve implantation (TAVI)

A substantial number of AS patients have reduced ejection fraction and severe coexisting conditions that preclude surgery. Recently transcatheter aortic-valve implantation (TAVI) has emerged as less invasive and saver alternative for those patients. TAVI can be performed either by a retrograde approach, in which a catheter is inserted through the common femoral artery, or by an antegrade, transapical approach, in which a catheter is inserted through the apex of the left ventricle with the use of an anterolateral thoracotomy. (Lazar, 2010) Initially single-center, nonrandomized trials have shown the feasibility of TAVI in patients who are not suitable candidates for surgical replacement of the aortic valve. (Himbert et al. 2009, Webb et al. 2009)

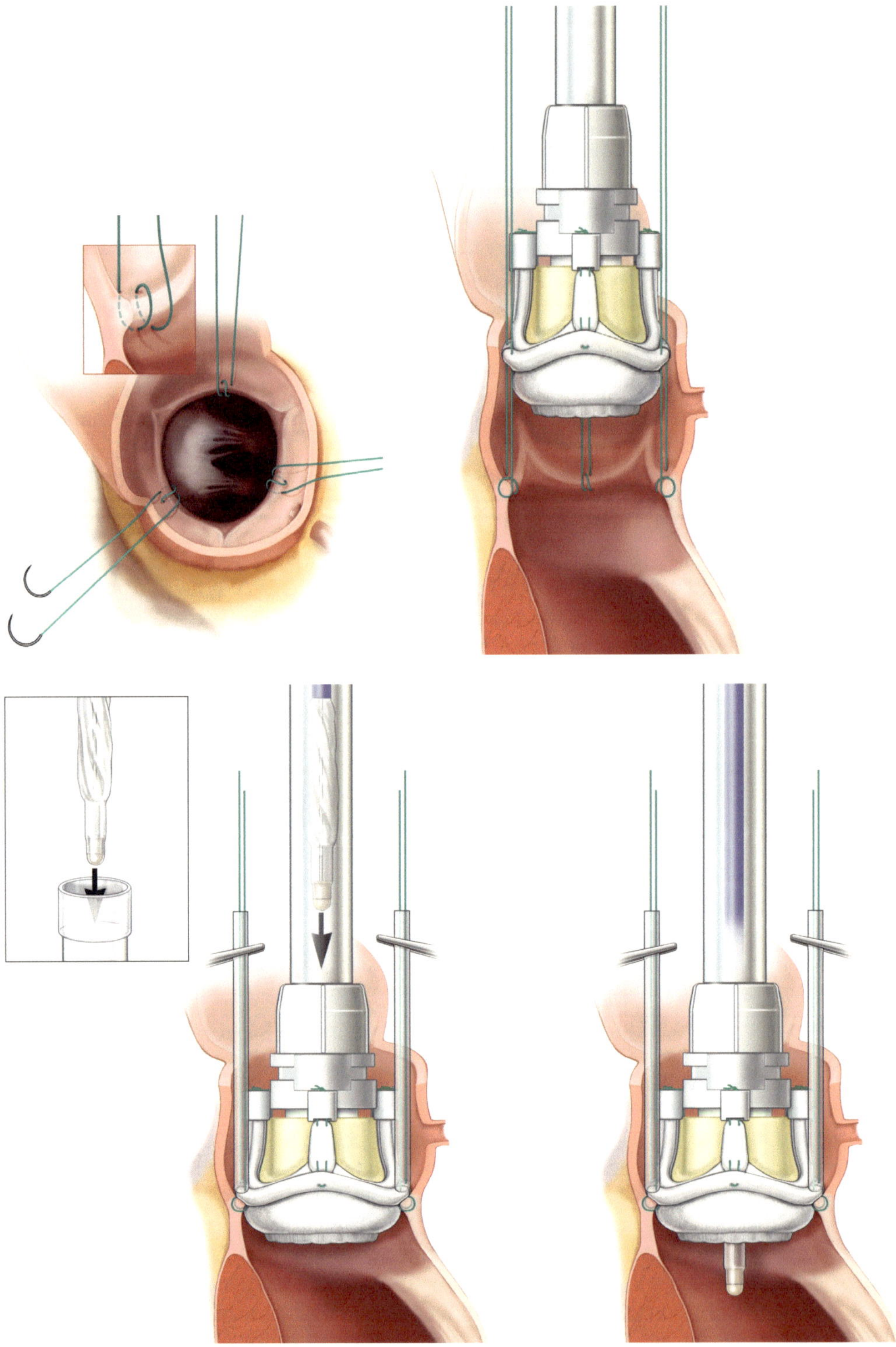

Fig. 8. Implantation of an Aortic Quick Connect Bioprosthetic valve (Edwards Lifesciences)

In 2011 Leon and his coauthors report the results of the placement of Aortic Transcatheter Valves (PARTNER) trial, a prospective, randomized, multicenter trial to determine the optimal method of treating patients with critical aortic stenosis who are considered not to be suitable candidates for surgery. This revealed promising results showed a 20% reduction in mortality in comparison to medical treatment alone in patients with significant aortic stenosis not suitable for surgery. Furthermore the trial revealed that TAVI can achieve similar results as surgery in high risk patients. (Leon 2011)

4.5.2 Sutureless aortic valve bio prostheses

Another step towards reduction of operative time and thus lowering the burden of surgical intervention for the patient is the invention of sutureless aortic bioprosthesis. Currently there are 3 different valve types on the market: Perceval (Sorin), Enable (ATS, Medical) and Aortic Quick Connect (Edwards Lifesciences). They require only three stitches at the nadirs of the annulus to navigate the valve into the right plane prior to deployment of the nitinol stent. Initial clinical experience with these valves was satisfactory revealing promising results. In case of the Perceval valve the study investigators were able to implant a well-functioning sutureless stent-mounted valve in the aortic position in less than 20 minutes of aortic crossclamping. This was associated with excellent early clinical and hemodynamic outcome in high-risk patients. (Flameng et al. 2011). The sutureless valve implantation technique is also feasible and safe with the ATS 3f Enable Bioprosthesis. Valve implantation resulted in excellent hemodynamics and significant clinical improvement. Overall, these data confirm the safety and clinical utility of the Enable(®) Bioprosthesis for aortic valve replacement. (Martens et al., 2011) Data for the most recent sutureless valve to appear on the market, the Aortic Quick Connect, are also excellent. (Kocher et al., 2011)
The quick implantation procedure shortens the operative time, in particular the cross clamp time. Which has been shown to be a variable for poor outcome after aortic valve replacement.

5. Conclusion

Aortic-valve replacement or transcatheter aortic valve implantation are the most effective treatments to alleviate symptoms and improve survival in patients with critical aortic stenosis. Aortic valve disease especially stenosis is on the rise as it is primarily a disease of the elderly. Patients with decreased EF are clearly a high risk population, demonstrating both increased morbidity and mortality after aortic valve surgery. However in this chapter we could show that the cardiovascular medical community has so far responded to this challenge by devising new strategies to cope with the problem of an ever sicker patient population. A substantial number of these patients with coexisting conditions that used to preclude surgery are nowadays treated by less invasive approaches like TAVI. Furthermore there is progress on many fronts: Serum markers like BNP will help to time the intervention, levosimendan is already employed to precondition the patients prior to surgical interventions. New technologies like sutureless valves and TAVI significantly reduced the burden of the intervention. Apart from these new inventions one of the most important strategies to improve the outcome of patients undergoing aortic valve replacement with and without impaired left ventricular function is meticulous surgical performance.

Patients with an aortic valve pathology and a severely reduced ejection fraction constitute a significant challenge. However, in light of the recent inventions, innovations, new technologies and strategies for this patient cohort we are positive that the scientist and medical professionals in the field of cardiovascular medicine will be able to tackle this problem.

6. References

Ali A. et al. 2006 Are Stentless Valves Superior to Modern Stented Valves? A prospective Randomized trial; Circulation. 2006; 114[suppl I]:I-535-I-540.

Bonow R. et al. 2006. ACC/AHA 2006 Guidelines for the Management of Patients with Valvular Heart disease; Journal of the American College of Cardiology Vol. 48, No. 3, 2006

Bottio T. et al. 2007. Heart valve surgery in a very high-risk population: a preliminary experience in awake patients. J Heart Valve Dis. 2007 Mar; 16(2):187-94.

Carabello B., Walter P. 2009 Aortic Stenosis; Lancet 2009; 373:956-66

Chaliki HP, et al. 2002 Outcomes after aortic valve replacement in patients with severe aortic regurgitation and markedly reduced left ventricular function. Circulation. 2002 Nov 19; 106(21):2687-93.

Clavel MA et al. 2008 Predictors of Outcome in Low-Flow, Low Gradient Aortic Stenosis Results of the Multicenter TOPAS Study; Circulation 2008; 118 [Suppl I]:S234-S242

Fedoruk L, et al. 2008 Statin Therapy Improves Outcomes After Valvular Heart Surgery; Ann Thorac Surg 2008; 85:1521-1526

Flameng W et al. 2011 Effect of sutureless implantation of the Perceval S aortic valve bioprosthesis on intraoperative and early postoperative outcomes. J Thorac Cardiovasc Surg. 2011 Apr 5

Grossi E, et al. 2008 High-Risk Aortic Valve Replacement: Are the Outcomes as Bad as Predicted? Ann Thorac Surg 2008; 85:102-7

Hannan E, et al. 2009 Aortic Valve Replacement for Patients with severe aortic stenosis: Risk Factors and Their Impact on 30-Month Mortality; Ann Thorac Surg 2009; 87:1741-50

Hashimoto K et al. 2006 Patient-Prosthesis Mismatch: The Japanese Experience; Ann Thorac Cardiovasc Surg. 2006 Jun; 12 (3):159-65

Himbert D et al. 2009 Results of transfemoral or transapical aortic valve implantation following a uniform assessment in high-risk patients with aortic stenosis. J Am Coll Cardiol 2009; 54:303

Järvelä K et al. 2008 Levosimendan in aortic valve surgery: cardiac performance and recovery. J Cardiothorac Vasc Anesth. 2008 Oct; 22(5):693-8.

Kocher A et al. 2011 Technical consideration regarding the implantation of a novel sutureless valve, 2011 ISMIC meeting

Lazar, L et al. Transcatheter Aortic Valves — Where Do We Go from Here? N Engl J Med 2010; 363:1667-1668 October 21, 2010

Leon M.B., et al. 2010. Transcatheter aortic-valve implantation for aortic stenosis in patients who cannot undergo surgery. N Engl J Med 2010;363:1597-1607

Martens S. et al. 2011. Clinical experience with the ATS 3f Enable(®) Sutureless Bioprosthesis. Eur J Cardiothorac Surg. 2011 Feb 20

Mascherbauer J. et al. 2008. Moderate patient-prosthesis mismatch after valve replacement for severe aortic stenosis has no impact on short- and long-term mortality. Heart 2008; 94:1639–1645.

Mihaljevic T. et al. 2008. Survival after valve replacement for aortic stenosis: Implications for decision making; J Thorac Cardiovasc Surg. 2008 Jun; 135(6):1270-8

Monin J.L. et al. 2003. Low-gradient aortic stenosis: operative risk stratification and predictors for long-term outcome: a multicenter study using dobutamine stress hemodynamics. Circulation. 2003 Jul 22; 108(3):319-24.

Nozohoor S. et al. 2009. B-type natriuretic peptide as a predictor of postoperative heart failure after aortic valve replacement. J Cardiothorac Vasc Anesth. 2009 Apr; 23(2):161-5.

Petracca F, et al. 2009. Usefulness of NT-proBNP in the assessment of patients with aortic or mitral regurgitation. J Cardiovasc Med (Hagerstown). 2009 Dec; 10(12):928-32

Rossebø AB, et al. 2008. Intensive lipid lowering with simvastatin and ezetimibe in aortic stenosis. N Engl J Med. 2008 Sep 25; 359(13):1343-56.

Ruel M, et al. 2006. Prosthesis-patient mismatch after aortic valve replacement predominantly affects patients with preexisting left ventricular dysfunction: effect on survival, freedom from heart failure, and left ventricular mass regression. J Thorac Cardiovasc Surg 2006; 131:1036–1044.

Scognamiglio R., et al. 2005. Long-term survival and functional results after aortic valve replacement in asymptomatic patients with chronic severe aortic regurgitation and left ventricular dysfunction. J Am Coll Cardiol. 2005 Apr 5; 45(7):1025-30.

Sharony R et al. 2003. Aortic valve replacement in patients with impaired ventricular function; Ann Thorac Surg 2003 Jun; 75(6):1808-14

Sionis A et al. 2010. Severe aortic regurgitation and reduced left ventricular ejection fraction: outcomes after isolated aortic valve replacement and combined surgery; J Heart Lung Transplant. 2010 Apr; 29(4):445-8

Subramanian H. et al. 2008. Is it ever worth contemplating an aortic valve replacement on patients with low gradient severe aortic stenosis but poor left ventricular function with no contractile reserve? Interactive Cardiovascular and Thoracic Surgery 7 (2008) 301-305

Talwar S, et al. 2001. Plasma N-terminal pro BNP and cardiotrophin-1 are elevated in aortic stenosis. Eur J Heart Fail. 2001 Jan; 3(1):15-9.

Urso S, et al. 2009. Patient-prosthesis mismatch in elderly patients undergoing aortic valve replacement: impact on quality of life and survival. J Heart Valve Dis. 2009 May; 18(3):248-55.

Vahanian A, et al. 2007. Task Force on the Management of Valvular Hearth Disease of the European Society of Cardiology; ESC Committee for Practice Guidelines. Guidelines on the management of valvular heart disease: the Task Force on the Management of Valvular Heart Disease of the European Society of Cardiology. Eur Heart J. 2007 Jan; 28(2):230-68.

Webb et al. 2009. Transcatheter aortic valve implantation: impact on clinical and valve-related outcomes. Circulation 2009; 119:3009-3016
Yap CH, et al. 2007. Prosthesis-patient mismatch is associated with higher operative mortality following aortic valve replacement. Heart Lung Circ 2007; 16:260–264.

10

Relationship Between Aortic Valve Replacement and Old Age

Jean-Michel Maillet[1] and Dominique Somme[2]
[1]*Centre Cardiologique du Nord, Saint-Denis,*
[2]*Hopital Européen Georges Pompidou, Paris,*
France

1. Introduction

Many factors can explain the most important increase of human life expectancy during the XXth century: better socioeconomic conditions, improved working conditions, development of preventive measures, less alcoholism, appearance of antibiotics, advances in medical practices, etc… At present, the fastest growing age group in western countries is people >80 years old; they will represent 9–10.5% of the population in those countries in 2050. Today, life expectancy at 80 years is, on average, 10 years for a woman and 7 years for a man in western countries (Health at a glance OECD indicators). This population is at high risk of cardiovascular disease (Assey, 1993). More specifically, aortic stenosis (AS) is the most frequent valvulopathy in adults ≥ 75 years old, being present in as many 4.6% (Nkomo et al., 2006). Progress made in anesthesia, surgery and intensive care explain why doctors, surgeons and cardiologists are less-and-less reluctant to propose aortic valve replacement (AVR) for older-and-older patients.
However, for this very specific population, many questions remain to be answered before such surgery can be undertaken:

- What is the spontaneous evolution of the disease?
- Is there a therapeutic option other than surgery?
- What are the postoperative results in terms of morbidity and mortality?
- Will surgical treatment relieve the symptoms and improve the quality of life (QOL) at intermediate and long term?
- What are the complications and constraints associated with the prosthesis?
- Are those results universal?
- Will my patient become frail or disabled after surgery?

2. Rationale for proposing surgical AVR for the elderly

2.1 Natural history of severe AS

Above all, the natural history of severe aortic stenosis (SAS) has a dismal prognosis. Once symptoms appear, life expectancy is 5 years for angina, 3 years for dyspnea or syncope and 2 years for cardiac failure (Chizner et al., 1980; Ross and Braunwald, 1968). Even though those results were obtained from old studies conducted during the 1960s and 1970s (Chizner et al., 1980; Horstkotte & Loogen, 1988; Ross & Braunwald, 1968), concerned young patients

(20 and 60 years old) and included small numbers of patients (15–55), more recent publications continue to emphasize the very poor natural history of SAS (Schueler et al., 2010; Varadarajan et al., 2006).

2.2 Failure of medical treatment

The introduction of medical treatments, such as beta-blockers, statins and angiotensin-converting–enzyme inhibitors, has not specifically modified SAS prognosis (Schueler et al., 2010). Recently, Schueler et al. prospectively compared the prognoses of medically treated elderly SAS patients (mean age: 86 years) at high surgical risk to age- and sex-matched patients with non-severe AS; at 2 years, 41.8% and 59.8%, respectively, were survivors. Independent factors associated with death of SAS patients were Society Thoracic Surgeons predicted risk of mortality (STS-PROM) score (Shroyer et al., 2003), pulmonary arterial pressure >30 mm Hg, creatinine and diabetes (Schueler et al., 2010). Scharwz et al. (1982) compared the prognoses of 135 SAS patients treated surgically with AVR versus 19 denied surgery: at 3 years, 87% of the surgical group were alive vs 21% of medically treated group ($p<0.001$). Varadarajan et al. (2006) showed that conservatively treated SAS patients had poorer outcomes, with respective 1-, 5- and 10-year survival rates of 62%, 32% and 18%.

2.3 Failure of balloon aortic valvuloplasty

Although balloon aortic valvuloplasty (BAV) acutely increases the aortic valve area and attenuates symptoms, neither change significantly improved prognosis, with high mortality and complication rates (NHLBI Balloon Valvuloplasty Registry participants, 1991). Moreover, its restenosis rate at 1 year was >80% (Eltchaninoff et al., 1995). Current indications for BAV are very limited, with valvuloplasty primarily considered a bridge to surgery or transvalvular aortic implantation (TAVI) in hemodynamically unstable patients (Vahanian and Otto, 2010).

Thus, for the time being, surgical AVR remains the treatment of choice for SAS. Notably, the international recommendations do not provide any specific guidelines concerning age (Bonow et al., 2006; Vahanian et al., 2007).

2.4 Age, aging and prognosis

Age is a known independent risk factor for in-hospital mortality after admission to the intensive care unit after cardiac surgery (Knaus et al., 1993; Roques & Nashef, 2003). However, although disease severity assessed with APACHE III can explain 80% of in-hospital deaths, age can explain only 13% (Knaus et al., 1993). The mechanism of excess death independent of elderly patients' disease severity has not yet been clearly elucidated. Setting aside the excess mortality linked to less intensive treatment of the elderly, it could be intrinsic, because of the greater vulnerability to disease, or extrinsic, attributable to a poorer response or even poorer tolerance of the therapeutic modalities used in intensive care. For both hypotheses, physiological particularities specific to the older patient are implicated. From a global perspective, Bouchon (1984) proposed a model in which morbidity of elderly patients resulted from 3 components (Figure 1).

Clinically detectable morbidity is usually the sum of organ aging, possible organic deterioration resulting from more-or-less quiescent chronic disease and deterioration appended by acute disease. We cannot detail here all those deteriorations organ-by-organ (Somme et al., 2009), but retain the broad lines that transcend organ specificities. First, the role of aging itself on organ decline is difficult to demonstrate. Indeed, a study on elderly individuals in very good health (old senior athletes) often had physiological cardiovascular system performances quite close to those of younger athletes but that is not the case for their osteoarticular system! Thus, the descriptions of so-called changes 'linked' to aging (i.e., frequent or typical of the old-old), be they histological or physiological performances, are the means of populations heterogeneous in terms of life style, exposures to personal or environmental risk factors and pathologies. When an attempt was made to show the same 'age-linked' changes exclusively in healthy aged or physically fit subjects, none was found (Somme et al., 2009). Hence, defining the slope of line 1 for individuals is difficult (Fig. 1), as it depends, organ by organ, on personal and environmental factors. Nevertheless, it could be useful to predict vulnerability, like an old person's response to treatment or knowing his/her level of physical activity, which is probably a better marker of physiological cardiovascular aging than chronological age. It is widely accepted that, for the young subject, cardiac function is the main parameter conditioning the maximal stress level, whereas for the elderly subject, it seems more often to be limited by respiratory function (Chan & Welsch, 1998). Finally, physiological aging can be represented as the functional state of adaptation mechanisms (or reserves) that are overwhelmed during stress or effort. These physiological particularities render the elderly more susceptible to acute diseases. This frailty should not limit access to intensive care for old patients, but should rather plead in favor of their adapted and early management.

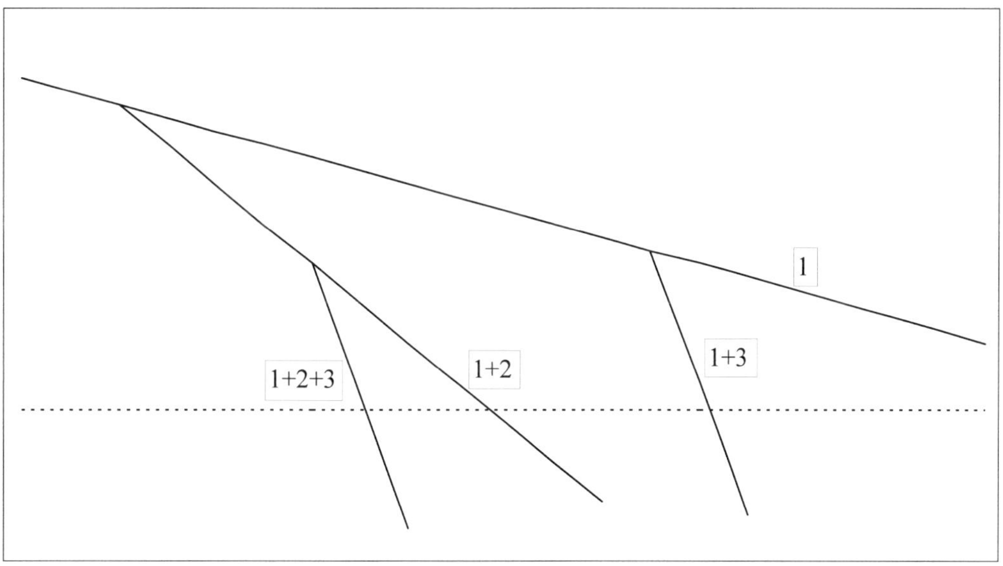

Fig. 1. Organ decline (regardless of the organ) due to aging is represented by slope 1. Two types of events are able to shift this organ under the threshold (dashed line) of organ insufficiency: a chronic (according to slope 2) or acute disease (the steepest slope 3). Adapted from 1+2+3: how to be effective in geriatrics? (Bouchon, 1984)

2.5 Threshold of old age

In practice, old age is defined 2 ways: that set by a chronological age and a dynamic approach taking into consideration the evolution of the health of the population.

The fixed chronological age definition (around 65–75 years for young-old; between 75–80 and 85–90 for the old-old, and >85–90 for the oldest-old) is the most extensively used in the medical literature. It has the advantages of enabling comparisons between published historical data and not encouraging interpretation. However, it does not account for the evolution of life expectancy at 60 years and, even less, its evolution without handicap(s). Indeed, life expectancy for a 60-year-old man in France increased from 15.4 to 21.7 years between 1950 and 2010. This prolongation obviously has an impact on the premonitory usefulness of aggressive therapies, like cardiac surgery after 60 years during that interval.
A dynamic definition of the old-age threshold can take those aspects into consideration. Several can be proposed but one seems readily accessible: survival at life expectancy at birth (Table 1). If we accept this definition, the percentage of 'aged' individuals (so defined) in France did not increase between 1950 (~11%) and 2010 (~9%), because life expectancy rose more quickly than the number of aged persons.

	1950	2010
Life expectancy at birth for males, years	63.4	78.1
Life expectancy at birth for females, years	69.2	84.8
Persons >65 years old in the population	11.4%	
Persons >75 years old in the population		9%

Table 1. 1950 to 2010: Evolution of life expectancy in France and the aged population

Age has always been identified as a major risk factor for mortality after cardiac surgery (Roques et al., 2003; Shroyer et al., 2003), but the mean age of operated patients is rising. Indeed, surgery on octogenarians is performed daily in western countries. Are there some limits for age and cardiac surgery? Florath et al. (2010) identified >84 years as an important independent risk factor for mortality 6 months after AVR for octogenarians. However, some publications indicated that surgeons seem less-and-less reluctant to operate on nonagenarians (Edwards et al., 2003; Praschker et al., 2006). During the 1980s, the age limit for cardiac surgery was progressively increased >80 years without drama considering outcomes (Edmunds et al., 1988). Should the story repeat itself for nonagenarians or even centenarians in the future?

2.6 Postoperative outcomes of surgical AVR for octogenarians

Surgical AVR results for octogenarians are acceptable and compare favorably with those of younger patients (Alexander et al., 2000; Thourani et al., 2008). Table 2 summarizes the early postoperative mortality (≤30 days) rate after AVR for octogenarians.
De facto, studies during the 1990s and 2000s included more patients than during 1980s. For example, in the UK, between 1996 and 2003, the rate of surgery performed on octogenarians increased 2-fold, from 4.1% to 9.8% (Stoica et al., 2006). For the studies with >200 patients, early in-hospital mortality (≤30 days) ranged from 6.6% to 10.1%. Very few studies included only patients with isolated AVR (Table 2). Most studies included AVR with and without coronary-artery bypass graft (CABG). Postoperative mortality rates were higher when CABG was combined with AVR compared to AVR alone.
However, the postoperative morbidity rate was very high for octogenarians after AVR (Melby et al., 2007; Thourani et al., 2008) and more than two-thirds of octogenarians will develop ≥1 postoperative complications (Collart et al., 2005; Kolh et al., 2007; Maillet et al.,

2009). Descriptions of the complications, their definitions, their characteristics and rates varied widely from one study to another. The most frequent complications are transfusion (48.8-81.4%), new onset supraventricular arrhythmia (31.2-45.2%), low cardiac output (16.7-35.7%), prolonged mechanical ventilation (≥24 hours) (22-26%), reoperation for bleeding (6-9%), permanent strokes (3-6%), acute renal failure (4.6-12%), infections (2.4-5.6%) and heart block requiring a pacemaker (2.3-5%) (Collart et al., 2005; Kohl et al., 2007; Maillet et al., 2009; Melby et al. 2007; Sundt et al., 2000; Thourani et al., 2008).

First Author	Year	N	Study period	I AVR	Mean age, yr	Overall operative mortality	Operative mortality	
							I AVR	AVR+CABG
Edmunds	1988	50	1976-1987	66%	81	NR	30%	23.5%
Levinson	1989	64	1974-1987	50%	82	9.4%	3.2%	16.1%
Bashour	1990	24	1983-1986	50%	83	12.5%	8.3%	16.6%
Culliford	1991	71	1976-1988	50%	82	12.7	5.7%	19.4%
Freeman	1991	87	1982-1986	50%	82	15.7%	9.6%	17.9%
Olsson	1992	44	1981-1989	100%	82	14%	14%	
Elayda	1993	152	1975-1991	45%	83	17.5%	5.2%	27.7%
Tsai	1994	132	1982-1992	42%	83	4.5%	1.8%	6.6%
Asimakopoulos	1997	1100	1986-1995	100%	82	6.6%	6.6%	
Sundt	2000	133	1993-1998	33.1%	84	11%	NR	NR
Sjögren	2004	117	1990-1993	NR	82	3.4%	NR	NR
Collart	2005	215	1993-2003	74%	83	8.8%	NR	NR
Chiappini	2004	115	1992-2003	62.1%	82	8.5%	NR	NR
Langanay	2004	771	1978-2003	85.2%	83	10.1%	NR	NR
Langanay	2006	442	2000-2004	77.8%	83	7.5%	NR	NR
Stoica	2006	706	1996-2003	27.2%	83	9.8%	9.4%	9.7%
Melby	2007	245	1993-2005	57%	84	9%	10%	NR
Kolh	2007	220	1992-2004	76%	83	13%	9%	24%
Huber	2007	136	1999-2003	25%	82	4.4%	NR	NR
Thourani	2008	88	1996-2006	100%	83	5.7%	5.7%	
Leonteyv	2009	282	1995-2006	100%	82	9.2%	9.2%	
Maillet	2009	84	1998-2003	49%	84	16.7%	10.2%	25.7%
Florath	2010	493	1996-2006	51%	83	8.4%	7.6%	9.5%
Folkmann	2010	154	2005-2007	52%	83	7.8%	NR	NR

AVR = aortic valve replacement; I AVR = isolated AVR;
CABG = coronary artery bypass graft; NR = not reported.

Table 2. Postoperative mortality rates after AVR with/without CABG for octogenarians between 1976 and 2010

2.7 Intermediate-term AVR results

At intermediate term, all studies documented impressive symptom regression, with 73.2-92.5% of the survivors being in New York Heart Association (NYHA) classification I or II (Collart et al., 2005; Kolh et al., 2007; Maillet et al., 2009,). The mean NYHA classification of survivors fell from 3.1 to 1.7 ($p<0.001$) (Sundt et al., 2000). Lastly, 91% of survivors were angina-free (Kolh et al., 2007).

Concerning the intermediate-term prognosis, crude results were good (Table 3), particularly compared with the natural course of SAS (Schwarz et al., 1982). At 5 years, survival ranged from 52% (Florath et al., 2010) to 82% (Stoica et al., 2006) for populations whose mean age at surgery was 83 years. Some authors reported a 30% 10-year survival rate with a Kaplan–Meier median-survival estimate of 7.4 years (Thourani et al., 2008). Many studies also showed that, compared to an age- and sex-matched population, prognoses were comparable in different western countries: France (Maillet et al., 2009) and Sweden (Sjögren & Thulin, 2004). Stoica et al. (2006) found that the standardized mortality ratio (observed postAVR mortality/observed mortality for matched population) was 45.6% in favor of the surgical population in the UK, with 5-year survival rates of 82.1% for the surgical group versus 55.9% for a general population with the same age–sex distribution ($p<0.001$). The most common causes of late death were dominated by malignancy (20.5%), non-valve related cardiac failure (18.5%), valve-related stroke (18%) and pneumonia (11%) in a cohort of 1100 elderly patients included in the UK Heart Valve Registry. It must be kept in mind that one-third of the patients with malignancy died within 18 months after cardiac surgery. That observation emphasizes the improved preoperative cancer screening of elderly patients before AVR (Asimakopoulos et al., 1997).

First Author	Year	N	Study period	I AVR	Age at surgery	Survival at 1 year	3 years	5 years	8 years
Elayda	1993	171	1975-1991	45%	83	90.8%	84.2%	76%	
Tsai	1994	132	1982-1992	42%	83	82%		62%	
Asimakopoulos	1997	1100	1986-1995	100%	82	89%		69%	45.8%
Sundt	2000	133	1993-1998	33.1%	84	80%		55%	
Chiappini	2004	115	1992-2003	62.1%	82	86.4%		69.4%	
Sjögren	2004	117	1990-1993	NR	82	92.3%		65%	
Collart	2005	215	1993-2003	74%	83	84%		56%	
Stoica	2006	706	1996-2003	27.2%	83	83.7%		82.1%	
Huber	2007	136	1999-2003	25%	82	94%	94%	75%	
Kolh	2007	220	1992-2004	76%	83	85.5%	80.8%	73.2%	
Melby	2007	245	1993-2005	57%	84	82%	70%	56%	
Thourani	2008	88	1996-2006	100%	83	87%	68.2%	61%	
Leontyev	2009	282	1995-2006	100%	83	81%	71%	57%	
Florath	2010	493	1996-2006	51%	NR	82%		52%	30%

AVR = aortic valve replacement; I AVR = isolated AVR; NR = not reported

Table 3. Intermediate-term AVR outcomes of octogenarians

2.8 Impact of AVR on QOL among octogenarians

Improving QOL is one of the most important aims of AVR especially for octogenarians. Authors of retrospective studies concluded that QOL was good after AVR at intermediate term but, in many studies, preoperative QOL had not been evaluated (Maillet et al., 2009; Sundt et al., 2000). Using the medical outcomes study Short Form-36 (SF-36), Sundt et al. (2000) showed that the QOL of a surgical population with a mean age of 84 years was comparable to that predicted for the general population >75 years old. Olsson et al. (1996), prospectively compared QOL evolution for 2 groups of patients referred for isolated AVR; 30 octogenarians vs 30 patients 65–75 years old. At 1-year postAVR, octogenarians, despite their more compromised preoperative status, had markedly regressed symptoms, and their physical abilities and general well-being were of a similar magnitude to those of the younger patients. Those improvements appeared as of 3 months. With mean follow-up of 8.3±1.9 years, Sjögren & Thulin (2004) found long-term postoperative QOL to be comparable to that of an age-matched population. In addition, Huber et al. (2007) showed that 97% of the survivors lived in their own homes. Finally, 81% had no or few self-perceived restrictions in their daily activities (Kohl et al., 2007), 93% felt much better after the operation and 81% of octogenarians had few disabilities in daily activities (Huber et al., 2007). Also, QOL was not affected by the constraints entailed by treatment(s) associated with the type of prosthesis. Indeed, after postoperative month 3, >90% who had received a bioprosthesis were in sinus rhythm and were taking only low-dose aspirin. Vicchio et al. (2008) compared the QOL of 62 octogenarians with bioprosthetic valves vs 98 with mechanical valves during a mean follow-up of 3.4 ± 2.8 years and found that the prosthesis type had no impact on their QOL.

2.9 Limitations of those studies

However, all those studies had some limitations. Indeed, all of them were retrospective except for Olsson et al. (1996). Only those by Asimakopoulos et al. (1997) and Stoica et al. (2007), representing UK registry results, were multicenter investigations. Very few studies specifically and exclusively evaluated the outcomes of isolated AVR for SAS (Asimakopoulos et al., 1997; Leonteyv et al., 2009; Thourani et al., 2008). Some studies mixed AVR with CABG or other operations, whereas others mixed AVR for SAS or severe aortic insufficiency (i.e., Stoica et al., 2006; Sundt et al., 2000). The sample sizes also varied widely from one study to another: ranging from 24 (Bashour et al., 1990) to 1100 patients (Asimakopoulos et al., 1997). Lastly, those studies retrospectively covered long periods, lasting 5 (Sundt et al., 2000) to 16 years (Elayda et al., 1993).

2.10 Decision-making

Those results must be interpreted carefully, keeping in mind that octogenarians with SAS referred to a surgeon are highly selected, as that decision-making is complex. Bouma et al. (1999) showed that only 59% of the patients who should have had an AVR according to international guidelines (Bonow et al., 2006) were actually offered surgical treatment. They were mainly symptomatic, >80 years old and had high transaortic valve gradients. On the other hand, Iung et al. (2005) observed that a decision not to operate was made for 33% of SAS patients. Multivariate analyses retained left ventricular ejection fraction and age (OR 1.84 for 80–85 year olds, OR = 3.38 for those ≥85 years) as being significantly and independently associated with the decision not to operate. Neurological dysfunction was the only comorbidity associated with that decision. During 2007, Freed et al. (2007) retrospectively studied the outcomes of SAS patients referred to their echocardiography laboratory. Among the 106 SAS patients, only 31% underwent surgery. The most common reasons symptomatic SAS patients did not undergo AVR were: their symptoms were thought to be unrelated to AS, too high surgical risk and/or patients refused (Freed et al., 2010).

3. Promises of a new approach: TAVI

In light of increasing life expectancy, the high incidence of AS in the elderly, the fact that many SAS patients are denied surgery, and because of improved endovascular technology, a new therapeutic approach using new devices is rapidly evolving, becoming widespread and would revolutionize AS treatment: TAVI.

After successful animal experimentation, Cribier et al. (2002) successfully performed the first human implantation of a balloon-expandable aortic valve prosthesis. Two TAVI devices are now under postmarketing surveillance in Europe: the balloon expandable Edwards SAPIEN™ prosthesis (Edwards Life-Sciences, CA) and the self-expandable CoreValve Revalving prosthesis™ (Medtronic Inc, MN). Two approaches are used: anterograde with transapical (TA) access or retrograde with transfemoral (TF) access. Two videos illustrating the TAVI procedures are available at www.NEJM.com.

3.1 Postoperative and short-term TAVI results

The first step in the development of these devices was to demonstrate a high rate of successful implantation that is improving with time, from 88% to >98% (Grube et al., 2007; Tamburino et al., 2011; Webb et al., 2009). At 30 days, outcome was good with 9–18% mortality (Zajarias & Cribier, 2009) for high-risk patients for whom surgery was denied (octogenarians, high Logistic EuroSCORE ≥20% (Roques & Nashef, 2003), STS-PROM ≥10% (Shroeyr et al., 2003) or specific surgical contraindication(s) (e.g. porcelain aorta, history of mediastinal radiotherapy). In all studies, the observed mortality was below those predicted by STS-PROM or Logistic EuroSCORE.

Surgery relieved symptoms with systematically lower NYHA classification and impressive decreases of the mean transvalvular gradient from 46 mm Hg preoperatively to 10 mm Hg thereafter, associated with increased aortic surface from 0.6 to 1.6 cm^2, respectively, for example, in the study by Webb et al. (2009). The NYHA classification and echocardiographically detected improvement of the mean gradient and aortic surface were sustained at 1 year (Tamburino et al., 2011; Webb at al., 2009). Survival at 1 year ranged from 73.8% (Webb et al., 2009) to 85% (Tamburino et al., 2011) and compared favorably with the spontaneous SAS evolution.

Prognosis at 1 year seems mostly related to comorbidities rather than cardiac status (Webb et al., 2009). In an Italian multicenter study, independent risk factors associated with late death were: prior stroke (hazard ratio (HR) 5.4; 95% confidence interval (CI) 1.47–20.39; p=0.01), prior acute pulmonary edema (HR 2.7; 95% CI, 1.1–6.7: p=0.03), chronic kidney disease (HR 2.5; 95% CI 1.0–6.4; p=0.048) and postprocedural paravalvular leak ≥2+ (HR 3.8; 95% CI 1.6–9.1: p=0.03) (Tamburino et al., 2011).

A landmark multicenter, prospective, randomized trial compared SAS patients, who surgeons considered unsuitable surgical candidates and were given standard treatment (including BAV) or TF transcatheter implantation of a balloon-expandable bovine pericardial valve (Leon et al., 2010). At 1 year, the death rate from any cause was 30.7% with TAVI and 50.7% with standard therapy (TAVI HR 0.55; 95% CI 0.4–0.74; p<0.001).

A principal concern of TAVI for octogenarians is its impact on QOL, for which data are scarce. At 3 months postTAVI, Krane et al. (2010) used SF-36, and found significantly improved QOL concerning the physical health summarized score, while the mental health summarized score remained unchanged. For a population ≥81 years, comparison of 6 months postTAVI to preoperative SF-36 data, Bekeredjian et al. (2010) obtained significantly improved physical and mental component summary scores from 28.4±10 to 46.8±9.2 ($p<0.001$) and from 37.3±10.8 to 50.6±10.1 ($p<0.001$), respectively.

3.2 Specific TAVI-related complications

The results of all studies demonstrated that TAVI can be implanted safely, with intraprocedural mortality now a mean of 1% (Webb et al., 2009; Tamburino et al., 2011). Implantation failure is becoming rare, with the successful implantation rate ≥98% in the most recent studies (Bleiziffer et al., 2009; Tamburino et al., 2011). Changing the surgical approach during the intervention has also become very rare.
Coronary obstruction rarely complicates valve implantation (<1%). Valve positioning is challenging, particularly when the distance between the annulus and the coronary artery is short, as the native valve may be pushed against the coronary ostium (Lefèvre et al., 2011).
Some complications seem to be related to the access route used. With TF access, major vascular complications occur in 6.8–11.7% of the cases (Bleiziffer et al., 2009; Webb et al., 2009). However, technological advances have permitted sheath-size reduction from 24F to 18F, thereby allowing a percutaneous procedure with locoregional anesthesia and fewer vascular injuries. Improved screening, case selection and experience should surely lower the vascular injury rate further.
Second, 10% of the patients suffer clinical strokes (Grube et al. 2007). In a recent diffusion-weighted, magnetic resonance imaging study on TAVI patients, the risk of diffuse cerebral embolism was 72.7%, with patients frequently having multiple new but clinically silent brain lesions. Although cerebral embolism was extremely common in the TF-TAVI cohort, the clinical stroke rate was 3.6% (Ghanem et al., 2010). It was suggested that TA-TAVI might be associated with fewer cerebral embolic events. However, results are controversial and further studies with larger cohorts are needed. Two mechanisms are involved: aortic atheroemboli and valvular calcific emboli. The elderly are at particularly high risk for perioperative neurological events because of advanced cerebral ischemic disease present preoperatively (Wang et al., 2010).
For both accesses, annulus measurement is challenging. Indeed, no gold standard currently exists for aortic annular measurement but transesophageal echocardiography provides accurate data to guide valve sizing before implantation (Messika-Zeitoun et al., 2010). Paravalvular aortic regurgitation is common after TAVI but remains stable at late follow-up (Webb et al., 2009). In the PARTNER study, moderate-or-severe perivalvular leakage was present in 11.8% of the patients at 30 days and 10.5% at 1 year (Leon et al., 2010). However, postprocedural paravalvular aortic regurgitation ≥2+ (HR 3.79) mainly affected later outcomes between 30 days and 1 year (Tamburino et al., 2011).
Conduction abnormalities are frequent after TAVI (Roten et al., 2010). The occurrence of atrioventricular block requiring pacemaker insertion at 30 days seems lower with the Edwards SAPIEN™ (<5%) (Lefèvre et al., 2011) than the CoreValve™ (up to 30%) (Jilaihawi et al., 2009). One possible explanation could be that the CoreValve™ was designed to be seated lower than the SAPIEN™ valve and might compress the underlying conduction system. However, based on a cohort of 67 patients (41 received CoreValve™ and 26 SAPIEN™), Roten et al. showed that the sole independent risk factor for complete atrioventricular block after TAVI was preexisting right bundle branch block (Roten et al., 2010). Because prosthesis sizing is a critical issue, to avoid perivalvular leakage and valve migration, "over sizing" of TAVI might have increased the risk of atrioventricular block (Bleiziffer et al., 2009). Further investigations are mandatory.

The results of some studies showed that the postoperative and short-term outcomes were worse for patients treated with TA than TF access, because the former were more severely ill and had more severe comorbidities. The Logistic EuroSCORE predicted risk was significantly higher for TA than TF, respectively: 35% vs 25% (p=0.01), as did STS-PROM 10.3% vs 8.7% (Webb et al., 2009). In-hospital mortality was 8% for the TF group vs 27% for TA group, with respective 1-year survival rates of 74±11% vs 60±13% (Al-attar et al., 2009). At 1 year, the European PARTNER study results were comparable (Lefèvre et al., 2011).

3.3 Risk assessment and patient selection

TAVI development has highlighted the complexity of risk assessment and patient selection. At present, TAVI is indicated only for SAS patients ineligible for conventional AVR, but the definition of "ineligible" remains vague. TAVI was initially designed to treat old-old patients, mean age 81–86 years (Bleiziffer et al., 2009; Tamburino et al., 2011), with high Logistic EuroSCORE predicted risk ≥20%, mean range 22–29% (Grube et al., 2007; Webb et al., 2009) or STS-PROM score ≥10%, mean range 16–23% (Al-attar et al., 2009; Bleiziffer et al., 2009) or with contraindication(s) for surgery.

Logistic EuroSCORE and STS-PROM scores are increasingly being used to estimate operative mortality based on cardiac and extracardiac factors. The STS-PROM score appears to be more reliable than the EuroSCORE for predicting outcomes of high-risk AVR patients. However, STS-PROM tends to underestimate mortality (Dewey et al., 2007). A meta-analysis showed EuroSCORE to have low discrimination ability for valve surgery and it slightly over predicted risk (Parolari et al., 2010), particularly for octogenarians referred for AVR (Leontyev et al., 2009). Both scores share the same limitations: predictive ability is limited for high-risk patients, who represented only a small proportion of the population used to derive them. They do not take into account the surgical results in a given institution, relationship between volume and mortality, and the impact of progress concerning surgical techniques, cardiopulmonary bypass, anesthesia and intensive care. The scores also fail to evaluate fully the high-risk patient because they do not integrate a very important element: clinical judgment. Indeed, many factors that negatively influence prognosis are not considered: cirrhosis, impact of body mass index, chest irradiation, chest deformation, multivalve surgery, porcelain aorta, previous CABG and vascular tortuosity for TAVI. It is estimated that neither the Logistic EuroSCORE nor STS-PROM would have classed approximately one-quarter of the patients at high risk and yet they were refused surgery because of such factors (Webb et al., 2009).

For the specific SAS octogenarian population, it seems that the development of a new specific scoring classification is necessary (Florath et al., 2010), especially one including demographic variables, such as nutritional status, disability, dementia and frailty.

3.4 Unanswered questions concerning TAVI

TAVI is not suitable for all patients ineligible for conventional AVR and patients referred for TAVI are also highly selected. In a cohort of 469 SAS patients referred for participation in a TAVI trial, 362 (77.1%) patients did not meet the inclusion/exclusion criteria. The main exclusion criteria were low STS-PROM score <10% (72 patients), peripheral vascular or aorta disease (58 patients), aortic valve area >0.8 cm^2 (54 patients), significant coronary artery disease (43 patients) and renal failure (25 patients). Among those 362 patients, 75 (20.7%) had 2 exclusion criteria and 26 (7.1%) had 3 exclusion criteria. Eighty-eight patients underwent surgery and 274 were treated medically, 177 of whom had BAV. At 2 years, the mortality rate was significantly lower for the surgical group vs the medically treated group, respectively, 28.1% vs 53.4% ($p<0.001$) (Ben-Dor et al., 2010). Another TAVI limitation is also the high incidence of severe coronary artery disease among elderly SAS patients that also influences prognosis and requires specific treatment.

Long-term durability of TAVI must now be demonstrated. TAVI provides acceptable hemodynamic results up to 3 years (Webb et al., 2009). At present, outcomes reflect comorbidities rather than cardiac status (Tamburino et al., 2011). Patient selection is a major concern for long-term durability evaluation of TAVI. Future studies should include patients with expected life expectancy unrelated to cardiac disease >5 years. At 2 years, survival was 60.9% in the study by Webb et al. (2009); what will the sample size be at 5 years?

With the learning curve, technological improvement and better patient selection, TAVI-related morbidity should decline, particularly concerning vascular injuries, strokes, pacemaker implantation and perivalvular leakage.

The next step for TAVI for SAS management should be its direct comparison with surgery for high-risk patients without contraindication(s) for surgery, and then for intermediate- and low-risk patients. Historical comparisons, case-control studies, propensity-score matching (Johansson et al., 2011) or comparison with spontaneous evolution are not able to answer these questions adequately. Multicenter, randomized-controlled trials should answer them (prognosis, durability, specific morbidity, etc…) in few years, thereby allowing the widespread development of this very promising technique.

4. Frailty and geriatric evaluation of octogenarians for SAS management

4.1 Frailty

To evaluate better an individual's situation on which the final therapeutic decision generally depends, the concepts of frailty or vulnerability are the themes of several international gerontology publications. We highlight that, at present, no consensual definition of frailty exists (Bergman et al., 2007; Karunananthan et al., 2009). However, the various authors agree that frailty is a state of susceptibility to aggression, which explains that, for a given health event, despite the same management and apparently sufficiently similar health status, the individuals will have very different outcomes. Thus, frailty is always defined as a function of the event that serves as the judgement criterion: falls, loss of autonomy, institutionalization, death… It is also defined by the time at which it is assessed. Therefore, an effective definition over the long term (Province et al., 1995) might not be operative to distinguish individuals in terms of consequences of hospitalization (Gill et al., 2004).

Regardless of the definition retained, the authors defined a certain number of common characteristics (Rockwood, 2005): frailty is a continuous state that is not simply present or absent; it is not the consequence of single organ involvement; the clinical manifestations are multiple. It can be recognized clinically, with that identification being considered the threshold of entry into frailty, the occurrence of the negative event marking the end of frailty in relationship to this factor (institutionalization or handicap, for example). The definitions of frailty are multiple (Ferrucci et al., 2004), but the most used are those that refer to the diminished physiological reserves, with a core event being the development of sarcopenia. This type of definition has shown its efficacy to predict the loss of autonomy, institutionalization or death in a cohort of patients with cardiovascular diseases but not initially handicapped and followed for 1 year (Fried et al., 2004). Its effect can be associated

with those of a disability and comorbidity, even though none of these 3 dimensions is superimposable or sufficient alone to explain the outcome (Fried et al., 2004).
According to those authors' definition (Fried et al., 2004), at least 3 criteria among the following must be satisfied to be qualified as 'fragile': diminished gripping force of the dominant hand, the feeling of fatigue/exhaustion, slower walking speed and non-intentional weight loss. Each of the elements is evaluated according to precise criteria. Such a definition could prove useful to study the long-term outcome of patients after cardiac surgery. In addition, this type of definition conceptually excludes the cognitive, sociofamilial and psychological dimensions of frailty (Fried et al., 2004). To take those dimensions into account, 2 types of solutions are proposed: an inventory of the situations at risk that can be extremely complex and overall clinical judgment, whose pertinence concerning loss of autonomy and death were recently validated (Jones et al., 2005).

4.2 Frailty and cardiac surgery

The concept of frailty and its clinical use in surgery in general and, more specifically, cardiac surgery, has recently appeared in the literature. Two recent studies (Afilalo et al., 2010; Lee et al., 2010) documented that frailty increased the risk of complications after cardiac surgery independently of age and included information from standard prognostic scores. Pertinently, those 2 studies are complementary.
Indeed, Afilalo et al. (2010) defined frailty as requiring assistance to accomplish at least one essential life activity, a diagnosis known of dementia or limited mobility. Although their definition can be debated on a conceptual level, because it mixes disability and fragility, it has the advantage of being clinically operational. The existence of a frailty phenotype, as defined, was independently associated with mortality (OR 1.8 [95% CI 1.1-3.0]), institutionalization and discharge from that facility (OR 6.3 [95% CI 4.2-9.4]) and intermediate-term survival (OR 1.5 [95% CI 1.1-2.2]).
Lee et al. (2010) defined frailty more precisely and more sensitively: walking speed tested as a mean time needed to go 5 m during 3 consecutive tries (limited to 6 seconds). Their definition is directly in line with the conceptual frailty-sarcopenia model. In their study, the risk of postoperative morbidity-mortality was multiplied by 3.05 [95% CI 1.23-7.64] for frail patients, even after adjustment for the STS-PROM score. In addition, frailty defined in this way doubled the risk of institutionalization or a prolonged stay there. Finally, in a manner not entirely clear, the risks linked to frailty are greater for women than men.
The results of those studies confirmed the findings of others concerning non-cardiac surgery, i.e., that such a definition of frailty is associated with "geriatric syndromes" (Robinson et al., 2009), sarcopenia (Makary et al., 2010) or a more holistic score-based definition (Dasgupta et al., 2009). In all those cases, the frailty phenotype was independently associated with age and other known prognostic factors of higher risk of morbidity and/or mortality.
Only authors of rare studies have envisaged frailty's appearance as a surgical consequence. Researchers of a single center study supported that hypothesis and strongly recommended that the appearance of that phenotype should be considered in future outcome investigations because this fragility is linked even more strongly to QOL than self-reported overall assessments of "health status" (Maillet et al., 2009).
We would also like to underscore the areas of uncertainty that persist today and that represent as many research projects. Afilalo et al.'s (2010) and Lee et al.'s (2010) examinations of potential relationships between a frailty phenotype and outcomes after cardiac surgery

were based on large majorities of patients (>60%) who underwent simple coronary artery bypass surgery. Even though the type of intervention was entered into the model, the phenotype's effect on valve-surgery complications (and even more so for the newer interventional techniques) warrants further clarification. The models currently used in cardiac surgery are mainly based on the frailty–sarcopenia concept. The contributions of other frailty dimensions to explaining outcome (biological, psychological, environmental and social) are also worthy of more detailed exploration. Finally, the available studies focused on subjects who were certainly old (>70 years), but the usefulness of the scores and the thresholds applied undoubtedly need to be adapted for the oldest-old (>85–90 years).

4.3 Contribution of geriatric evaluation to AVR decision-making

All of the above underscore the complexity of decision-making and follow-up of the oldest-old when AVR becomes necessary, and support an interdisciplinary approach bringing together cardiologists, surgeons, geriatricians, anesthesiologists and intensivists. However, convincing data on the impact of a geriatric approach in this setting are still lacking. The geriatrician is most probably in an ideal position, in terms of professional competence, to detect frailty, but the impact of this identification on the decisions to be made and, even more so, on the outcomes are not yet documented. As we have seen, it is also likely that the consequences of cardiac surgery, beyond its cardiovascular impact, are multidimensional (Maillet et al., 2009). It seems highly probable that an overall approach, like that proposed by geriatricians in another context (Rydwik et al., 2008), would contribute to improving the outcomes of individuals, not only in functional terms but also nutritional, psychological, social and even cognitive aspects.

4.4 Adapted rehabilitation

Rehabilitation after cardiac surgery is not less effective in the elderly than young patients (Macchi et al., 2007; Pasquali et al., 2001) and improves the outcome, even though information on the oldest-old are scarce (Pasquali et al., 2001). Indeed, it seems, for the aged patient, that rehabilitation after cardiac surgery should not be postponed and should be prolonged (Macchi et al., 2009). This is especially true for women >80 years who achieve a gain in functional autonomy 1 year after the intervention (Barnett & Halpin, 2003). Some authors recommend particular preoperative precautions, notably respiratory. The preoperative identification of frail patients could also be a pertinent way to select patients likely to benefit the most from specific programs, e.g., early mobilization in the intensive care unit (Needham, 2008). Multidimensional rehabilitation programs also achieved favorable results (Eder et al., 2010; Mazza et al., 2007; Opasich et al., 2010), which, in addition, proved their safety and efficacy in terms of rehabilitation, nursing needs, mobility capability, muscle force, equilibrium and, last but certainly no least, duration of stay.

5. Conclusion

Surgical AVR for SAS in octogenarians is the treatment of choice and is performed daily, with good intermediate-term results, despite high postoperative morbidity. In the very near future, TAVI should profoundly modify the treatment strategy for SAS. Despite all the improvements since the beginning of cardiac surgery, much progress remains to be achieved in all the steps: improving patient selection, more accurately stratifying the risks, choosing the best treatment, limiting morbidity regardless of the technique used, and proposing a personalized and adapted rehabilitation program. New scoring systems, including specific markers for elderly patients (disability, frailty, etc…), should be developed. A multidisciplinary approach, including surgeons and cardiologists, along with geriatricians, intensivists and rehabilitation specialists, would contribute to achieving all those improvements. The scarcity of scientific literature on the link between age (and particularly old-old age >85 years), outcomes and the frailty-syndrome subset opens vast avenues for future research.

6. References

Afilalo, J., Eisenberg, M.J., Morin, J.F., Bergman, H., Monette, J., Noiseux, N., Perrault, L.P., Alexander, K.P., Langlois, Y., Dendukuri, N., Chamoun, P., Kasparian, G., Robichaud, S., Gharacholou, S.M., & Boivin, J.F. (2010). Gait speed as an incremental predictor of mortality and major morbidity in elderly patients undergoing cardiac surgery. *J Am Coll Cardiol*, 56, 1668–1676, ISSN 0735-1097

Al-Attar, N., Himbert, D., Descoutures, F., Iung, B., Raffoul, R., Messika-Zeitoun, D., Brochet, E., Francis, F., Ibrahim, H., Vahanian, A., & Nataf, P. (2009). Transcatheter aortic valve implantation: selection strategy is crucial for outcome. *Ann Thorac Surg*, 87, 1557–1563, ISSN 0003-4975

Alexander, K., Anstrom, K.J., Muhlbaier, L.H., Grosswald, R.D., Smith, P.K., Jones, R.H., & Peterson, E.D. (2000). Outcomes of cardiac surgery in patients ≥ 80 years: results from the national cardiovascular network. *J Am Coll Cardiol*, 35, 731–738, ISSN 0735-1097

Asimakopoulos, G., Edwards, M.B., & Taylor, K.M. (1997). Aortic valve replacement in patients 80 years of age and older: survival and cause of death based on 1100 cases: collective results from the UK Heart Valve Registry. *Circulation*, 96, 3403–3408, ISSN 0009-7322

Assey, M.E. (1993) Heart disease in the elderly. *Heart Dis Stroke*, 2, 330–334, ISSN 1058–2819

Barnett, S.D., & Halpin, L.S. (2003). Functional status improvement in the elderly following coronary artery bypass graft. *J Nurs Care Qual*, 18, 281–287, ISSN 1057-3631

Bashour, T.T., Hanna, E.S., Myler, R.K., Mason, D.T., Ryan, C,. Feeney, J., Iskikian, J., Wald, S.H., Antonin, C., Sr., & Malabed, L.L. (1990). Cardiac surgery in patients over the age of 80 years. *Clin Cardiol*, 13, 267–270, ISSN 0160-9289

Bekeredjian, R., Krumsdorf, U., Chorianopoulos, E., Kallenbach, K., Karck, M., Katus, H.A., & Rottbauer, W. (2010). Usefulness of percutaneous aortic valve implantation to improve quality of life in patients > 80 years of age. *Am J Cardiol*, 106, 1777–1781, ISSN 0002-9149

Ben-Dor, I., Pichard, A., Gonzalez, M.A., Weissman, G., Li, Y., Goldstein, S.A., Okubagzi, P., Syed, A.I., Maluenda, G., Collins, S.D., Delhaye, C., Wakabayashi, K., Gaglia, M.A., Torguson, R., Xue, Z., Satler, L.F., Suddath, W.O., Kent, K.M., Lindsay J., & Waskman R. (2010). Correlates and causes of death in patients with severe symptomatic aortic stenosis who are not eligible to participate in a clinical trial of transcatheter aortic valve implantation. *Circulation*, 122 (Suppl 1), S37–S42, ISSN 0009-7322

Bergman, H., Ferrucci, L., Guralnik, J., Hogan, D.B., Hummel, S., Karunananthan, S., & Wolfson, C. (2007). Frailty: an emerging research and clinical paradigm – issues and controversies. *J Gerontol A Biol Sci Med Sci*, 62, 731–737, ISSN 1079-506

Bleiziffer, S., Ruge, H., Mazzitelli, D., Schreiber, C., Hutter, A., Laborde, J.C., Bauernschmitt, R., & Lange, R. (2009). Results of percutaneous and transapical transcatheter aortic valve implantation performed by a surgical team. *Eur J Cardiothorac Surg*, 35, 615–621, ISSN 1010-7940

Bonow, R.O., Carabello, B.A., Chatterjee, K., de Leon, A.C., Faxon, D.P., Freed, M.D., Gaasch, W.H., Lytle, B.W., Nishimura, R.A., O'Gara, P.T., O'Rourke, R.A., Otto, C., Shah, P.M., Shanewise, J.S., Smith, S.C., Jacobs, A.K., Adams, C.D., Anderson, J.L., Antman, E.M., Faxon, D.P., Fuster, V., Halperin, J.L., Hiratzka, L.F., Hunt, S.A., Lytle, B.W., Nishimura, R., Page, R.L., & Riegel, B. (2006). ACC/AHA 2006 practice guidelines for the management of patients with valvular heart disease: a report of the American College of Cardiology/American Heart Task Force on Practice Guidelines (Writing Committee to revise the 1998 guidelines for the management of patients with valvular heart disease). *J Am Coll Cardiol*, 48, e1–e148, ISSN 0735-1097

Bouchon, J.P. (1984). 1 + 2 + 3. Comment être efficace en Gériatrie. *Rev Prat*, 34, 888–892, ISSN 0035-2640

Bouma, B.J., van der Brink, R.B.A., van der Meulen, J.H.P., Chereix, E.C., Hamer, H.P.M., Dekker, E., Lie, K.I., & Tijssen, J.G.P. (1999). To operate or not on elderly patients with aortic stenosis: the decision and its consequences. *Heart*, 82, 143–148, ISSN 1355-6037

Chan, E.D., & Welsh, C.H. (1998). Geriatrics respiratory medicine. *Chest*, 114, 1704–1733, ISSN 0012-8703

Chiappini, B., Camurri, N., Loforte, A., Di Marco, L., Di Bartolomeo, R., & Marinelli, G. (2004). Outcome after aortic valve replacement in octogenarians. *Ann Thorac Surg*, 78, 85–89, ISSN 0003-4975

Chizner, M.A., Pearle, D.L., & deLeon, A.C. (1980). The natural history of aortic stenosis in adults. *Am Heart J*, 99, 419–424, ISSN 0002-8703

Collart, F., Feier, H., Kerbaul, F., Mouly-Bandini, A., Riberi, A., Mesana, T.G., & Metras, D. (2005). Valvular surgery in octogenarians: operative risks factors, evaluation of EuroSCORE and long term results. *Eur J Cardiothorac Surg*, 27, 276–280, ISSN 1010-7940

Cribier, A., Eltchaninoff, H., Bash, A., Borenstein, N., Tron, C., Bauer, F., Derumeaux, G., Anselme, F., Laborde, F., & Leon, M.B. (2002). Percutaneous transcatheter implantation of an aortic valve prosthesis for calcific aortic stenosis: first human, case description. *Circulation*, 106, 3006–3008, ISSN 0009-7322

Culliford, A.T., Galloway, A.C., Colvin, S.B., Grossi, E.A., Baumann, G., Esposito, R., Ribakove, G.H., & Spencer, F.C. (1991). Aortic valve replacement for aortic stenosis in persons aged 80 years and over. *Am J Cardiol*, 67, 1256–1260, ISSN 0002-9149

Dasgupta, M., Rolfson, D.B., Stolee, P., Borrie, M.J., & Speechley, M. (2009). Frailty is associated with postoperative complications in older patients with medical problems. *Arch Gerontol Geriatr*, 48, 78–83, ISSN 0167-4943

Dewey, T.M., Brown, D., Ryan, W.H., Herbert, M.A., Prince, S.L., & Mack, M.J. (2007). Reliability of risk algorithms in predicting early and late operative outcomes. *J Thorac Cardiovasc Surg*, 135, 180–187, ISSN 0022-5223

Eder, B., Hofmann, P., von Duvillard, S.P., Brandt, D., Schmid, J.P., Pokan, R., & Wonisch, M. (2010). Early 4-week cardiac rehabilitation exercise training in elderly patients after heart surgery. *J Cardiopulm Rehabil Prev*, 30, 85–92, ISSN 1932-7501

Edmunds, L.H., Jr., Stephenson, L.W., Edie, R.N., & Ratcliffe, M.B. (1988). Open-heart surgery in octogenarians. *N Engl J Med*, 319, 131–136, ISSN 0028-8614

Edwards, M.B, Taylor, M.P., & Taylor, K.M. (2003). Outcomes in nonagenarians after heart valve replacement operation. *Ann Thorac Surg*, 75, 830–834, ISSN 0003-4975

Elayda, M.A., Reul, R.M., Alonzo, D.M., Gillette, N., Reul, G.J., Jr., & Cooley, D.A. (1993) Aortic valve replacement in patients 80 years and older. Operative risks and long term results. *Circulation*, 88, II11–II16, ISSN 0009-7322

Eltchaninoff, H., Cribier, A., Tron, C., Anselme, F., Koning, R., Soyer, R., & Letac, B. (1995). Balloon aortic valve valvuloplasty in elderly patients at high risk for surgery, or inoperable: an alternative to valve replacement? *Eur Heart J*, 16, 1079–1084, ISSN 0195-668X

Ferrucci, L., Guralnik, J.M., Studenski, S., Fried, L.P., Cutler, G.B., Jr., & Watson, J.D. (2004). Designing randomized controlled trials aimed at preventing or delaying functional decline and disability in frail, older persons: a consensus report. *J Am Geriatr Soc*, 52, 625–634, ISSN 0002-8614

Florath, I., Albert, A., Boening, A., Ennker, I.C., & Ennker, J. (2010). Aortic valve replacement in octogenarians: identification of high-risk patients. *Eur J Cardiothorac Surg*, 37, 1304–1310, ISSN 1010-7940

Folkmann, S., Gorlitzer, M., Weiss, G., Harrer, M., Thalmann, M., Poslussny, P., & Grabenwoger, M. (2010). Quality of life in ocotogenarians one year after aortic valve replacement with or without coronary artery bypass surgery. *Interact Cardiovasc Thorac Surg*, 11, 750–753, ISSN 1569-9293

Freed, B.H., Sugeng, L., Furlong, K., Mor-Avi, V., Raman, J., Jeevanandam, V., & Lang, R.M. (2010). Reasons for nonadherence to guidelines for aortic valve replacement in patients with severe aortic stenosis and potential solutions. *Am J Cardiol*, 105, 1339–1342, ISSN 0002-9149

Freeman, W.K., Schaff, H.V., Orszulak, T.A., & Tajik, A.J. (1991). Cardiac surgery in the octogenarian: outcome and clinical follow-up. *J Am Coll Cardiol*, 18, 29–35, ISSN 0735-1097

Fried, L.P., Ferrucci, L., Darer, J., Williamson, J.D., & Anderson, G. (2004). Untangling the concepts of disability, frailty, and comorbidity: implications for improved targeting and care. *J Gerontol A Biol Sci Med Sci*, 59, 255–263, ISSN 1079-5006

Ghanem, A., Muller, A., Nähle, C.P., Kocurek, J., Werner, N., Hammerstingl, C., Schild, H.H., Schwab, J.O., Mellert, F., Fimmers, R., Nickenig, G., & Thomas, D. (2010). Risk and fate of cerebral embolism after transfemoral aortic valve implantation. *J Am Coll Cardiol*, 55, 427–432, ISSN 0735-1097

Gill, T.M., Allore, H.G., Holford, T.R., & Guo, Z. (2004). Hospitalization, restricted activity and the development of disability among older persons. *JAMA*, 292, 2115–2124, ISSN 0098-7484

Grube, E., Schuler, G., Buellesfeld, L., Gerckens, U., Linke, A., Wenaweser, P., Sauren, B., Mohr, F.W., Walther, T., Zickmann, B., Iversen, S., Felderhoff, T., Cartier, R., & Bonan, R. (2007). Percutaneous aortic valve replacement for severe aortic stenosis in high-risk patients using the second- and the current third-generation self-expanding CoreValve prosthesis. *J Am Coll Cardiol*, 50, 69–76, ISSN 0735-1097

Health at a glance OECD indicators. www.sourceoecd.org/socialissues/9789264061538

Horstkotte, D., & Loogen, F. (1988). The natural history of aortic valve replacement. *Eur Heart J*, 9 (Suppl E), 57–64, ISSN 0195-668X

Huber, C.H., Goeber, V., Berdat, P., Carrel, T., & Eckstein, F. (2007). Benefits of cardiac surgery in octogenarians - a postoperative quality of life assessment. *Eur J Cardiothorac Surg*, 31, 1099-1105, ISSN 1010-7940

Iung, B., Cachier, A., Baron, G., Messika-Zeitoun, D., Delahaye, F., Tornos, P., Gohlke-Bärwolf, C., Boersma, E., Ravaud, P., & Vahanian, A. (2005). Decision-making in elderly patients with severe aortic stenosis: why are so many denied surgery? *Eur Heart J*, 26, 2714-2720, ISSN 0195-668X

Jilaihawi, H., Chin, D., Vasa-Nicotera, M., Jeilan, M., Spyt, T., Ng, G.A., Bence, J., Logtens, E., & Kovac, J. (2009). Predictors for permanent pacemaker requiring after transcatheter aortic valve implantation with the CoreValve bioprosthesis. *Am Heart J*, 157, 860-866, ISSN 0002-8703

Johansson, M., Nozohoor, S., Kimblad, P.O., Harnek, J., Olivecrona, G.K., & Sjögren, J. (2011). Transapical versus transfemoral aortic valve implantation: a comparison of survival and safety. *Ann Thorac Surg*, 91, 57-63, ISSN 0003-4975

Jones, D., Song, X., Mitnitski, A., & Rockwood, K. (2005). Evaluation of a frailty index based on a comprehensive geriatric assessment in a population based study of elderly Canadians. *Aging Clin Exp Res*, 17, 465-471, ISSN 1594-0667

Karunananthan, S., Wolfson, C., Bergman, H., Beland, F., & Hogan, D.B. (2009). A multidisciplinary systematic literature review on frailty: overview of the methodology used by the Canadian Initiative on Frailty and Aging. *BMC Med Res Methodol*, 12, 68, ISSN 1471-2288

Knaus, W.A., Wagner, D.P., Zimmerman, J.E., & Draper, E.A. (1993). Variations in mortality and length of stay in intensive care units. *Ann Intern Med*, 118, 753-761, ISSN 0003-4819

Kolh, P., Kerzmann, A., Honore, C., Comte, L., & Limet, R. (2007). Aortic valve surgery in octogenarians: predictive factors of operative and long-term results. *Eur J Cardiothorac Surg*, 31, 600-606, ISSN 1010-7940

Krane, M., Deutsch, M.A., Bleizziffer, S., Schneider, L., Ruge, H., Mazzitelli, D., Schreiber, C., Brockmann, G., Voss, B., Bauernschmitt, R. & Lange, R. (2010). Quality of life among patients undergoing transcatheter aortic valve implantation. *Am Heart J*, 160, 451-457, ISSN 0002-8703

Langanay, T., De Latour, B., Ligier, K., Derieux, T., Agnino, A., Verhoye, J.P., Corbineau, J., & Leguerrier, A. (2004). Surgery for aortic stenosis in octogenarians: influence of coronary disease and other comorbidities on hospital mortality. *J Heart Valve Dis*, 13, 545-552, ISSN 0966-8519

Langanay, T., Verhoye, J.P., Ocampo, G., Vola, M., Tauran, A., De La Tour, B., Derieux, T., Ingels, A., Corbineau, H., & Leguerrier, A. (2006). Current hospital mortality of aortic valve replacement in octogenarians. *J Heart Valve Dis*, 15, 630-637, ISSN 0966-8519

Lee, D.H., Buth, K.J., Martin, B.J., Yip, A.M., & Hirsch, G.M. (2010). Frail patients are at increased risk for mortality and prolonged institutional care after cardiac surgery. *Circulation*, 121, 973-978, ISSN 0009-7322

Lefèvre, T., Kappetein, A.P., Wolner, E., Nataf, P., Thomas, M., Schächinger, V., De Bruyne, B., Eltchaninoff, H., Thielmann, M., Himbert, D., Romano, M., Serruys, P., & Wilmmer-Greinecker, G., on behalf PARTNER EU Investigator Group. (2011). One year follow-up of the multi-centre European PARTNER transcatheter heart valve study. *Eur Heart J*, 32, 148-157, 0195-668X

Leon, M.B., Smith, C.R., Miller, M.M., Moses J.W., Svensson, L.G., Tuzcu, E.M., Webb, J.G., Fontana, G.P., Makkar, R.R., Brown, D.L., Block, P.C., Guyton, R.A., Pichard, A.D.,

Bavaria, J.E., Herrmann, H.C., Douglas, P.S., Peterson, J.L., Akins, J.J., Anderson, W.N., Wang, D., & Pocock, S., for the PARTNER Trial investigators. (2010). Transcatheter aortic-valve implantation for aortic stenosis in patients who cannot undergo surgery. *N Engl J Med*, 363, 1597–1607, ISSN 0028-8614

Leonteyv, S., Walther, T., Borger, M.A., Lehmann, S., Funkat, A.K., Kempfert, J., Falk, V., & Morh, F.W. (2009). Aortic valve replacement in octogenarians: utility of risk stratification with EuroSCORE. *Ann Thorac Surg*, 87, 1440–1445, ISSN 0003-4975

Levinson, J.R., Akins, C.W., Buckley, M.J., Newell, J.B., Palacios, I.F., Blosk, P.C., & Fifer, M.A. (1989). Octogenarians with aortic stenosis. Outcome after aortic valve replacement. *Circulation*, 80, 49–56, ISSN 0009-7322

Macchi, C., Fattirolli, F., Lova, R.M., Conti, A.A., Luisi, M.L., Intini, R., Zipoli, R., Burgisser, C., Guarducci, L., Masotti, G., & Gensini, G.F. (2007). Early and late rehabilitation and physical training in elderly patients after cardiac surgery. *Am J Phys Med Rehabil*, 86, 826–834, ISSN 0894-9115

Macchi, C., Polcaro, P., Cecchi, F., Zipoli, R., Sofi, F., Romanelli, A., Pepi, L., Sibilo, M., Lipoma, M., Petrelli, M., & Molino-Lova, R. (2009). One-year adherance to exercise in elderly patients receiving postacute inpatient rehabilitation after cardiac surgery. *Am J Phys Med Rehabil*, 88, 727–734, ISSN 0894-9115

Makary, M.A., Segev, D.L., Pronovost, P.J., Syin, D., Bandeed-Roche, K., Patel, P., Takenaga, R., Dervgan, L., Holzmueller, C.G., Tian, J., & Fried, L.P. (2010). Frailty as a predictor of surgical outcomes in older patients. *J Am Coll Surg*, 210, 901–908, ISSN S1072-7515

Maillet, J.M., Somme, D., Hennel, E., Lessana, A., Saint-Jean, O., & Brodaty, D. (2009). Frailty after aortic valve replacement in octogenarians. *Arch Gerontol Geriatr*, 48, 391–396, ISSN 0167-4943

Mazza, A., Camera, F., Maestri, A., Longoni, F., Patrignani, A., Gualco, A., Opasich, C., & Cobeli, F. (2007). Elderly patient-centered rehabilitation after cardiac surgery. *Monaldi Arch Chest Dis*, 68, 36–43, ISSN 1112–0643

Melby, S.J., Zierer, A., Kaiser, S.P., Guthrie, T.J., Keune, J.D., Schuessler, R.B., Pasque, M.K., Lawton, J.S., Moazami, N., Moon, M.R., & Damiano, R.J., Jr. (2007). Aortic valve replacement in octogenarians: risk factors for early and late mortality. *Ann Thorac Surg*, 83, 1651–1657, ISSN 0003-4975

Messika-Zeitoun, D., Serfaty, J.M., Brochet, E., Ducrocq, D., Lepage, L., Detaint, D., Hyafil, F., Himbert, D., Pasi, N., Laissy, J.P., Iung, B., & Vahanian, A. (2010). Multimodal assessment of the aortic annulus diameter: implications for transcatheter aortic valve implantation. *J Am Coll Cardiol*, 55, 186–194, ISSN 0735-1097

Needham, D.M. (2008). Mobilizing patients in the intensive care unit: neuromuscular weakness and physical function. *JAMA*, 300, 1685–1690, ISSN 0098-7484

NHLBI Balloon Valvuloplasty Registry participants. (1991). Percutaneous balloon aortic valvuloplasty: acute and 30-day follow-up results from the NHLBI Balloon Valvuloplasty Registry. *Circulation*, 84, 2383–2397. ISSN 0009-7322

Nkomo, V., Gardin, J.M., Skelton, T.N., Gottdiener, J.S., Scott, C.G., & Enriquez-Sarano, E. (2006). Burden of valvular heart diseases: a population-based study. *Lancet*. 368, 1005–1011, ISSN 0140-6736

Olsson, M., Granstrom, L., Lindblom, D., Rosenqvist, M., & Ryden, L. (1992). Aortic valve replacement in octogenarians with aortic stenosis: a case study. *J Am Coll Cardiol*, 20, 1512–1516, ISSN 0735-1097

Olsson, M., Janfjall, H., Orth-Gomer, K., Unden, A., & Rosenqvist, M. (1996). Quality of life in octogenarians after valve replacement due to aortic stenosis. *Eur Heart J*, 17, 583–589, 0195-668X

Opasich, C., Patrignani, A., Mazza, A., Gualco, A., Cobelli, F., & Pinna, G.D. (2010). An elderly-centered, personalized, physiotherapy program early after cardiac surgery. *Eur J Cardiovasc Prev Rehabil*, 17, 582–587, ISSN S1741-8267

Parolari, A., Pesce, L.L., Trezzi, M., Cavallotti, L., Kassem, S., Loardi, C., Pacini, D., Tremoli, E., & Alamanni, F. (2010). EuroSCORE performance in valve surgery: a meta-analysis. *Ann Thorac Surg*, 89, 787–793, ISSN 0003-4975

Pasquali, S.K., Alexander, K.P., & Peterson, E.D. (2001). Cardiac rehabilitation in the elderly. *Am Heart J*, 142, 748–755, ISSN 0002-8703

Praschker, B.G.L., Leprince, P., Bonnet, N., Rama, A., Bors, V., Liévre, L., Pavie, A., & Gandjbakch, I. (2006). Cardiac surgery in nonagenarians: hospital mortality and long-term follow-up. *Interact Cardiovasc Thorac Surg*, 5, 696–700, ISSN 1569-9293

Province, M.A., Hadley, E.C., Hornbrook, M.C., Lipsitz, L.A., Miller, J.P., Mulrow, C.D., Ory, M.G., Sattin, R.W., Tinetti, M.E., & Wolf, S.L. (1995). The effects of exercise on falls in elderly patients. A preplanned meta-analysis of the FICSIT trials. Frailty and Injuries: Cooperative Studies of Intervention Techniques. *JAMA*, 273, 1341-1347, ISSN 0098-7484

Robinson, T.N., Eiseman, B., Wallace, J.L., Church S.D., McFann, K.K., Pfister, S.M., Sharp, T.J., & Moss, M. (2009). Redefining geriatric preoperative assessment using frailty, disability and co-morbidity. *Ann Surg*, 250, 449–455, ISSN 0003-4932

Rockwood, K. (2005). Frailty and its definition: a worthy challenge. *J Am Geriatr Soc*, 53, 1069–1070, ISSN 0002-8614

Roques, F., Michel, P., Goldstone, A.R., Nashef, S. (2003). The Logistic EuroSCORE. *Eur Heart J*, 24, 881–882, ISSN 0195-668X

Ross, J., & Braunwald, E. (1968). Aortic stenosis. *Circulation*, 38(Suppl I), I61–I67, ISSN 0009-7322

Roten, L., Wenaweser, P., Delacretaz, E., Hellige, G., Stortecky, S., Tanner, H., Pilgrim, T., Kadner, A., Eberle, B., Zwahlen, M., Carrel, T., Meier, B., & Windecker, S. (2010). Incidence and predictors of atrioventricular conduction impairment after transaortic valve implantation. *Am J Cardiol*, 106, 1473–1480, ISSN 0002-9149

Rydwik, E., Lammes, E., Frändin, K., & Akner, G. (2008). Effects of a physical and nutritional intervention program for a frail elderly people over age 75. A randomized controlled pilot treatment trial. *Aging Clin Exp Res*, 20, 159–170, ISSN 1594-0667

Scharwz, F., Baumann, P., Manthey, J., Hoffmann, M., Schuler, G., Mehmel, H.C., Schmitz, W., & Kübler, W. (1982). The effect of aortic valve replacement on survival. *Circulation*, 66, 1105–1110, ISSN 0009-7322

Shroyer, A.L., Coombs, L.P., Peterson, E., Eiken, M.C., DeLong, E.R., Chen, A., Ferguson, T.B., Grover, F.L., & Edwards, F; Society of Thoracic Surgeons. (2003). The Society of Thoracic Surgeons: 30-day operative mortality and morbidity risk models. *Ann Thorac Surg*, 75, 1856–1865, ISSN 0003-4975

Schueler, R., Hammersting, C., Sinning, J.M., Nickenig, G., & Omran, H. (2010). Prognosis of octogenarians with severe aortic valve stenosis at high risk for cardiovascular surgery. *Heart*, 96, 1831–1836, ISSN 1355-6037

Sjögren, J., & Thulin, L.I. (2004). Quality of life in the very old elderly after cardiac surgery: a comparison of SF-36 between long term survivors and an age-matched population. *Gerontology*, 50, 407–410, ISSN 0304-324X

Somme, D., Maillet, J.M., & Fagon, J.Y. (2009). Particularités physiologiques du sujet âgé, In: *Réanimation Médicale* sous l'égide du Collége National des Enseignants de Réanimation Médicale, pp. 218–225, Masson, Paris, ISBN 978-2-294-08855-1

Stoica, S.C., Cafferty, F., Kitcat, J., Baskett, R.J.F., Goddard, M., Sharples, L.D., Wells, F.C., & Nashef, S.A.M. (2006). Octogenarians undergoing cardiac surgery outlive their peers: a case for early referral. *Heart*, 92, 503–506, ISSN 1355-6037

Sundt, T.M., Bailey, M.S., Moon, M.R., Mendeloff, E.N., Huddleston, C.B., Pasque, M.K., Barner, H., & Gay, Jr, W.C. (2000). Quality of life after aortic valve replacement at the age of > 80 years. *Circulation*, 102 (Suppl III), III70–III74, ISSN 0009-7322

Tamburino, C., Capodanno, D., Ramondo, A., Petronio, A.S., Ettori, F., Santoro, G., Klugmann, S., Bedogni, F., Maisano, F., Marzocchi, A., Poli, A., Antoniucci, D., Napodano, M., De Carlo, M., Fiorina, C., & Ussia, G.P. (2011). Incidence and predictors of early and late mortality after transcatheter aortic valve implantation in 663 patients with severe aortic stenosis. *Circulation*, 123, 299–308, ISSN 0009-7322

Thourani, V.H., Myung, R., Kilgo, P., Thompson, K., Puskas J.D., Lattouf, O.M., Cooper, W.A., Vega, J.D., Chen, E.P., & Guyton, R.A. (2008). Long-term outcome after isolated aortic valve replacement in octogenarians: a modern perspective. *Ann Thorac Surg*, 86, 1458–1465, ISSN 0003-4975

Tsai, T.P., Chaux, A., Matloff, J.M., Gray, R.J., DeRobertis, M.A., & Khan, S.S. (1994). Ten-year experience of cardiac surgery in patients aged 80 years and over. *Ann Thorac Surg*, 58, 445–450, ISSN 0003-4975

Vahanian,A. & Otto, C.M.(2010). Risk stratification of patients with aortic stenosis. Eur Heart J, 31, 416–423, ISSN 0195-668X

Vahanian, A., Baumgartner, H., Bax, J., Butchard, E., Dion, R., Filippatos, G., Flachskampf, F., Hall, R., Iung, B., Kasprzak, J., Nataf, P., Tornos, P., Torracca, L., & Wenink, A. (2007). Guidelines on the management of valvular heart disease. The Task Force on the Management of Valvular Heart Disease of the European Society of Cardiology. *Eur Heart J*, 28, 230–268, ISSN 0195-668X

Varadarajan, P., Kapoor, N., Bansal, R.C., & Pai, R.G. (2006). Clinical profile and natural history of 453 non surgically managed patients with severe aortic stenosis. *Ann Thorac Surg*, 82, 2111–2115, ISSN 0003-4975

Vicchio, M., Della Corte, A., De Santo, L.S., De Feo, M., Caianiello, G., Scardone, M., & Cotrufo, M. (2008). Tissue versus mechanical prostheses: quality of life in octogenarians. *Ann Thorac Surg*, 85, 1290–1295, ISSN 0003-4975

Wang, P., Acker, M.A., Bilello, M., Melhem, E.R., Stambrook, E., Ratcliffe, S.J., & Floyd, T.F.; DENOVO (determining neurologic outcomes from valve operations) investigators. (2010). Sex, ageing and preexisting cerebral ischemic disease in patients with aortic stenosis. *Ann Thorac Surg*, 90, 1230–1235, ISSN 0003-4975

Webb, J.G., Altwegg, L., Boone, R.H., Cheung, A., Ye, J., Lichtenstien, S., Lee, M., Masson, J.B., Thompson, C., Moss, R., Carere, R., Munt, B., Nietlispach, F., & Humphries, K. (2009). Transcatheter aortic valve implantation. Impact on clinical and valve-related outcomes. *Circulation*, 119, 3009–3016, ISSN 0009-7322

Zajarias, A. & Cribier, A.G. (2009). Outcomes and safety of percutaneous aortic valve replacement. *J Am Coll Cardiol*, 53, 1829–1836, ISSN 0735-1097

11

Neurological Complications in Aortic Valve Surgery and Rehabilitation Treatment Used

M. Paz Sanz-Ayan[1], Delia Diaz[1],
Antonio Martinez-Salio[2], Francisco Miguel Garzon[1],
Carmen Urbaneja[1], Jose Valdivia[1] and Alberto Forteza[3]
[1]*Department of Rehabilitation, University Hospital 12 de Octubre, Madrid*
[2]*Department of Neurology, University Hospital 12 de Octubre, Madrid*
[3]*Department of Cardiac Surgery, University Hospital 12 de Octubre, Madrid*
Spain

1. Introduction

Around the second decade of the twentieth century there was speculation about the possibility of cardiac surgery and its possible consequences in the central nervous system. To reduce these potential consequences as much as possible, research was carried out into three different approaches: systemic hypothermia, by placing the patient in a bath of ice-cold water, cross circulation between two people, and cardiopulmonary bypass (CPB) with a roller pump and an artificial oxygenator (Clau Terré, 2009). Shortly after using these procedures, it became clear there was an advantage provided by the CPB technique with an independent oxygenator and normal systemic flows that neither cross-circulation nor surface hypothermia could provide. It thus became possible to address increasingly complex congenital heart disease and ventricular septal defects, tetralogy of Fallot and other more complex examples. With the introduction of CPB, early neurological complications such as coma, cognitive impairment, strokes, etc. began to appear.

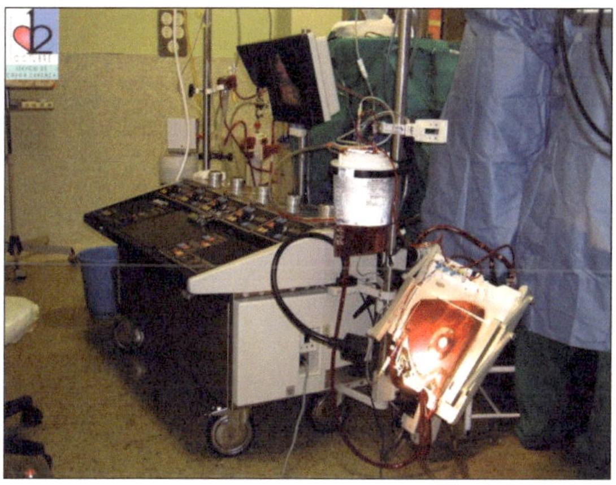

Fig. 1. Extracorporeal (CPB) blood pump

Neurological complications (NC) associated with postoperative aortic valve surgery are relatively frequent in spite of technical advances in surgery and CPB systems, and they give rise to an increase in morbidity and mortality, increased lengths of stays in hospital and rising costs after discharge from hospital. Therefore, the main purpose of the medical team responsible for assessing and treating patients who require cardiac surgery is to conduct a proper assessment and preventive measures for these complications and, once they have occurred, to minimise the physical, psychological, social and economic consequences for the patient and their family.

2. Changes in cerebral blood flow during CPB with extracorporeal pump

The brain weighs about 2% of total body weight. Cerebral blood flow accounts for 10 to 15% of cardiac output. Cerebral blood flow in normothermia is 50 millilitres (ml)/100 grams (g) of tissue per minute (min) and oxygen consumption is 3.5 ml/100 g tissue / min. Cerebral circulation is unusual in its self-regulating ability performed through the arteries of medium and large size. The ability for self-regulation acts at between 50 and 155 millimetres of mercury (mm Hg) for systolic blood pressure in normal conditions, but below 50 mm Hg brain irrigation is directly dependent on the amount of flow to this area. In cases of severe hypertensive disease or cerebral vascular disease, the lower limits can be much higher (Sotaniemi et al., 1986, Caplan et al., 1999).
At normothermia, there is permanent neurological damage when there is a cerebral perfusion defect or flow is less than 125 ml/min for more than 7 minutes. Vascular territories with little reserve, such as the border zones of cerebral arteries, the spinal cord and basal ganglia are the most sensitive and most affected by a situation of ischemia. The hippocampal cells and cerebellar Purkinje cells are also particularly sensitive to ischemia.

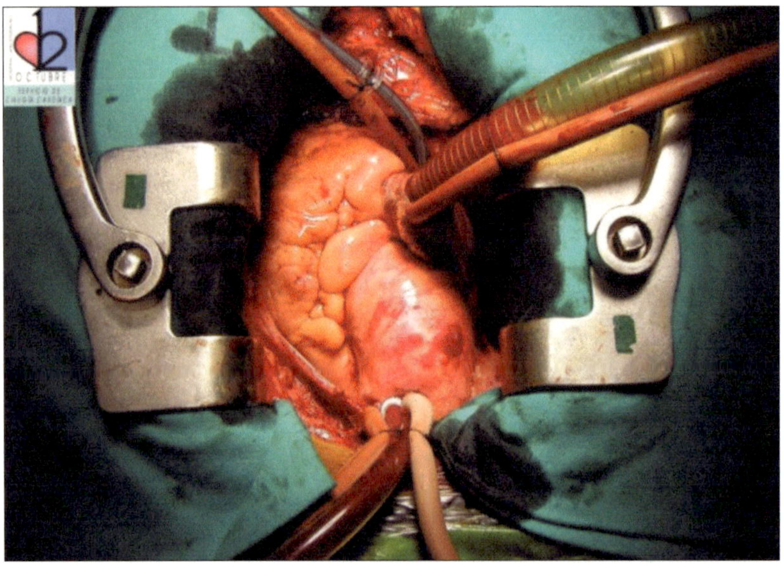

Fig. 2. Cannulation in ascending aorta and right atrium in preparation for using cardiopulmonary bypass. Similarly, the coronary sinus is cannulated to administer cardioplegic solution

The average cerebral blood flow in adult CPB is 25 ml/100g/min, which is approximately 6% of systemic flow. The ability for self-regulation with normotension persists, even in cases of hypothermia, ranging between 50 and 155 mm Hg. A decrease below 40 mm Hg may cause a significant decrease in cerebral oxygen delivery.

3. Etiological classification of neurological complications

The series that we can see in the bibliography show that there is a greater number of NCs in valve replacement surgery than in coronary artery bypass grafting, with an incidence of stroke or transient ischemic attack of 1.7% in patients undergoing coronary artery bypass grafting, 3.6% in those with a simple valve replacement, 3.3% in those undergoing both procedures and 6.7% in those who undergo a multiple valve replacement (Boeken et al., 2005)

The NCs in these patients may affect the brain, the spinal cord and peripheral nerves, and the most common of these are often strokes, anoxic-ischemic encephalopathy, epilepsy and brachial plexus injuries

Among the many threats to which the Nervous System is subjected during cardiovascular surgery, we can highlight the following: embolism, CPB, general anaesthetics, hypothermia, aortic clamping, and in some cases circulatory arrest. (Mills, 1995; Roach et al., 1996; Hallow et al, 1999).

According to the guidelines of the American College of Cardiology / American Heart Association as regards heart surgery for 1999, neurological complications are classified as type I deficiency, including focal lesions such as stroke and stupor or coma, and type II when intellectual functioning and memory are affected, and seizures. However, there are intermediate forms that are difficult to classify (Roach et al., 1996).

Strokes or **cerebrovascular accidents** are on the whole 80% ischemic and 20% hemorrhagic (use of anticoagulants). 50% of the ischemic ones are usually caused by atherothrombotic reasons, 25% are lacunar (associated with chronic arterial high blood pressure), 20% are cardioembolic, and the remaining 5% involve the ones we usually include in cardiac surgery: heart attacks in the border zone area between the anterior cerebral artery and the middle cerebral artery (called man-in-the-barrel syndrome due to its clinical consequences), and between the latter and the posterior cerebral artery. (Sanz et al., 2008)

In cardiac surgery, the incidence of stroke ranges from 0.7 to 3.8% when assessed retrospectively or between 4.8 to 5.2% if assessed prospectively (Bocerius, 2004). This is the main cause of morbidity in people undergoing cardiac surgery. Its frequency is 5% higher in patients with valvular disease, either due to an increased frequency of atrial fibrillation in these cases or because the valve surgery requires opening the heart chambers and increases the likelihood of air embolization, unlike in coronary surgery.

It may appear early on, occurring during surgery, and become apparent when the patient awakes, or later after normal awakening with no focal neurological damage apparent. Both the early and late kinds have a high hospital mortality of 41% and 13% respectively. (Hogue et al, 1999).

Strokes cause major disability and high rehabilitation costs because these patients most often require the use of different technical aids or orthotics for walking, wheelchairs, adaptation of their home due to architectural barriers, help from third parties and in some cases the everyday need for health care staff, requiring admission to specialised homes.

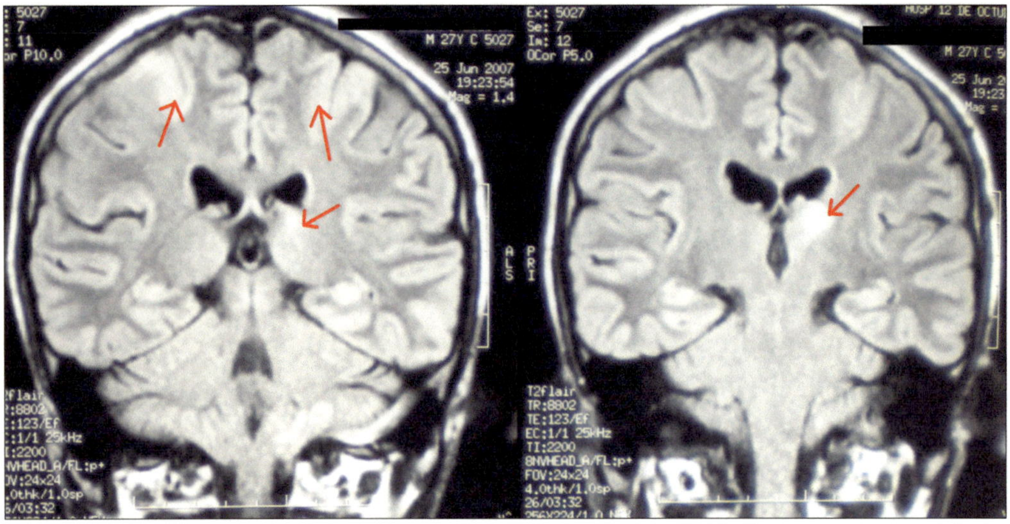

Fig. 3. Sagittal cross-section MRI image showing effects firstly on the cortex of both hemispheres of the brain in the superior fronto-parietal regions and bilaterally. Bilateral basal ganglia are also affected, especially in the left thalamus and both heads of the caudate nuclei. Infarction in the border zone. Man in a barrel syndrome

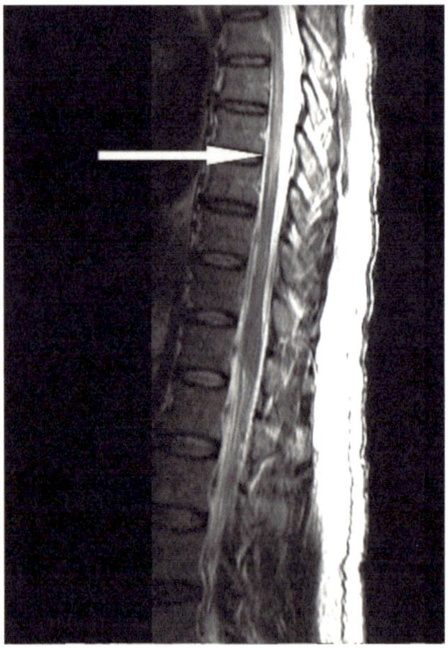

Fig. 4. Sagittal cross-sectional MRI image showing a hyperintense lesion in T2 (which was T1 hypointense) from D7 to L2, compatible with secondary spinal cord ischemia with aortic arch surgery. (Taken from Martin C et al, 2007)

Encephalopathy is usually secondary to a diffuse cerebral injury, and is believed to originate from multiple microembolic events or hypoperfusion (Jacobs et al, 1998). This clinical situation manifests itself in various ways, but it is diagnosed as a state of global impairment of cognitive functions, a reduced level of consciousness that is sometimes prolonged, hallucinations, and increased or decreased psychomotor activity. Its incidence ranges from 3 to 12% and though it involves high mortality (7.5%) this is usually lower than that of a stroke, and has an average hospital stay double that of the usual stay. Encephalopathy in these patients may be metabolic (disorders in the internal environment), pharmacological (drug toxicity), hypoxic ischemic (hypotension) or due to multiple causes (the aforementioned ones plus sepsis, use of balloon counterpulsation).

Epilepsy usually occurs as a result of diffuse encephalopathy, a stroke, and in patients with previous epilepsy, and is usually related to the presence of metabolic disorders (generalized epilepsy) or a structured lesion (focal epilepsy). It occurs in 0.3 and 10% of cases and does not often lead to epilepsy.

Effects on the **spinal cord** are usually diagnosed by the appearance of paraparesis in connection with a spinal cord infarction related to hypotension in the border zone or clamping of the aorta. The effects appear most often in reconstructive aortic aneurysms, dissections or traumatic rupture, as well as in valve repairs and the use of intra-aortic balloon counterpulsation.

The most common injuries to the **Peripheral Nervous System** are **brachial plexus neuropathy**, **recurrent laryngeal nerve injury** and **phrenic nerve injury**, almost all related to compression neuropathy of a mechanical nature, due to fracture of the first rib by excessive intraoperative traction exerted on the sternum and chest wall.

- Brachial plexus trauma injury is related to trauma during jugular cannulation, plexus stretching and during the dissection of the internal mammary artery that requires extreme retraction of the chest wall. The incidence ranges between 2.6 and 13%. Most of the deficits are usually transient. (Benecke et al, 1988).
- Phrenic nerve injuries are usually related to local hypothermia for myocardial protection (Beran et al, 2008).
- Injuries to the radial or ulnar nerve are usually associated with puncturing or hematoma when cannulating arteries for intraoperative pressure monitoring.
- Recurrent laryngeal nerve injuries occur in surgery affecting the convexity of the aortic arch.
- The facial nerve is usually affected by hypothermia or direct mechanical injury.
- Peroneal nerve compression resulting from incorrect and prolonged support of the fibular head on a hard surface.

We must rule out other types of polyneuropathy such as ICU, produced by malnutrition or deficits such as phosphorus.

Extrapyramidal system damage: especially choreoathetosis, whose frequency ranges from 1-12% of patients with neurological complications. This is most often associated with hypothermia and total cardiac arrest. It appears between the 2nd and 6th days after surgery and usually decreases in intensity over time, although it may leave significant hypotonia.

Neuropsychological disorders: these are assessed by means of memory, intelligence, visual acuity and motor tests. Diffuse disorders can appear in up to 80% of cases in the immediate postoperative period and up to 20-40% still persist two months after surgery. They are more common at older ages. They appear as the patient's subjective sensation of loss of concentration, alertness, memory, learning etc. (Asenbaum et al, 1991; Bendszus et al, 2002).

Table 1 shows a summary of the most common complications in cardiac surgery in general.

SYNDROME	DIAGNOSTICS	MECHANISMS
Diffuse encephalopathy	Anoxo-ischemic encephalopathy Metabolic encephalopathy Encephalopathy for various reasons	- Hypotension - Drug toxicity - Disorders in the internal medium - Sepsis
Focal defect	Stroke Cerebral Haemorrhage	- Embolism - Hypotension (hemodynamic infarction) - Clotting factor consumption - Anticoagulants
Epilepsy	Diffuse encephalopathy STROKE Prior epilepsy	- Metabolic disorder (generalized epilepsy) - Structural lesion (focal epilepsy)
Paraparesis	·Spinal cord infarction	- Hypotension (border zone) - Aortic clamping
Peripheral neuropathy	Brachial plexus neuropathy Recurrent laryngeal lesion Injury of the phrenic nerve	- Compression neuropathy

Table 1. Major neurological complications in cardiac surgery

4. Prevention of neurological damage in aortic valve surgery

Identifying patients at high risk of neurological damage is as important as the techniques to prevent it.

Pre-operative prevention: achieving adequate metabolic control, especially in hypertensive and diabetic patients, optimizing treatment for each patient (antihypertensive, anti-anginal), hemodynamic stabilisation and prevention of the patient's previous arrhythmias, and attempting to reduce postoperative atrial fibrillation. It is also important to carry out a prophylaxis to minimise perioperative stress through suitable information for the patient on the surgery they are to undergo.

Intraoperative prevention: the possibility of embolisation is the main cause of postoperative stroke, especially as regards the ascending aorta's atheromatous plaques, so it is important to conduct a pre- and post-operative transesophageal echocardiography to diagnose these plaques. In this way one can locate and change the cannulation site, location and type of clamping. Another region from which the embolisations come is the left atrial appendage, above all the flap, and the risk of embolisation here may be reduced by ligature of the same. In valve surgery, delicate mobilization of the heart is particularly important as well as adequate purging of the cavities.

CPB may cause injury to the central nervous system in various ways: it is a cause of embolism and a stimulus for the activation of systemic inflammatory response. This is why

membrane oxygenators are used, as well as arterial line filters and smaller circuits coated with heparin. These circuits also attempt to maintain the functioning of platelets, preventing the formation of procoagulants, fibrinolysis, reducing bleeding and the need for transfusion.
Proper control of temperature is important (avoiding cerebral hyperthermia), metabolic control and correctly maintaining the acid-base status so as not to increase the possibility of neurological effects.
Cerebral hypoperfusion may reduce purging of microemboli, thereby encouraging neighbouring infarcts. This is why hemodynamic stability should be maintained throughout the surgery. Although autoregulation of cerebral blood flow during cardiopulmonary bypass occurs within a wide range of pressures, hypertensive and diabetic patients may require higher average pressures to maintain perfusion (90 mm Hg). Therefore, although the optimal level is not firmly established, one attempts to apply more pressure than usual to reduce neurological damage in high-risk patients.
Non-CPB surgery does not remove medical complications since the inflammatory response is also triggered, though to a lesser degree. This is associated with a relative reduction in the risk of stroke by 50%.
It is important to try to avoid haematomas on the central or peripheral vascular accesses and pressure zones in order to decrease potential injury to the peripheral nervous system.
Post-operative prevention: metabolic control should be continued as regards blood glucose and adequate oxygenation, and anticoagulation and antiagregation should be started immediately. Arrhythmias should be avoided as much as possible, especially atrial fibrillation, usually by using beta blockers.
One should continue avoiding zones of compression or of excessive pressure in order to decrease injury to the peripheral nervous system.
It is very important at this stage to control all that has been mentioned above since all of this may prolong the time in intensive care units, possibly leading to polyneuropathy in the critical patient with a pattern of axonal damage that would cause long-term consequences similar to those caused by the side effects of a stroke. It is therefore important to get the patient to sit up as soon as possible.

5. Rehabilitation treatment for neurological complications after aortic valve surgery

The **rehabilitative treatment** for NCs arising from aorta surgery ranges from prevention of possible complications to restoring the motor control of walking, improving limb functions and increasing the patient's participation in and return to daily life.
In patients with stroke and severe postoperative NCs, rehabilitation treatment in the **acute phase** is:

- Reducing **respiratory complications** such as atelectasis, retention of secretions, respiratory infections, pleural effusions or those generated by phrenic nerve palsy causing paresis or diaphragmatic paralysis. In any patient on whom a median sternotomy or thoracotomy is performed, active and passive chest physiotherapy protocols are carried out. These patients are protected with a sternal compression vest to avoid pain with the movements induced by Valsalva manoeuvres such as coughing.
  A technique of expectoration, chest expansion, postural drainage and chest vibrations could be added to techniques such as incentive spirometry and airflow acceleration techniques.

The typical respiratory pattern of patients undergoing median sternotomy is: low tidal volume, high respiratory rate, absence of sighing, restrictive pattern [reduced vital capacity, reduced inspiratory capacity and reduced functional residual capacity produced by both anesthesia (18%) and decubitus (30%)]. Apart from altering the exchange of gases, it is also beneficial in that there are cases where there is aspiration as this decreases mucociliary activity, decreases cough reflex, and produces a hyper-reactive and altered alveolar surfactant.

- **Swallowing, hydration and nutrition:** the incidence of dysphagia in strokes is 50% with a high risk of aspiration and pneumonia. Early sitting up is essential. If there are signs of impaired swallowing as tolerance to food increases, liquids should be thickened and if necessary nasogastric tubes should be put in place to avoid choking. In this event, patients should be referred to medical specialists in dysphagia rehabilitation.
- **Urinary incontinence** is common (30-50%) in the early days, due to lack of sphincter control, immobility, communication problems, prior prostate or gynaecological diseases, urinary tract infection and confusional states. The bladder catheter must be removed when possible, because this is usually resolved in the first few days. If it is not resolved, it is necessary to carry out a urodynamic study to determine the exact cause of the incontinence.
- 5% of stroke cases also present **deep vein thrombosis**, and **pulmonary embolism** is the leading cause of death between the 2nd and 4th week after the stroke. Early mobilisation and low molecular weight heparin are the two possibilities for prevention. Medium compression stockings are used for patients at high risk of developing this.
- **Contractures and spasticity:** Immobilization in shortened positions is the main mechanism of contracture with limited passive movement. Prevention is based on passive exercises involving the complete joint range of motion and prolonged muscle stretching. If spasticity appears, one may consider using braces to keep up the stretching and functional postures.

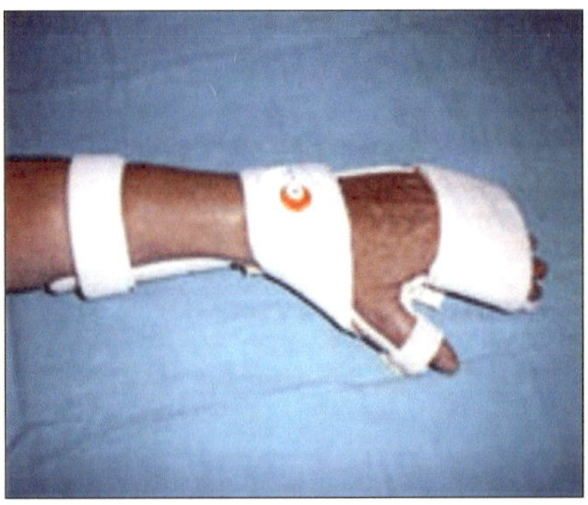

Fig. 5. Postural night splint

- **Early mobilisation:** Beginning activities early on such turning over in the bed or transfer to the seated position. Helping to gain control over the trunk in the sitting position as an essential step to the standing position. The patient should use their non-plegic limbs for basic hygiene and begin to resume everyday activities.
- **Shoulder pain:** With stroke, subluxation may appear in the first weeks as a result of the flaccid stage and it may also appear solely due to immobilization. The appearance of

this shoulder pain may delay the recovery process. Prevention is based posture and movement guidelines given by the patient's medical staff and family. Transcutaneous neuromuscular stimulation can prevent and treat pain but is not recommended as a standard guideline.

- **Perception, cognitive and communication deficits:** Orientation, contact and communication with people and the environment is to be helped. Speech therapy treatment is to begin as soon as possible when the patient's condition permits this.

In the **subacute phase** of postoperative neurological complications, work is done directly on the motor deficit and physical disability using different techniques involving: compensation, facilitation, task-oriented rehabilitation, technology applied to rehabilitation programmes geared towards tasks (e.g. walking on a treadmill with part of the body weight suspended), therapy by movement induced by the healthy side being restricted, muscle strengthening techniques and aerobic exercise. Intervention in the perceptual and cognitive area and emotional disturbances.

Technical aids such as braces, walking sticks, walking frames, botulinum toxin and occupational therapy are also used.

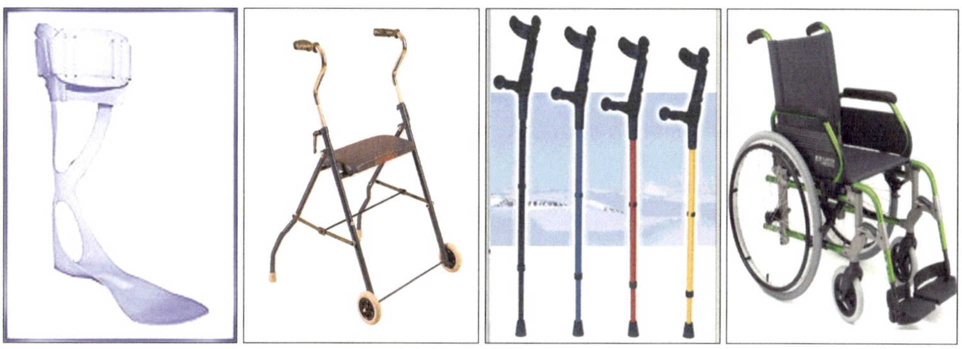

Fig. 6. Different technical aids and ortheses used for hemiplegics

There follows an analysis of the impact of different NCs in aortic valve surgery, including both early and late complications from 2008 to 2010 in the University Hospital 12 de Octubre (Madrid). The study includes single and multiple aortic valve replacements, aortic valve replacement plus coronary artery bypass grafting and aortic valve replacement plus tube graft due to root aneurysm (techniques: Bentall (Kirali et al, 2002), David (modified) (Forteza et al, 2010) and 2nd aortic valve replacement).

6. Objectives

1. To assess the clinical risk factors for NC developing.
2. To assess the different NCs and their impact/frequency.
3. To analyse the different rehabilitation techniques that have been used in the treatment of NCs.

7. Materials and methods

452 patients who underwent aortic valve surgery were retrospectively analyzed by being divided into the following groups: single and multiple aortic valve replacements, aortic

valve replacement plus coronary artery bypass grafting and aortic valve replacement plus tube graft due to root aneurysm between January 2008 and November 2010.

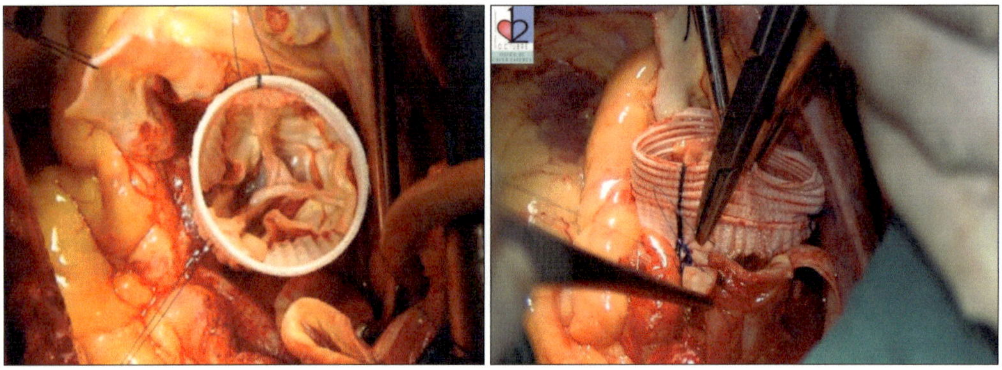

Fig. 7. Reimplantation using the inclusion (David) technique

An NC was defined as the occurrence of a cerebrovascular accident (STROKE) (ischemic or hemorrhagic), transient ischemic attack (TIA), spinal cord injury, peripheral neuropathy, seizure, stupor, coma, polyneuropathy of critically ill patient, dementia, acute delirium or encephalopathy.

A comparative analysis was carried out on the incidence of NCs according to a series of preoperative and postoperative clinical variables: arterial hypertension, diabetes mellitus, dyslipidemia, chronic obstructive pulmonary disease, heart failure, renal failure, prior STROKE, smoker, drinker, calcified valves, endocarditis, peripheral arterial disease, previous revascularization, aortic atherosclerosis, acute myocardial infarction within 3 months prior to surgery, left ventricle ejection fraction, aortic clamping time and CPB time, postoperative arrhythmia, number of transfusions required, whether resuscitation techniques were required, drugs the patients were taking, surgical priority (scheduled, priority and urgent) and type of surgery performed.

An attempt was made to determine which of these variables was more important statistically in relation to the others.

7.1 Definitions used

- **Prior STROKE:** a documented history of STROKE with side-effects such as impaired motor, speech or sight functions.
- **STROKE:** sudden onset of one or more neurological symptoms caused by ischemia or haemorrhage persisting longer than 24 hours or which leaves side-effects.
- **TIA:** loss of neurological function caused abruptly by ischemia persisting less than 24 hours and with no side-effects.
- **Spinal Cord Injury:** alteration of the spinal cord that can cause loss of sensation and mobility
- **Seizures:** sudden, short event duration in relation to excessive abnormal cortical neuronal activity. This is usually transient with convulsive movements and with or without loss of consciousness.
- **Stupor:** decreased activity of intellectual functions together with immobility and mutism.

- **Coma:** complete lack of consciousness with no evidence of voluntary motor reactivity, no response to verbal or visual stimuli.
- **Critical illness polyneuropathy:** generalised effects on the peripheral nervous system responsible for muscle weakness that occurs during the care and recovery of patients in intensive care units and which delays withdrawal of ventilator and leads to prolonged immobilization.
- **Acute confusional state:** altered mental state characterized by being acute and reversible.
- **Encephalopathy:** a set of brain disorders that cause deterioration in general, in terms of motor functions, seizures and psychiatric disorders
- **Arterial hypertension (AHT):** a previous history of hypertension that has been diagnosed or treated with medication, a diet or exercise by a doctor
- **Diabetes Mellitus (DM):** a previous history of DM that has been diagnosed or treated by a doctor with medication, a diet or exercise.
- **Dyslipidemia (DL):** a previous history of DL that has been diagnosed or treated by a doctor with medication, a diet or exercise.
- **Chronic obstructive pulmonary disease (COPD):** a prior history of COPD that has been diagnosed or treated with medication or chest physiotherapy.
- **Heart failure (CHF):** at least one of the following medical history cases must be present: paroxysmal nocturnal dyspnea, pulmonary rales, pulmonary congestion in the chest x-ray, dyspnea, or ventricular gallop.
- **Renal failure:** serum creatinine greater than 2 mg/dl.
- **Regular smoker:** any person who has smoked tobacco daily, regardless of the amount, for at least the last month. Our country, Spain, is currently among the highest per capita consumers of cigarettes (>2500 cigarettes/person/ year).
- **Drinker:** harmful alcohol consumption between 40-57gr/day depending on whether female or male or 35 to 50 units of a standard drink meaning 8-10 grams of absolute alcohol.
- **Endocarditis:** infectious inflammatory process located in the natural or prosthetic valves that were operated on.
- **Peripheral arterial disease (PAD):** This is considered to be present when the patient has intermittent claudication or underwent peripheral vascular surgery or non-traumatic amputation.
- **Ejection fraction of left ventricle (EF):** Normal>59%, Light 50-58%, 30-49% moderate, severe <30%.
- **Priority of the surgery: scheduled** (stable patients who undergo surgery on a scheduled basis), **priority** (the clinical picture does not allow for medical discharge even though one could wait a few days) and **urgent** (patients admitted to operating theatre with a cardiovascular emergency).
- **Kinesitherapy:** These are the different treatment techniques based on moving different parts of the body and they must be performed by a physiotherapist through medical prescription. Kinesitherapy can be passive, active-assisted, with resistance, or hydro-kinesitherapy.
- **Occupational Therapy:** This is the set of techniques and therapies used to prevent, restore and maintain the physical, mental and social state of individuals, helping in performing daily activities that are important for the patient's health and welfare.

- **Bentall technique:** This is a surgical technique that replaces the aortic root and aortic valve with a valved conduit (dacron graft*, which has a mechanical aortic valve prosthesis). It requires reimplanting the coronary arteries in the graft.
- **Inclusion (David) technique:** This is also called "aortic valve reimplantation" and consists of replacing the entire aortic root and reimplanting the coronary arteries while preserving the patient's aortic valve. This technique avoids the complications of mechanical prostheses and the anticoagulant treatment they need.
- **Electrotherapy:** This is the application of various types of electric currents for therapeutic purposes.
- **ASIA: American Spinal Injury Association.** The ASIA classification provides basic definitions for terms used in the assessment of spinal cord injury (SCI) and describes the neurological examination: **A:** complete SCI with lack of sensory and motor functions that extends to the sacral segments S4-S5. **B**: incomplete, with preservation of sensory function below the neurological level of injury, extending to sacral segments S4-S5 with absence of motor function. **C:** incomplete, with preservation of motor function below the neurological level and more than half of the key muscles below the neurologic level having a muscle grade lower than 3. **D:** incomplete, with preservation of motor function below the neurological level and more than half of the key muscles below the neurologic level having muscle grade of 3 or more. **E:** normal.
- **Key muscle groups:** 10 muscle groups that are assessed as part of the spinal cord standardized test (5 on the upper limb and 5 on the lower limb)

8. Results

8.1 Descriptive analysis

Of the 452 patients, 261 (57.7%) were men and 191 (42.3%) women. The overall average age was 66 years. The types of surgery carried out were divided into: aortic valve replacement + coronary artery bypass grafting (n=71, 15.7%; biological 57.7% and mechanical 42.3%), aortic valve replacement (n=227; biological 50.2%, mechanical 44.5%), aortic valve replacement and another valve (n=72, 15,9%; biological 9.7%, mechanical 90.3%), aortic valve replacement with insertion of tube due to aortic root aneurysm (Bentall's technique) (n=58; 12.8%) (Modified inclusion (David) technique) (n=10, 2,2%), aortic valve replacement (n=12; 2.6% 16.6% biological, 83.4% mechanical), by endoscopy (n=2; 0.4% 100% mechanical). 4% had a history of previous coronary artery bypass grafting. 94.7% of the surgery was scheduled, 2.65% was priority and 2.65% was urgent.

Of the 452 patients, 62.8% (284 patients) had hypertension, 20.8% (94 patients) DM, 48.4% (219 patients) DL, 7.5% (34 patients) COPD, 58.2% (263 patients) CHF with NYCA dyspnea classifications: I - 5.4%, II – 41.6%, III - 45% and IV – 7.8%. CRI was present in 8.4% (38 patients). 37.6% were smokers and 4.4% drinkers. 29.6% had calcified valves, and of these 57.4% were Ao, 18% were mitral, 2.2% were tricuspid, 0.7% were pulmonary and 23.1% had more than one. 4.2% had PAD. 21.2% had a history of chronic atrial fibrillation and 1.5% had had AMI within 3 months prior to the valvular surgery.

The average aortic clamping time was 101 minutes and the CPB was 125.2 minutes. On average 2 packed red cell transfusions were performed per patient.

There were 22 cases of Ao valve replacement for endocarditis due to multiple causes, including Arthrographis Kalrae Fungi, Streptococcus viridans (2 cases), Streptococcus bovis, Streptococcus mitis, Coxiella burnetii (Q fever), Enterococcus faecalis (3 cases), lactococcus, actinomyces odontolyticus, Granulicatella, pseudomonas aeruginosa, staphylococcus epidermidis, S. pneumoniae, 2 cases reported as Gram strains and two other cases as undetermined.

Drugs	Anti AHT	Sintrom	Diuretics	Hypolipemiant	Antiplatelet	OAD/Insulin
%	67	18.1	34.3	42.5	29.9	17.5

Table 2. Drugs used by patients with operation on the Ao valve

NC	STROKE	TIA	SCI	PN	Seizure	Stupor	Coma	CIP	ACS	Encephalopathy
%	1.5	0.67	0.4	0.2	1.3	1.3	0.4	1.1	6.6	5

Table 3. Percentages of NCs (neurological complications): TIA (transient ischemic attack), SCI Spinal Cord Injury, PN (peripheral neuropathy), CIP (critical illness polyneuropathy), ACS (confusional syndrome)

Table 3 shows the percentages of different NCs in Ao valve surgery. The rate of strokes was 1.5%, corresponding to 7 cases. Of these 7 cases, 2 came from the 71 patients who underwent valve replacement + CABG AO (2.8%), 3 were from the 227 patients that underwent single Ao valve replacement surgery (1.3%), one case was from the 72 patients who underwent multiple valve replacement (1.4%) and finally there was one case from the 12 patients who underwent a 2nd Ao valve replacement (8.3%). Table 4 shows the three most common NCs that have been seen in this study according to the different surgical techniques and the average times for CPB and Ao clamping measured in minutes.
Of the 23 cases of encephalopathy, 17.4% had a metabolic cause, in 56.5% the cause was hypoxic-ischemic and 26% had various causes. Of the strokes, 57.1% were right hemisphere and 42.9% were on the left. There was only one case in which the stroke was haemorrhagic. Of the ischemia (6 cases - 85.7%), 4 were of cardioembolic origin (66.6%), 2 border territory (33.3%) (Man in the Barrel Syndrome) and one was lacunar (16.6%).

Type of surgery	n	Stroke	ACS	Encephalopathy	T. CPB	T. Clamp
Replacement + CBPG	71	2(2.8)	8(11.3)	5(7)	128.5	105.7
1 Ao valve replacement	227	3(1.3)	12(5.3)	6(2.6)	96.5	75.4
Multiple vv replacement	72	1(1,4)	4(5.5)	5(6,9)	151.2	126.8
Ao root repl. (Bentall)	58	0	5(8.6)	5(8.6)	148.2	118.2
Ao root repl. (David)	10	0	0	0	133.6	129.2
2nd Ao valve repl.	12	1(8,3)	3(25)	2(16.6)	166.2	127.3
Endoscopic valve repl.	2	0	0	0	-	-

Table 4. Most common NC percentages according to the different techniques used. Ao (aorta), vv (valve), repl (replacement), n: total number of patients, ACS (acute confusional syndrome). T. CPB (cardiopulmonary bypass time measured in minutes), T. Clamp (aortic clamping time measured in minutes). CBPG (coronary artery bypass grafting)

There are only 2 cases described of spinal cord injury. One was a side effect of Ao valve replacement surgery and the other came after surgery for aortic arch replacement using the Bentall technique. The two cases were side effects to a spinal cord ischemia. One was a ASIA

A, D6 D7 Spinal Cord Injury Syndrome and the other was an ASIA C, D7-D8 spinal cord injury syndrome. Both patients were taken to a hospital specializing in spinal cord injury (National Hospital for Paraplegics in Toledo).
Overall mortality was 1.7% and in no way associated with cases of stroke, or with patients who suffered acute confusional state. There were, however, two deaths of patients with hypoxi-ischemic encephalopathy and multiple causes.
The average time of hospitalization was 18.7 days. Table 5 specifies the different durations of hospital stay depending on the surgery performed and the most common NCs suffered.

Type of surgery	Hospital stay without NCs	Stroke	Hospital stay	ACS	Hospital stay	Encephalopathy	Hospital stay
Replacement + CBPG	16	2	39	8	23	5	63.5
1 Ao valve replacement	12	3	23.3	12	21	6	58.2
Multiple v replacement.	18	1	68	4	17.7	5	60.5
Ao root repl. (Bentall)	16	0	16	5	24.8	5	33.1
Ao root repl. (David)	14.5	0	14.5	0	14.5	0	14.5
2nd AO v replacement	14	1	41	3	30	2	26.5
Endoscopic v. repl.	9	0	9	0	9	0	9

Table 5. Average hospitalization time measured in days in the most common NCs.
ACS = Acute confusional state

The most common risk factors associated with NCs are shown in Table 6.
As regards rehabilitation for these patients, 97.3% underwent pulmonary rehabilitation before and after surgery, aiming to prevent respiratory complications. 43.8% of patients had some type of neurological complication and needed kinesitherapy techniques. 3.5% required occupational therapy. 1.75% of patients with NCs underwent electrotherapy techniques. During this period, no patient required any type of orthosis and only one of them needed to use a walker at home.

RFs	AHT	DM	DL	COPD	CHF	CRI	Prior stroke
STROKE	85.7%	14.2%	42.8%	28.6%	85.7%	14.2%	42.8%
ACS	53.1%	34.3%	31.2%	6.2%	46.9%	15.6%	12.5%
Encephal.	73.9%	21.7%	39.1%	-	65.2%	21.7%	17.4%
	Smokers	Drinkers	PAD	AT	AF	AMI	-
STROKE	42.8%	14.2%	14.2%	14.2%	28.6%	-	-
ACS	28.1%	6.25%	6.25%	-	21.9%	3.1%	-
Encephal.	43.5%	4.3%	-	4.3%	34.8%	-	-

Table 6. Risk factors for NC in Ao valve surgery in %. RFs (risk factors), AHT (arterial hypertension), DM (Diabetes Mellitus), DL (dyslipidemia), COPD (chronic obstructive pulmonary disease), CHF (heart failure), CRF (chronic renal failure), PAD (peripheral arterial disease), AT (atheromatous plaques in Ao), AF (a history of chronic atrial fibrillation), AMI (history of acute myocardial infarction in the last three months)

9. Discussion

NCs are still a common cause of morbidity and mortality in postoperative patients who have undergone aortic valve surgery. Although much has been achieved, there are still many issues to resolve. The research is complex because of the many variables to be considered.

Recent neuropsychological studies have shown that over 50% of patients undergoing cardiac surgery suffer brain injury, as evidenced by a CT scan or MRI (Mc Khan et al., 1997; Hallow et al, 1999).

As regards the sex of the patients, the percentages are fairly balanced (57.7% men and 42.3% women), which is a difference compared to other studies where the male sex clearly prevails over females (Hallow et al, 1999).

Our study evaluates the type of technique used in aortic valve surgery, focusing on the paradigm that with strokes as a neurological complication fewer complications have arisen than in other studies (Zabala, 2005). These averages in Ao valve replacement surgery + coronary artery bypass grafting were 2.8% compared to 3.3%, and in patients undergoing single Ao valve replacement they came to 1.3% compared to 3.3%. In the patients who underwent multiple valve replacement the percentage was 1.4% as opposed to 6.7%, and finally out of the patients that underwent a 2nd Ao valve replacement the percentage was 8.3%. (Table 4.)

The NCs evident in postoperative aortic surgery are in keeping with the big series: 0.4% for coma, 6.6% for ACS, 1.5% for STROKE and 5% for encephalopathy (Murkin, 1993, Harrison, 1995; Filsoufi et al, 2008), although there are others in which the incidence is higher (Bucerius et al, 2004).

Identifying predictors for NCs is important for understanding the pathogenesis of these complications as well as for developing preventive strategies (Mornals K et al, 1998; Tjang YS et al, 2007). According to the results of our study, the most influential risk factors in the development of intraoperative and postoperative NCs in aortic valve surgery are: arterial hypertension, heart failure, smoking, having a previous stroke, dyslipidemia and atrial fibrillation in this order, with lesser importance attached to COPD, diabetes mellitus, CRF, being a heavy drinker and peripheral arterial disease. The CPB and aortic clamping time is seen to be longer in cases where there is a NC but with no clearly significant relationship.

As regards strokes, we found that 85.7% were ischemic, as in other studies (Zabala, 2005), but the percentages into which the ischemic strokes are usually divided are not what we found in this study. 4 were of cardioembolic origin (66.6%), 2 border territory (33.3%) (Man in the Barrel Syndrome) and one lacunar (16.6%), whereas in the recorded literature 50% are usually due to atherothrombotic causes, 25% are lacunar (related to a chronic hypertension), 20% cardioembolic, and there remain 5% in which we most often include border zone infarctions in cardiac surgery.

The aortic valve surgery that proportionately produces the most NCs is 2nd aortic valve replacement followed by Ao valve replacement + coronary artery bypass grafting, aortic root replacement (Bentall) (17.2%), multiple valve replacement and finally single Ao valve replacement. Table 4.

As for the 22 cases of endocarditis, 50% occurred in single aortic valve replacement, followed by 27.2% in multiple replacement surgery, and 9% in both second valve replacement and aortic arch replacement. Of these 22 cases, 2 of them had a stroke, one an acute confusional syndrome and 3 suffered encephalopathy. 11 of them were operated on a valve and 11 on a prosthetic valve. The bacteria that produced it and the complications are

similar to other work associated with the incidence of endocarditis (Arauz-Gongora et al, 1998).
The average times for aortic clamping and CPB were 101 and 125.2 minutes respectively. This is somewhat higher in some of the surgeries with more NCs such as in 2nd valve replacement, followed by multiple valve replacement and aortic arch replacement (Bentall). Table 4.
Overall mortality was 1.7% and in no way associated with cases of stroke, or with patients who suffered acute confusional state. There were, however, two deaths of patients with hypoxi-ischemic encephalopathy and multiple causes. These results are similar to other publications. However, in our work the appearance of a neurological complication did not significantly increase mortality (Redmond et al, 1996). There are groups with no mortality although the number of patients is lower (n=118) (Mutarelli EG et al, 1993).
The length of hospital stay increases dramatically when there are NCs, as evidenced in other works. Table 5.
The data provided in connection with rehabilitation techniques carried out fall far short because many patients were referred to another hospital area in Madrid or another province of Spain and continued the rehabilitation in places near their original home.
This study is limited mainly in that it is a retrospective study and this prevents us from knowing the exact time of the onset of the NC and therefore we cannot draw valid conclusions regarding the type of NC, the rehabilitation treatment carried out and the prognosis.

10. Conclusions

According to the results of our study, cardiovascular aortic valve surgery has similar incidence of postoperative NC when compared with bypass surgery or combined surgeries. The risk factors in order of importance were: a history of arterial hypertension, heart failure, dyslipidemia, having a previous stroke and being a smoker.
NCs after aortic valve surgery have been associated with increased morbidity and mortality, with increased hospitalization time and rehabilitation costs, and they thus contribute to decreased quality of life. The incidence of NCs has remained unchanged in recent years, despite increasing age and comorbidity. The improvement in technical advances has contributed to keeping these percentages up.
Although most complications can be associated with cardiopulmonary bypass, other factors are also involved. Identifying high-risk patients may reduce the incidence of complications in high risk groups, but this seems to be a poor prevention strategy.
In an increasingly aging population and with a growing number of diseases, prevention strategies should focus on three aspects: firstly, technical improvements in cardiac surgery and cerebral protection, secondly, identifying reliable techniques to assess neuropsychological dysfunction after cardiac surgery, and finally carrying out technical training in rehabilitation to avoid or minimize the side effects as a result of NCs arising from aortic surgery.

11. References

Arauz-Góngora AA, Souta-Meiriño CA, Cotter-Lemus LE, Guzman-Rodriguez C, Méndez Dominguez A. The neurological complications of infectus endocarditis. Arch Inst Cardiol Mex. 1998 68(4): 328-32

Asenbaum S, Zeitlhofer J, Spiss C, Wolner E, Deecke L. Neurologic and psychiatric complications after heart surgery. *Klin Wochenschr.* 1991; 69(8):368-73

Bendszus M, Reents W, Franke D, Mullges W, Babin-Ebell J, Koltzenburg M, et al. Brain damage after coronary artery bypass grafting. Arch Neurol. 2002;59:1090-5

Benecke R, Klingelhöfer J, Rieke H, Conrad B, de Vivie R. Form of manifestations and course of brachial plexus lesions following medial sternotomy. *Nervenarzt.* 1988; 59(7):388-92.

Beran E, Marzouk JF, Dimitri WR. Bilateral phrenic nerve palsy following aortic valve surgery. *J Card Surg.* 202008 Nov-Dec; 23(6):691-2.

Bocerius J., Gummert J.F., Borger M.A., Walther T., Doll N., Onnasch J.F. et al. Stroke after cardiac surgery: a risk factor analysis of 16184 consecutive patients. *Ann Thorac Surg.* 2004; 78(2):755-6

Boeken U, Litmathe J, Feindt P, Gams E. Neurological complications after cardiac surgery: risk factors and correlation to the surgical procedure. *Thorac Cardiovasc Surg.* 2005; 53:33-6

Caplan L. R., Hurts J.W., Ghimowitz M.I. Clinical Naurocardiology, 1st edition: 226-257,1999.

Clau Terré F (2009) Estudio de la morbimortalidad de la cirugía cardiaca de revascularización coronaria. Efectos clínicos y repercusiones de la cirugía extracorpórea. [Doctoral Thesis], Zaragoza. Universidad de Zaragoza

Filsoufi F, Rahmanian PB, Castillo JG, Bronster D, Adams DH. Incedence, imaging analysis, and early and late outcomes of stroke after cardiac valve operation. *Am J Cardiol* 2008; 15; 101(10):1472-8

Forteza A, Prieto G, Centeno J, Cortina J. A modified David technique in endocarditis with multiple paravalvular abscesses. *J Heart Valve Dis.* 2010; 19(2):254-6.

Hallow L., Lanternier G., Diez M., Barbagelata A., Gabet E., García M. et al. Complicaciones neurológicas en el posoperatorio inmediato de una cirugía cardiovascular. Incidencia, pronóstico y factores de riesgo. *Revista Argentina de Cardiología.* 1999; 67: 617-23

Harrison MJG. Neurologic complications of coronary artery bypass grafting: Diffuse or focal ischemia? Ann Thorac Surg 1995; 59:1356-1358

Hogue Ch.W. Jr, Murphy S.F., Schechtman K.B, Dávila-Román V.C. Risk factors for early or delayed stroke after cardiac surgery. Circulation.1999; 100:642-7

Jacobs A, Neveling M, Horst M, Ghaemi M, Kessler J, Eichstaedt H, et al. Alterations of neuropsychological function and cerebral glucose metabolism after cardiac surgery are not related only to intraoperative microembolic events. *Stroke.* 1998; 29(3):660-7

Kirali K, Mansuroglu D, Omeroglu SN, Erentug V, Mataraci I, Ipek G, et al. Five-year experience in aortic root replacement with the flanged composite graft. Ann Thorac Surg. 2002;73(4):1130-7

Martin C, Forteza A, Navarro M, Cortina J. Isquemia medular aguda tras cirugía de disección de aorta ascendente tipo 1 de DeBakey. Rev Esp Cardiol 2007; 60: 1102-1103

Mc Khanan GM, Goldsborough MA, Borowicz LM. Predictors of stroke risk coronary artery bypass patients. Ann Thorac Surg.1997; 63:516-521

Mills SA. Risk factors for cerebral injury and cardiac surgery. *Ann Thorac Surg* 1995; 59:1296-1299

Mornals K, Santos J, Gonzalez-Prendes CM, Rodriguez F, García B, Sainz H. Disfunción neurológica en la cirugía cardiovascular: acercamiento al tema. Rev Cubana Cardiol Cardiovasc. 1998; 24(1):20-8

Murkin JM. Anesthesia, the brain, and cardiopulmonary bypass. *Ann Thorac Surg*. 1993; 56:1461-63

Mutarelli EG, GonÇalves MM, Bonetti E, Auler Jr JO, Carvalho MJ, Menezes VL et al. Neurologic evaluation of 118 patients in the first postoperative period of cardiovascular surgery. *Arq Neuropsiquiatr*. 1993; 51(2):179-82

Redmon JM, Greene P, Goldsborough MA. Neurologic injury in cardiac surgical patients with a history of stroke. *Ann Thorac Surg* 1996; 61:42-47

Roach GW, Kanchuger M, Mangano CM, Newman M, Nussmeier N, Wolman R, et al for the Multicenter Study of perioperative ischemia Research Group and the isquemia Research and Education Foundation Investigators. Adverse cerebral outcomes after coronary bypass surgery. *N Engl J Med*. 1996; 335:1857-63

Sanz-Ayán M.P, Rodríguez-Palero S, Garzón-Márquez F.M, Sánchez-Callejas S, Pérez-Novales D. Síndrome del "hombre en Barril". A propósito de un caso. Rehabilitación (Madr). 2008; 42 (5):256-9

Sotaniemi K.A., Monomen H., Hokkanen T.E. Longterm cerebral outcome after open heart surgery. A five year neurophysiological follows up study. *Stroke* 17: 410-416, 1986

Tjang YS, van Hees Y, Körfer R, Grobbee DE, van der Heijden GJ. Predictors of mortality after aortic valve replacement. Eur J Cardiothorac Surg. 2007; 32(3):469-74.

Zabala J.A. Complicaciones neurológicas de la cirugía cardiaca. *Rev Esp Cardiol*. 2005; 58(9):1003-6

Part 6

Congenital Anomaly Application

12

Correction of Transposition of Great Arteries with Ventricular Septal Defect and Left Outflow Tract Obstruction with Double Arterial Translocation with Preservation of the Pulmonary Valve

Gláucio Furlanetto and Beatriz H. S. Furlanetto
Furlanetto Institute
Brazil

1. Introduction

Transposition of the great arteries (TGA) was first recognized by Mathew Bailie in 1797. The term transposition of the aorta and pulmonary artery (PA) was applied by Farre in 1814. Van Praagh proposed that TGA was one variety of malposition of the great arteries secondary to aberrations in conotruncal development. The other tipes of malposition include double-outlet right ventricle, double-outlet left ventricle, and anatomically corrected malposition. According the Congenital Heart Surgery Nomenclature and Database Project (James 2000), TGA always has discordant ventriculoarterial alignment such that the aorta arises entirely or in large party from the right ventricle (RV), the PA arises entirely or in large part above the left ventricle (LV) and concordant atrioventricular alignment is nearly always present. The term simple TGA has come to be used to denote those patients without associated ventricular septal defect (VSD) or left ventricular outflow tract obstruction (LVOTO) and nearly 75% of TGA patients have the simple type. Usually in the simple form of TGA the left ventricle doesn't has subpulmonary conus, so there is fibrous continuity between pulmonary and mitral valves, and tha aorta is anterior and to the right of the PA. The VSD occur in 40-45% of TGA patients and about 30% of these defects will be very small. LVOTO occurs in 25% of patients and is rare in patients with intact ventricular septum, ocurring in 5%. Approximated 30% of patients with TGA-VSD have LVOTO. A subvalvar LVOTO can be dynamic, localized fibrous ring, diffuse tunnel-like obstruction, muscular obstruction related to malposition of the outlet septum and LVOTO result from malposition of the mitral apparatus on the interventricular septum.

TGA is the second more common cyanotic congenital heart disease (CHD) and represents approximately 5-7% of all CHD and has a incidence of 20-30 in 100.000 live births, with a male preponderance of approximately 2:1. In patients with TGA, VSD and LVOTO early survival reaches 70% at one year and 29% at 5 years. Neonates with TGA, VSD and severe LVOTO have diminished pulmonary blood flow and they represents 5-8% of neonatal TGA population. Clinical findings are similar to those in the infants with tetralogy of Fallot with severe pulmonar stenosis.

The physiologic abnormalitie in TGA is that systemic and pulmonary circulations function in parallel rather in series as in normal infance, the consequence is deficiency of oxygen supply to the tissues. The arterial oxigen saturation and the extend of intercirculatory mixing dependents on the number, size and position of the anatomic communications like atrial septal defect (ASD), VSD and persistent ductus arteriosus.
Infants with TGA, VSD and LVOTO have been successfully palliated with systemic-to-pulmonary anastomosis with a politetrafluorethilene (PTFE) modified Blalock-Taussig shunt. In these patients the intracardiac correction is carried out at later age. The optimal age for the performance of a corretive repair remains controversial because of the balance between palliation and correction. Palliation leads to the performance of Rastelli repair at an older age with larger conduits, therefore reducing the need for reoperations. However, palliation also leads to LV overloading, and cyanosis.
The conventional surgical technique to repair TGA, VSD and LVOTO is the Rastelli operation (Rastelli, 1969). This operation was described with the theoretic advantage of incorporating the left ventricle as the systemic ventricle for correction of TGA. This technique achieves redirection of the left ventricular outflows and relieves pulmonary stenosis by bypassing it. The repair consists of: 1) repair of the VSD with a patch in such a way to connect the LV with the aorta using the closure of the right ventricle outflow as part of the left ventricular outflow, 2) division of the pulmonary artery and oversewn the cardiac end and 3) reconstruction of the pulmonary artery with a valved conduit. However, the Rastelli operation is far from ideal because it is not feasible in many patients because of unfavorable intracardiac anatomy, it requires the use of a prosthetic conduit for the reconstruction of the pulmonary outflow tract and the intraventricular tunnel used at Rastelli operation is not ideal because it can show some degree of stenosis at medium follow-up.
The Lecompte procedure, or "reparation a l'etage ventriculaire" (Borromée, 1988) is a surgical procedure that resects the infundibular septum to creates a large communication between the LV and the aorta. The aim of this resection is to construct a straight and direct aortic outflow tract to the aortic valve. The aorta is connected to the LV with a patch smaller than in the Rastelli operation and the tunnel between the LV and aorta is situated just beneath the aorta orifice and occupies very little space in the RV cavity. The pulmonary artery is transected above the pulmonary valve and is translocated onto the subaortic ventricular incision and the pulmonary outflow tract was completed with an anterior patch and a monocusp pericardial valve.
Double-outlet LV is conventionally correct with an intraventricular tunnel or with an extracardiac conduit when pulmonary stenosis is present. Pulmonary root translocation with the pulmonary valve to the RV is an important alternative surgical technique to correct this CHD (Chiavarelli, 1992).
This concept was used to correct TGA, VSD and LVOTO (Silva, 2000). In this procedure the pulmonary artery and its branches were dissected from the aorta and its posterior connections. The pulmonary root was dissected from the LV with the pulmonary valve. Than the VSD is closed, diverting the blood from the LV to the aorta like in the Rastelli operation and the pulmonary root is translocated to the RV. The follow-up of two children showed that the pulmonary root diameter can grown.
The Nikaidoh procedure (Nikaidoh, 1984) changed the concept to treat the LVOTO. In this procedure, after dissection of the aorta and the main pulmonary artery, the ascending aorta was totally mobilized with the aortic valve and the coronary arteries, the pulmonary artery is transected just above the pulmonary valve. The pulmonary annulus, subpulmonic fibrous

tissue, and the crista supraventricularis is transected anteriorly into the superior corner of the VSD. The ascending aorta is moved posteriorly and sutured to the posterior pulmonary annulus. The large anterior defect is now closed, from the margin of the VSD to the aortic root. A large pericardial patch is utilized to reconstruct the continuity of the RV outflow without implant of pulmonary valve.

The Nikaidoh procedure was modified by Hu (Hu, 2007). In this procedure the ascending aorta and the pulmonary trunk were transected and the coronary arteries were detached. The pulmonary root and the ascending aortic with the aorta valve were dissected out of ventricles. The subvalvar stenosis was relieved by resecting the conal septum, the VSD is closed and the detached ascending aorta with the aortic valve is translocated posteriorly and coronary arteries was reimplanted. After the Lecompte maneuver the pulmonary root is translocated anteriorly to the RV outflow. The pulmonary root is incised and a monocusp bovine jugular vein was used to enlarge the RV outflow tract.

Direct surgical relief of severe LVOTO depends on the anatomic type and severity of obstruction. In patients with mild LVOTO it can be resected and the Jatene arterial switch operation (Jatene, 1976) can be done.

Another surgical approach is the aortic root translocation plus arterial switch (Bautista-Hernandez, 2007). In this surgical technique proposed by del Nido a segment of the ascending aorta was transected from the right ventricle. The coronary arteries were excised as circular shape from the ascending aorta than the main pulmonary artery was transected. The ampliation of the LVOTO was made like the Nilaidoh procedure from the pulmonary annulus toward the VSD. The aortic autograft was sewn to the LV outflow and to the ascending aorta after the Lecompte maneuver. Reimplantation of the coronary arteries was performed into the neoaorta. The RV to pulmonary arteries continuity was established by a homograft.

We proposed a new approach for correction of TGA, VSD and LVOTO performing the double arterial translocation with preservation of the pulmonary valve. In this surgical technique the ascending aorta is translocated with the aortic valve and the coronary arteries to the left ventricle, after correction of left outflow tract obstruction and correction of the VSD, associated to pulmonary root translocation to the right ventricle, conserving integrally the pulmonary valve (Furlanetto, 2010).

2. Double arterial translocation with preservation of the pulmonary valve, surgical technique

This procedure was achieved employing cardiopulmonary bypass with hypothermia at 25°C and myocardial protection with warm induction blood cardioplegic solution at a proportion of 3:1 followed by hypothermic cardioplegic solution and modified ultrafiltration. Initially an incision inferior to the aortic valve was made, excising the ascending aorta (including aortic valve and coronary arteries) beneath the annular level of aortic valve from the right ventricle. Then we performed the excision of the pulmonary root, including pulmonary valve, beneath the annular level of the pulmonary valve from the left ventricle [figure 1]. After section of the infundibular septum in direction to the VSD, the LVOT and the VSD was closed with glutharaldeide-fixed bovine pericardium patch [figure 2]. The resulting gap of the aortic translocation was partially closed with fresh autologous pericardium. Finally the ascending aorta with the aortic valve and the coronary arteries were sutured into the left ventricle outflow and the pulmonary root with the pulmonary valve was sutured into the right ventricular outflow [figure 3].

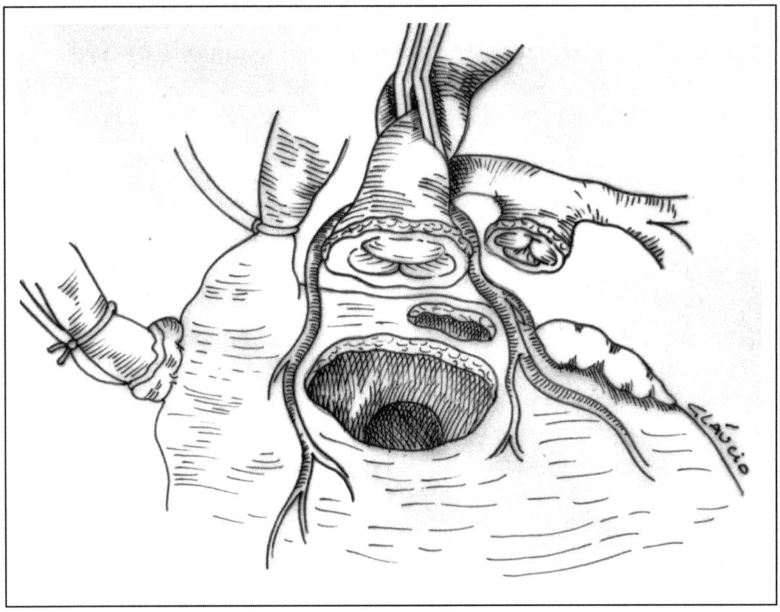

Fig. 1. Double arterial translocation with preservation of the pulmonary valve. Withdrawal of the ascending aorta with the aortic valve and coronary arteries from the right ventricle and removal of the pulmonary trunk with the pulmonary valve from the left ventricle

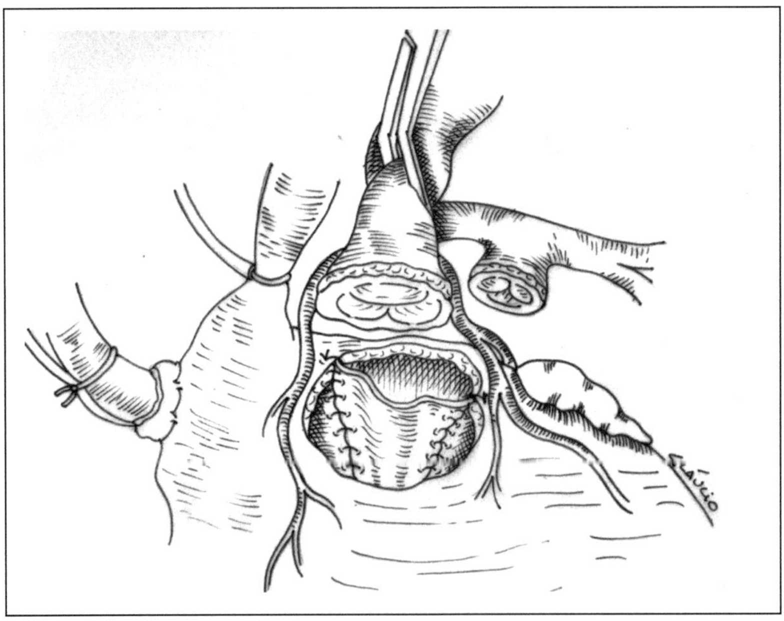

Fig. 2. Double arterial translocation with preservation of the pulmonary valve. After section of the pulmonary ring and infundibular septum toward the interventricular communication, an enlargement of the left ventricle outflow tract and a closure of interventricular communication was carried out using a glutaraldehyde-fixed bovine pericardium graft

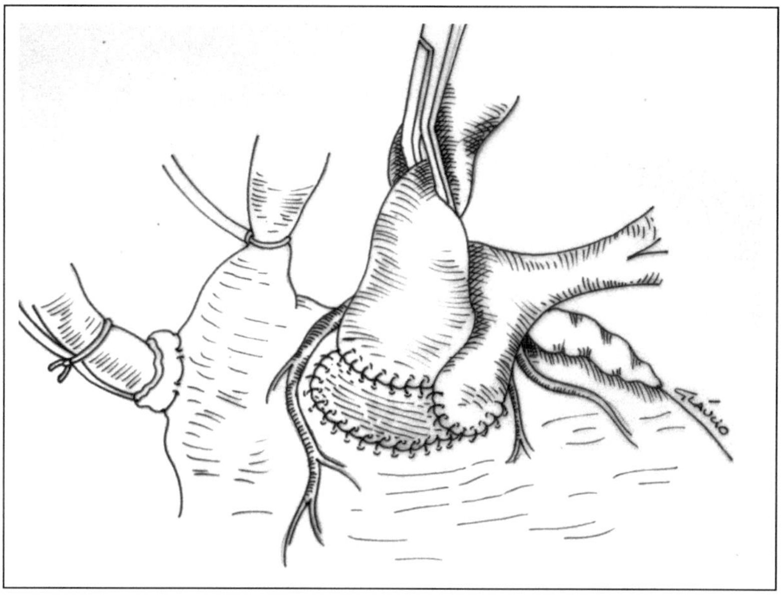

Fig. 3. Double arterial translocation with preservation of the pulmonary valve. The resulting opening from resection of the ascending aorta was partially closed to the right with a fresh autologous pericardial patch. The ascending aorta with the coronary arteries and the aortic valve was sutured to the left ventricle outflow tract and the pulmonary trunk with the pulmonary valve was sutured to the right ventricle outflow tract

2.1 Patients, general

Between November 1994 and June 2011, a total of 212 consecutive children with TGA were submitted to surgical treatment at the Hospital São Joaquim da Real e Benemérita Associação Portuguesa de Beneficência as follows: simple TGA (n = 110; 51,8%); TGA, VSD (n = 66; 31,1%); TGA, VSD and LVOTO (n = 34; 16,0%). The diagnosis was based on color echodopplercardiographic findings. The following procedures were used in children with TGA, VSD and LVOTO: modified BT shunt (n = 10), Rastelli procedure (n = 13), Jatene procedure (n = 3) and arterial translocation procedure (n = 8), with two further divisions - modified Nikaidoh (n = 5) and double arterial translocation with preservation of pulmonary valve (n = 3).

In the modified BT shunt group, the VSD was not committed in two patients. Two patients had mitral valve straddling. Two patients had sistemic-pulmonar collateral arteries and one patient had multiple VSD. Seven patients were neonates, one was 2 months old and two patients were 1 year old. The mean weight was 4,3 kg (range 1,8 kg - 8,8 kg). In the Rastelli group three patients had previous modified BT shunt. Two patients had restrictive VSD. One patient had mitral valve insuficience and one patient had right pulmonary artery stenosis. Five patients were neonates, five patients were younger than 1 year of age (mean age was 6,2 months; range 2 months-eleven months), three patients were older than 1 year of age (mean age was 5,6 years; range 3 years - ten years). The mean weight was 7,9 kg (range 3,0 kg - 28,0 kg). In the Jatene procedure two patients were neonates and one patient was 4 months old. The mean weight was 3,8 kg (range 2,9 kg - 5,2 kg). In the arterial translocation group two patients had previous modified BT shunt and one patient had two previous modified BT shunt. Three patients were neonates, one patient was 6 months old and four patients were older than 1 year of age (mean age was 1,6 years; range 1 year - 2 years). The mean weight was 7,0 kg (range 2,6 kg - 11,3 kg).

2.1.1 Patients, double arterial translocation with preservation of the pulmonary valve

Three children with TGA with perimembranous VSD and LVOTO type-fibromuscular tubular obstruction associated to hypoplasia of the pulmonary valve ring underwent doble arterial translocation with preservation of the pulmonary valve: Patient 1, female, aged two years, weighing 10.8 kg, underwent two previous Blalock-Taussig shunt surgeries. Preoperative color Doppler echocardiography revealed a LVOTO gradient of 40 mmHg. CPB time was 195 minutes and the aortic clamping time was 123 minutes. Pressure measurement after surgical correction revealed a ratio of systolic pressure between the RV and LV (RV/LV) of 0.6 and a pulmonary gradient of 25 mmHg. The postoperative Doppler echocardiography revealed a pulmonary transvalvular gradient of 42 mmHg; Patient 2, male, aged 6 months, weighting 7.3 kg. Preoperative Doppler echocardiography revealed LVOT gradient of 65 mmHg. CPB time was 184 minutes and aortic clamping time was 140 minutes. Pressure measurement after surgical correction revealed RV/LV systolic pressure of 0.8 and pulmonary transvalvular gradient of 30 mmHg. Postoperative Doppler echocardiography revealed a pulmonary transvalvular gradient of 31 mmHg. Heart computaticional angiotomography (CT) performed during the immediate postoperative period showed appropriate positioning of the pulmonary trunk, pulmonary artery and aorta in both patients (Figure 4).
Patient 3, male, aged 1 year, weighting 8.0 kg. Preoperative Doppler echocardiography revealed LVOT gradient of 31 mmHg. CPB time was 182 minutes and aortic clamping time was 155 minutes. Pressure measurement after surgical correction revealed RV/LV systolic pressure of 0.7 and pulmonary transvalvular gradient of 30 mmHg.

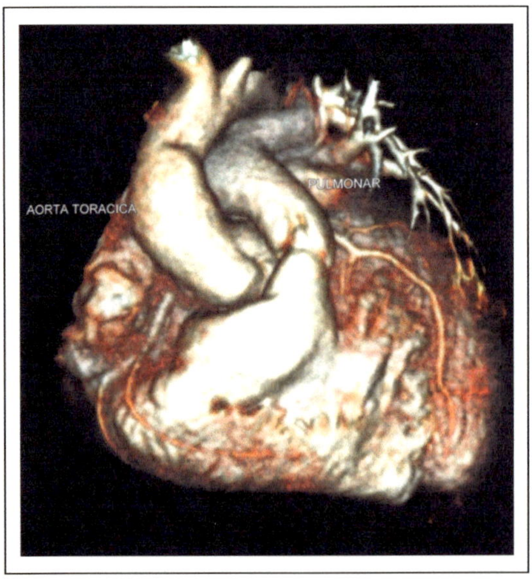

Fig. 4. Double arterial translocation with preservation of the pulmonary valve.
CT angiography performed in the immediate postoperative period showed appropriate positioning of the pulmonary artery and pulmonary branches as well as the ascending aorta

2.1.2 Surgical technique

The palliative BT shunt was made by median sternotomy in seven patients, by right thoracotomy in two patients and by left thoracotomy in one patient. The interposition of a polytetrafluoroethylene (PTFE) tube was made between the innominate artery and the right pulmonary artery in nine patients, and between the left subclavian artery and the left pulmonary artery in one patient. In seven patients the diameter of the PTFE tube was 4 mm, and in three patients it was 5 mm. The Rastelli, Jatene and modified Nikaido procedures and double arterial translocation with preservation of the pulmonary valve were made by median sternotomy and moderate hypothermic cardiopulmonary bypass and myocardial protection with warm cardioplegic induction, followed by hypothermic blood cardioplegic solution at a proportion of 3:1 every 20 minutes. In the Rastelli procedure, the VSD was repaired through the right ventriculotomy in such a way to connect the left ventricle to aorta. The reconstruction of the pulmonary artery was performed with a glutaraldehyde-fixed bovine pericardium valved conduit in eight patients and with a glutaraldehyde-fixed bovine-valved jugular vein in six patients. In the Jatene group, the LVOTO was a subvalvar fibromuscular ridge. After aorta transection was performed resection of the localized LVOTO. The pulmonary trunk was transected proximal to its bifurcation. After the LeCompte maneuver, a button of the left and right coronary artery was excised from its sinus, and was inserted into the neoaorta. Coronary type was Yacoulb I in all patients. The reconstruction of the neopulmonar was done with a single, fresh autologous pericardium patch. In the modified Nikaidoh group the aorta was translocated with the aortic valve and coronary arteries to the left ventricle, after an enlargement of the left ventricle outflow tract and closure of VSD with a single glutaraldehyde-fixed preserved bovine pericardium patch. In this series of patients we used a valved conduit to reconstruct the right ventricular outflow. This approach was different from the original technique, in which the pulmonary trunk is used without a valve. We used a glutharaldeide-fixed valved bovine jugular vein in three patients. In one patient a glutharaldeide-fixed valved bovine pericardium conduit was used, and in one patient a Lhydro porcine valved pulmonary trunk [8]. During the analyzed period there was a change in the surgical procedure. At first, modified BT technique prevailed; later, Rastelli operation and Jatene operation were performed, and finally the arterial translocation operation.

3. Results

Two patients died in the modified BT shunt group (20%), three patients died in the Rastelli group (23,0%) and one patient died in the arterial translocation group (20%). All patients in the Jatene group and in the double arterial translocation with preservation of the pulmonary valve all patients survived. The statistical analyses (Fisher's Exact Test) showed no difference between all groups ($p = 0.811$).

4. Comments

The surgical management of TGA with VSD and LVOTO is a surgical challenge. The Rastelli operation remains the most applied procedure for this congenital cardiopathy.

The most appropriate timing of the Rastelli operation is controversial. When it is performed during early infancy, it is a physiologic correction and avoids systemic hypoxemia. On the other hand, the palliative procedure of modified BT shunt performed during early infancy avoids early reoperation to change the valved conduit.

There is a significant incidence of late mortality after Rastelli procedure, with survival rate of 82% at 5 years and 52% at 20 years. In 25 years of experience, Kreutzer noticed that the most common cause of late death was left ventricular failure, present in 25% of patients (Kreutzer, 2000). The intraventricular tunnel from left ventricle to aorta is tortuous and can develop stenosis in the late follow-up, which can explain the left ventricle disfunction. The presence of valved conduit dysfunction and right ventricular dysfunction may be associated with ventricular tachycardia and sudden cardiac death. Therefore, all patients submitted to Rastelli procedure will need to change the right ventricle to pulmonary artery conduit once. In the Lecompte procedure, the resection of the infundibular septum creates a straight, direct tunnel between the left ventricle to aorta occupying little space in the right ventricle outflow tract, in order to improve the intraventricular tunnel from the left ventricle to aorta. This procedure presents a better solution to the left ventricle outflow tract reconstruction, but in the right ventricle outflow the monocuspid pericardial valve used will develop some dysfunction on medium-term follow-up. The percentage of reoperation in patients submitted to LeCompte procedure is lower when compared to Rastelli procedure. A very interesting option to correct TGA, VSD and LVOTO is the Nikaidoh procedure. In this procedure, aortic translocation with the aortic valve and coronary arteries to the left ventricle, after enlargement of the left ventricular outflow and closure of the VSD with a single patch, creates an anatomical left ventricle outflow, but reconstruction of the right ventricle outflow without the pulmonary valve will cause right ventricle dysfunction. The Hu procedure utilizes the aortic translocation like the Nikaidoh procedure but translocating the pulmonary root and amplificating the pulmonary valve with a bovine jugular vein monocuspid to the right ventricle after performing the LeCompte maneuver performed to reconstruction of the right ventricle outflow. This procedure corrects the left ventricle outflow in an anatomical way, but the amplification of the pulmonary valve with a bovine jugular vein monocusp will certainly cause dysfunction of the pulmonary valve at medium-term follow-up. The use of Silva procedure could avoid the reoperation to change the valved conduit. In this operation the pulmonary root is translocated with the pulmonary valve to the ventriculotomy on the right ventricle with expansion of the pulmonary root after dissection from the right ventricle. There is also the possibility of growth, because all the structures of the pulmonary root were preserved, but the correction of the left ventricle outflow tract is done like the Rastelli procedure with all disadvantages of this procedure. The surgery proposed by del Nido translocate a segment of the ascending aorta with anastomoses of the coronary arteries after enlargement of the left ventricle outflow tract employing a homograft to reconstruct the right ventricle outflow tract. Like in the Nikaidoh and Hu procedures the left outflow tract is anatomical but the use of a homograft at the right side will need change of the graft at medium follow-up.

The surgical technique that we performed, the double arterial translocation with preservation of the pulmonary valve, differs from all the other techniques used up to now because it corrects LVOTO through the aorta translocation with the aortic valve and coronary arteries after enlargement of the left outflow tract and closure of the VSD with a patch and corrects the right ventricle outflow with pulmonary root translocation with entire pulmonary valve to the right ventricle without the LeCompte maneuver and without right ventricolotomy. We believed that this procedure can be performed in patients with TGA, VSD and LVOTO when the pulmonary valve has an adequate annular diameter and the leaflets thickness is not too exacerbated. In these cardiopathies the LVOTO is subvalvar and valvar. The subvalvar stenosis is in the form of a localized fibrous ring, a tunnel-type fibromuscular or a muscular obstruction. The valvar stenosis is caused by annular hypoplasia and the valve could be bicuspid.

The use of prosthetic valves and of a connection without valve in the pulmonary position in children brings about dysfunction of the right ventricle on medium/late-term follow up. Based on this fact, the preservation of the native pulmonary valve with mild to moderate residual gradient has been accepted in the correction of tetralogy of Fallot by Voges (Voges 2008), who admit the size of the pulmonary valve with z-score superior to -4. This concept can also be used in the conservation of the pulmonary valve performed at double arterial translocation with preservation of the pulmonary valve. It is possible that the pulmonary root could grow and the use of this surgical technique could diminish reoperation rates in these patients, but a late follow-up will be necessary to verify the potential of valve growth.

In one child submitted to double arterial translocation with preservation of the pulmonary valve the preoperative color doppler echocardiography revealed a LVOTO gradient of 40mmHg. The transvalvar gradient between the right ventricle and the pulmonary trunk measured in the operating room after surgical correction was 25mmHg, and the postoperative doppler echocardiography revealed a pulmonary transvalvar gradient of 42mmHg. In another child, submitted to the same procedure, the preoperative color doppler echocardiography revealed a LVOTO gradient of 65mmHg. The transvalvar gradient between the right ventricle and the pulmonary trunk measured in the operating room after surgical correction was 30mm Hg and the postoperative doppler echocardiography revealed a pulmonary transvalvar gradient of 31mmHg. Heart computadorized angio-tomography performed during the immediate postoperative period showed appropriate positioning of the pulmonary trunk, the pulmonary artery and the aorta in both patients [Figure 4]. One third patient with preoperative Doppler echocardiography revealed a LVOT gradient of 31 mmHg. The pressure measurement after surgical correction revealed RV/LV systolic pressure of 0.7 and pulmonary transvalvular gradient of 30 mmHg.

5. Conclusion

We can conclude that there was an evolution in the approach of TGA, VSD and LVOTO. The modified BT shunt operation, the operation of Rastelli and more recently the Jatene operation, modified Nikaidoh and the double translocation with preservation of the pulmonary valve were responsible for part of this evolution. In spite of the increase of surgical difficulty, there was no significant difference in the mortality. A late follow-up of a larger series of children will be important to check the potential development of the pulmonary valve in the double arterial translocation with preservation of the pulmonary valve.

6. References

Jaggers, J. J.; Cameron, D. E.; Herlong, R. Et al. (2000). Congenital Heart Surgery Nomenclature and Database Project: transposition of the great arteries. *Ann Thorac Surg*, Vol 69 (3) suppl 1, PP. 205-235.

Rastelli, C. ; Wallace, R.B. & Ongley, A. (1969). Complete repair of transposition of the great arteries with pulmonary stenosis. A review and report of a case corrected by using a new surgical technique. *Circulation*, Vol.39, (Jannuary 1969), pp. 83-95.

Borroomee, L.; Batisse, A.; Lecompte, Y. et al. (1988). Anatomic repair of anomalies of ventriculoarterial connection associated with ventricular septal defect. II. Clinical results in 50 patients with pulmonary outflow tract obstruction. *J Thorac Cardiovasc Surg,* Vol.95, (January 1988), pp. 96-102.

Chiavarelli, M.; Boucek, M.; Bailey, L. (1992). Arterial correction of double outlet left ventricle by pulmonary artery translocation. *Ann Thorac Surg,* Vol.53, (January 1992), pp. 1098 –100.

Silva, P.; Baumgratz, F.; Fonseca, L. (2000). Pulmonary root translocation in transposition of great arteries repair. *Ann Thorac Surg,* Vol.69, (February 2000), pp643-5.

Nikaidoh, H. (1984). Aortic translocation and biventricular outflow tract reconstruction. A new surgical repair for transposition of the great arteries associated with ventricular septal defect and pulmonary stenosis. *J Thorac Cardiovasc Surg,* Vol.88, (September 1984), pp. 365-72.

Hu, S.; Li, J.; Wang, X. et al. (2007). Pulmonary and aortic root translocation in the management of transposition of the great arteries with ventricular septal defect and left ventricular outflow tract obstruction. *J Thorac Cardiovasc Surg,* Vol.133, (April 2007), pp. 1090-2.

Jatene, A.; Fontes, V.; Paulista, P. et al (1976). Anatomic correction of transposition of the great vessels. *J Thorac Cardiovasc Surg,* Vol.72, (March 1976), pp. 364-370.

Bautista-Hernandez, V.; Marx, G. R.; Bacha, E. A. et al. (2007). Aortic Root Translocation Plus Arterial Switch for Transposition of the Great Arteries With Left Ventricular Outflow Obstruction. JACC, Vol. 49, (January 2007), pp. 485-90.

Furlanetto, G.; Henriques, S.; Furlanetto, B. (2010). New technique: aortic and pulmonary translocation with preservation of pulmonary valve. *Rev Bras Cir Cardiovasc,* Vol.25, (January/March 2010), pp. 99-102.

Voges, I.; Fischer, G.; Scheewe, J. et al. (2008). Restrictive enlargement of the pulmonary annulus at surgical repair of tetralogy of Fallot: 10-year experience with a uniform surgical strategy. *Eur J Cardiothorac Surg,* Vol.34, (November 2008), pp. 1041-5.

Part 7

New Technology

13

An Expansible Aortic Ring for a Standardized and Physiological Approach of Aortic Valve Repair

Emmanuel Lansac[1], Isabelle Di Centa[2], Rémi Escande[3], Maguette Ba[3,4], Nizar Kellil[3], Eric Arnaud Crozat[5], Eric Portocarrero[6], Aicha Abed[3,4], Anthony Paolitto[7], Mathieu Debauchez[1] and Anne Meddahi- Pellé[3,4]
[1]*Institut Mutualiste Montsouris, Cardiovascular Surgery Department, Paris*
[2]*Vascular Surgery Department, Foch Hospital, Suresnes*
[3]*Inserm U698, Bioengineering for Cardiovascular Imaging and Therapy Team CHU Xavier Bichat, Paris*
[4]*IUT Saint Denis, Paris 13 University*
[5]*Cardiac Surgery Department, La Tronche Hospital,*
[6]*Cardiac Surgery Nancy Hospital, Nancy,*
[7]*CoroNéo Inc, Montreal*
[1,2,3,4,5,6]*France*
[7]*Canada*

1. Introduction

Dystrophy of the ascending aorta is the main etiology of thoracic aortic aneurysms and/or pure aortic insufficiency (tricuspid or bicuspid valves) operated in western countries (Iung et al., 2003; Roberts et al., 2006). It includes two phenotypes depending on whether the sinuses of Valsalva and/or supracoronary aorta are dilated: 1) isolated AI and/or supra-coronary aneurysm (sinuses of Valsalva<40 mm); 2) aortic root aneurysms (sinuses of Valsalva>45 mm) (Lansac et al., 2008). Until recently, prosthetic valve replacement was the only surgical option for AI, performing either isolated valve replacement, composite valve and graft replacement or supracoronary graft and/or valve replacement. However, none of the current valve substitutes are ideal options, since mechanical valves require life-long anticoagulation and bioprosthetic valves present the risk of reoperation (Houel et al., 2002). Inspired by mitral experience, reconstructive methods have been developed to treat AI, based on sparing or repairing the native aortic valve, while replacing or stabilizing the other components of the aortic root. The two original valve sparing procedures - remodeling of the aortic root and reimplantation of the aortic valve - focused on root reconstruction to reduce the dilated root diameters in order to restore proper valve function. "Remodeling" technique provides the most physiological reconstruction of the root, but it does not address the dilated annular base (Yacoub et al., 1983). Alternatively, the Reimplantation, as an inclusion technique, provides a subvalvular annuloplasty to the detriment of valve dynamics (David & Feindel, 1992). Numerous technical variations aimed to associate preservation of aortic root dynamics with the treatment of dilated native annulus (Aicher et al., 2010; Hopkins, 2003). This results in a lack of standardization and limits their widespread application.

Furthermore, most failures with valve sparing techniques are due to residual cusp prolapse, either as a primary unrecognized lesion or secondary to an induced prolapse after root reconstruction. Despite its more frequent detection intra operatively, cusp prolapse remains challenging to evaluate and treat.

As restorations of both root geometry and cusp coaptation are the prerequisite for a successful valve sparing procedure, we propose a standardized aortic valve repair approach addressing both the aorta and the valve, associating a physiological reconstruction of the aortic root, with cusp resuspension and subvalvular external aortic ring annuloplasty (Lansac et al., 2005a, 2006, 2009, 2010a, 2010b, 2010c, 2011a, 2011b). Depending on the phenotype of the ascending aorta, physiological reconstruction of the root will be achieved through to the Remodeling technique (root aneurysm, sinuses of Valsalva ≥45 mm), or a supracoronary graft (supracoronary aneurysm, sinuses of Valsalva <40 mm). Subvalvular aortic annuloplasty is achieved through external implantation of a calibrated expansible aortic ring that reduces dilated diameters in diastole in order to increase valvular coaptation height, while maintaining root systolic expansibility (Lansac et al., 2009).

2. Anatomical landmarks for aortic valve repair

2.1 The ascending aorta: Descriptive anatomy

The ascending aorta may be defined as the ensemble of two distinct entities, separated by the sinotubular junction (STJ): (1) the aortic root, initial portion of the aorta that includes the aortic valve with its crown-shaped annulus, interleaflet triangles, coronary arteries ostia and sinuses of Valsalva and (2) the supracoronary aorta extending above the STJ up to the brachiocephalic trunk (Fig. 1) (Anderson et al., 1991; Lansac & Di Centa, 2010c; Reid, 1970; Robicksek, 1991; Sutton et al., 1995). Coronary arterial ostia are more frequently located below the sinotubular junction, arising within the left and right sinuses of Valsalva and are named accordingly (Muriago et al., 1997; Tops et al., 2008; Turner & Navartnam, 1996). A recent study examining 169 patients using multislice computed tomography, showed that the mean distance from the basal attachment of the cusps to the left and right coronary ostia was 14.4 +/- 2.9 mm and 17.2 +/- 3.3 mm respectively (Tops et al., 2008).

The aortic annulus is not planar since it is formed by the semilunar insertion of the cusps that extend from their basal attachments within the left ventricle (aortic annular base) to their distal attachments at the STJ, forming the commissures (Anderson et al., 1991). This three-dimensional structure of the aortic annulus may be rationalized into two functional diameters of the aortic root, ensuring proper valve function, namely the aortic annular base and the STJ (Anderson et al., 1991; Lansac & Di Centa, 2010c, De Waroux et al., 2007) (Fig. 1). Echographic measurement of the aortic annulus corresponds to the aortic annular base diameter (Fig. 2) (Roman et al., 1987).

Cut-off point of "normal" diameters of the aortic root ensuring valve coaptation can be defined from analysis of main series as an aortic annular base diameter ranging from 21 to 24.5 mm (mean 22.9 mm) and a sinotubular junction diameter ranging from 27.5 to 28.1 mm (mean 27.5 mm) with a normal root ratio STJ/annular base of 1.2. Although difficult to assess precisely, the aortic annular base seems to present a systolic expansion of 6.2% (2.5-9.6%). Systolic expansion at the sinotubular junction level is reported to be 5.7% (2.8-9.8%) (Lansac & Di Centa, 2010c; Tamas & Nylander, 2007).

Out of main series describing dystrophic aortic roots, aortic annular base diameter superior to 25 mm and sinotubular junction diameter superior to 35 mm are reported and should be considered as dilated (Gallo et al., 1995; Lansac & Di Centa, 2010c).

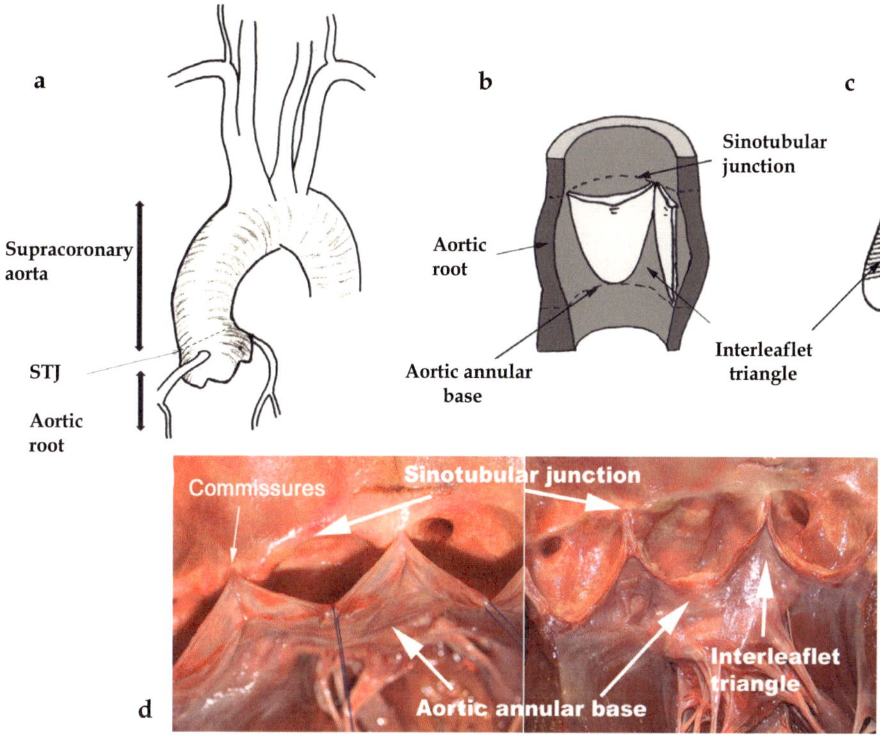

Fig. 1. Anatomy of the ascending aorta and detailed anatomy of the aortic root

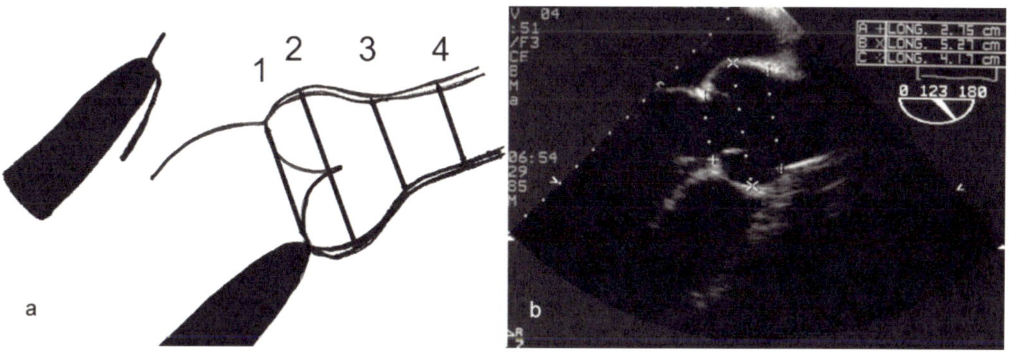

Fig. 2. Echocardiographic measurements of aortic root diameters, in long-axis. 1) Aortic annular base diameter (internal diameter), 2) Sinuses of Valsalva (external diameter, from leading edge to leading edge), 3) Sino-tubular junction (external diameter, from leading edge to leading edge), 4) Ascending aorta (external diameter, from leading edge to leading edge)

Aortic cusps dimensions vary from one patient to another, as well as from one cusp to another, in height, width, and surface area. In a study of 200 normal hearts, only five hearts were found to have cusps of equal size (Roberts, 1970; Silver & Roberts, 1985; Vollebergh & Becker, 1977). Cusp geometry determines cusp coaptation that depends on length of free margin and aortic insertion, intercommissural distance, and cusp height. These values are difficult or impossible to measure by echocardiography or intra-operative measurements. Bierbach et al. have proposed to use the relative height difference between insertion and free margin of the cusp (effective height) as a surrogate parameter of cusp coaptation. In their study effective height has a constant relationship to root dimensions and body size (Bierbach et al., 2010). Authors suggest to measure this parameter as the indicator of configuration and geometric height of a cusp and designed a specific calliper to measure it intra-operatively (Schäfers et al., 2006). Effective height revealed values in healthy adult individuals measured by transthoracic echocardiography in the range of 7 to 12 mm. The three interleaflet triangles are an extension of the left ventricular outflow tract and are composed of aorta's fibrous walls between the expanded sinuses of Valsalva. The two interleaflets triangles placed on both sides of the noncoronary cusp are in fibrous continuity with the menbranous septum, the fibrous trigones and the mitral valve (Sutton et al., 1995). The membranous interventricular septum extends downward and upward corresponding to the interleaflet triangles between the right and non coronary sinuses. It is in close relationship with the atrioventricular node. The bundle of His crosses the right fibrous trigone and passes along the lower edge of the membranous septum. This anatomical landmark is important when performing aortic valve surgery in order to avoid inducing intraventricular conduction abnormalities or heart block (Kunzelman et al., 1994).

2.2 The ascending aorta: A dynamic structure

Better understanding of aortic valve dynamics recently became a concern because of the increase use of stentless bioprostheses and aortic valve repair and sparing procedures. Although the relationship between the sinuses of Valsalva and the aortic valve had been intuitively shown by Leonardo da Vinci (Robicksek, 1991), the aortic valve has been for a long time regarded as a passive, tri-leaflet structure that moves back and forth according to pressure differences between the left ventricle (LV) and aorta. This concept has led to the development of all mechanical and stented bioprostheses. Several authors have questioned this simplistic view by showing that expansion of the aortic root actively participates in aortic valve opening, reducing shear stress on the cusps (Brewer et al., 1976; Pang et al., 2000; Thubrikar et al., 1977). In 1976, Brewer et al. described the interdependence of aortic valve opening and root expansion in an isolated aortic root model (Brewer et al., 1976). They showed that valve opening was related to the 16% radial displacement of the commissures, which was interpreted as a mechanism to reduce shear stress on the cusps. Using radio-opaque markers in dogs, Thubrikar et al. (Thubrikar et al, 1977, 1979) confirmed in vivo that aortic valve opening was related to commissural expansion prior to ejection. They suggested that the mechanism of aortic valve opening was related to the release of the inward pull of the commissures that occurs during isovolumic contraction. Although they did not measure it, they also suggested that the constraining effect of the annular base was part of the mechanism. Limited by their data-sampling rate (60 Hz), all calculations were made on abnormal cardiac cycles under the assumption that a non-ejecting extra systole was equivalent to the isovolumic contraction (IVC). Similarly, Vesely et al. interpreted aortic root dilation prior to valve opening as secondary to passive hemodynamic recoil of the aortic root (Hansen et al., 1995).

Three-dimensional (3D) digital sonomicrometry, characterized by a high rate of data acquisition (200 to 800 Hz), offers opportunity for a precise time-related study of the aortic root and valve dynamics within each phase of the normal cardiac cycle (Gorman et al., 1996; Hansen et al., 1995; Pang et al., 2000). Using this technique we intended to precise the mechanism of aortic root expansion and the shape of the aortic valve orifice at maximum opening on an ovine model.

A significant aortic root expansion occurs during isovolumic contraction and initiates the aortic leaflet separation prior to ejection (2.1 ± 0.5%). This opening is primarily due to commissural expansion, but it is also due to the expansion of the annular base. Both expansions are strongly related to the left ventricular pressure increase (r = 0.95) during IVC. The aortic root volume increases by 33.7 ± 2.7% with a maximal deformation happening during the systole at the commissural level, maximizing left ventricular ejection. These findings also confirm the study of Sutton et al. (Sutton et al., 1995), who described the interleaflet muscular triangles - located under the semilunar attachment of the cusps - as an essential component of the aortic annulus and part of the left ventricular outflow tract.

Indeed the aortic root is a junction between the left ventricular and the systemic circulation. Thin cusps separate these two compartments with different hemodynamic systems. The first, left ventricular compartment is situated below the cusps and includes the sigmoid-shaped cusp attachments (traditionally described as the annulus), the interleaflet triangles, and the commissures. These structures are related to the left ventricular hemodynamics. The second, aortic compartment, is situated above the cusps, includes the sinuses of Valsalva, the sinotubular junction and ascending aorta, and is related to aortic and coronary flow dynamics. During IVC, aortic root expansion starts at the left ventricular compartment due to volume redistribution in the left ventricular outflow tract. The aortic compartment expansion is delayed at the end of IVC due to a redistribution of volume above the cusps. Confirmation of these bi-compartmental volume dynamics is provided during end-diastole, by the observed re-expansion of the aortic root related to left ventricular compartment expansion during left ventricular filling.

The initiation of cusp separation (i.e., valve opening) is a dynamic process that occurs in the presence of a negative left ventricular –aorta pressure gradient (-8.5 ± 2.6 mmHg).

The shape of the aortic valve orifice remains speculative. Thubrikar et al. (Thubrikar et al., 1977, 1979, 1993), followed by Higashidate et al. (Higashidate et al., 1995), described it as initially stellate, then triangular and circular at maximal opening. These studies were limited by their low data sampling rate (60 Hz), which did not allow for continuous recording of the changes in valve orifice within each phase of the cardiac cycle. Sonometrics analysis at 200 to 800 Hz showed that the shape of the aortic valve orifice progressed from initially stellate to triangular then circular and finally clover shaped at maximum opening following the shape of the three sinuses of Valsalva (Figure 3). At that time, the cusp's free edge area exceeded the commissural area by +16.3 ± 2.0%. This behavior of the valve cusps might explain cases of early cusp deterioration following re-implantation of the aortic valve within a tubular conduit without sinuses of Valsalva (Gallo et al., 1995; Grande-Allen et al., 2000; Leyh et al., 1999) because cusp expansion beyond the commissural level would result in cusp impact against the wall of the cylindrical conduit.

Furthermore, as previously published, aortic root expansion is also asymmetric, and it induces a tilting dynamic of the aortic valve throughout the cardiac cycle (Dagum et al., 1999; Lansac et al., 2005b). In an ovine model, the aortic root tilt angle between the basal and commissural plane decreases in systole, aligning the left ventricular outflow tract with the ascending aorta in order to maximize ejection. As soon as the valve starts closing and during diastole, the angle tilts back (as a shock absorber), reducing stress on the cusps.

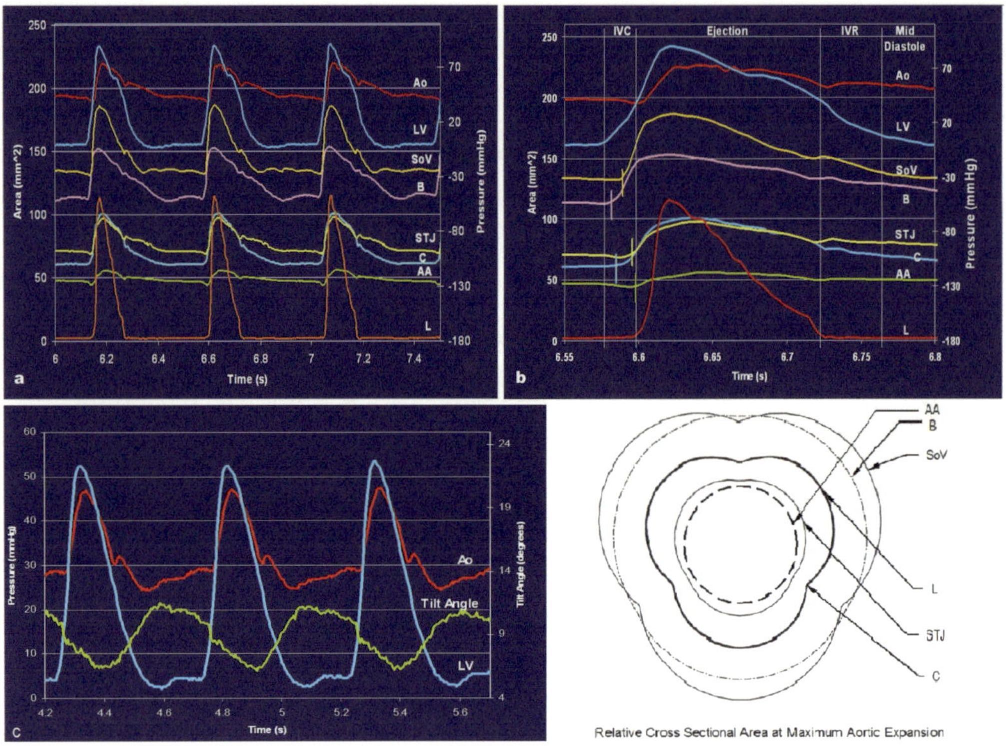

Fig. 3. Changes at each level of the aortic root time related to left ventricular and ascending aorta pressures in one sheep, a) during three cardiac cycles and b) detail of one cardiac cycle. c) Dynamic changes of tilt angle of the aortic root time related to left ventricular and aortic pressures. d) cross-sectional area diagram of the aortic root at maximum expansion during ejection (sonomicrometry) showing the clover-shaped orifice of the aortic valve. *Ao* aortic pressure, *LV* left ventricular pressure, *SoV* sinuses of Valsalva, *B* annular base, *STJ* sinotubular, *C* commissures, *AA* ascending aorta, *L* leaflet

Therefore, the durability of native aortic valve seems to rely on a dynamic triad associating 1) systolic expansion of the aortic root, 2) a clover-shaped aortic orifice that embraces the bulging sinuses of Valsalva, and 3) tilting dynamics of the aortic valve (Lansac et al., 2002). Aortic valve surgery should try to preserve these baseline dynamics as much as possible using more physiologically based surgical approaches.

3. Dystrophic aortic roots

3.1 Dystrophic aortic roots: A diameter disease

Dystrophic aortic roots are characterized by dilation of both functional diameters of the aortic root: the aortic annular base and sino-tubular junction (STJ) diameters (>25mm and >35 mm respectively), preventing coaptation of otherwise thin and pliable valves (De Waroux et al., 2007; La Canna et al., 2009; Lansac et al., 2008, 2010c). Cusp prolapse is often associated with root aneurysms and is the most common cause of isolated dystrophic aortic insufficiency (AI). On an echocardiographic study of patients with aortic root aneurysms (n=700) or isolated aortic insufficiency (n=595), average aortic annular base diameter was respectively 26.4mm (25-27.5mm) and 27.3mm (27-28mm), and average sinotubular junction was respectively 45.3mm (39.5-52.4mm) and 31mm (28-35mm). Ratio between the sinotubular junction and aortic annular base diameters was 1.7 in case of root aneurysms, whereas for isolated aortic insufficiency it was 1.1 (Lansac et al., 2008, 2010c).

3.2 Surgical indications

Surgical emergency operation is indicated in the setting of acute ascending aortic dissection or rupture into the pericardium (acute cardiac tamponade). Operative mortality remains significant and death is almost certain in the case of rupture or acute dissection if not surgically addressed.

Based on natural history of ascending aortic aneurysms, prophylactic surgery seems appropriate at 5 to 5.5 cm diameter depending on the etiology. Intervention criteria are summarized in Figure 4 (Hiratzka et al., 2010; Vahanian et al., 2007). Actually, elective surgery of the ascending aorta is much safer than emergency intervention (mortality 4.3%).

For patients with Marfan's syndrome and bicuspid valves size criterion is somewhat lower. In those patients, prophylactic repair is warranted for an intervention criterion of 4.5 to 5.0 cm diameter for most authors (Bentall & De Bono, 1968; Yacoub et al., 1998). Dissection or rupture have been stated at sizes less than 5.0 cm in several cases, and an increase rate of aneurysm dilatation greater than 5mm/y is known to lead to an 4.1-fold risk of complications.

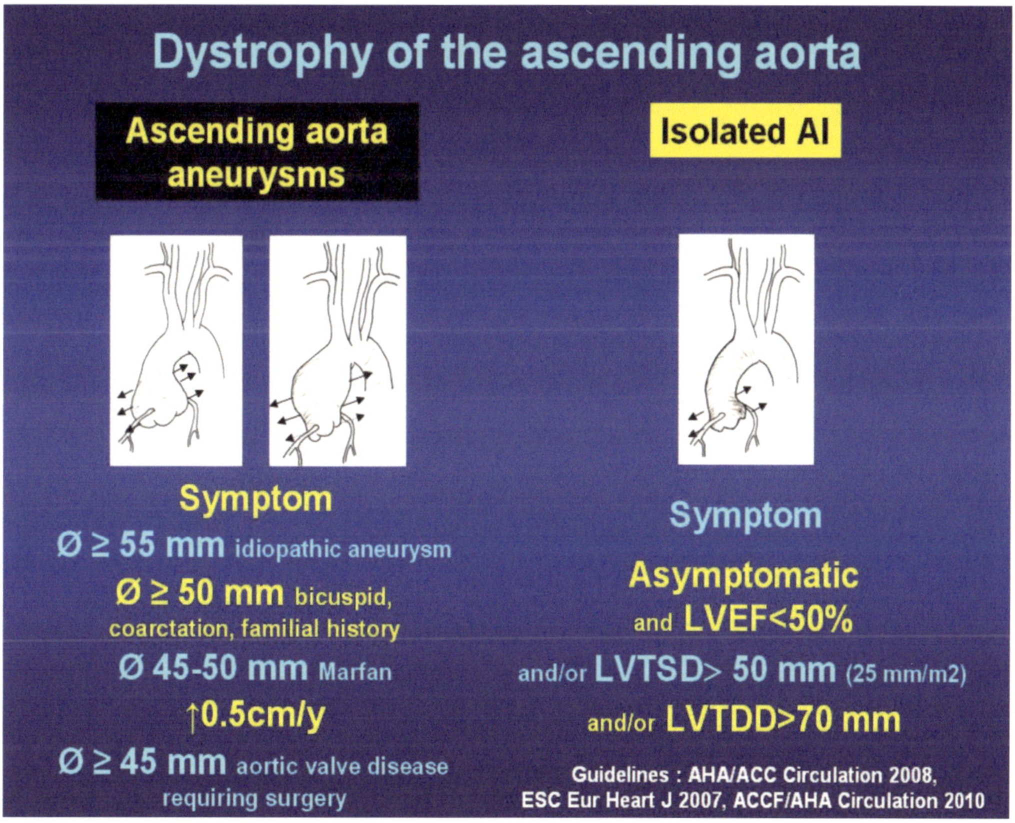

Fig. 4. Surgical indications for ascending aorta aneurysms and/or aortic insufficiency

Other risk factors for aortic dissection in patients with Marfan syndrome include familial history of aortic dissection and a ratio between observed diameter and predicted diameter above 1.3. Women with Turner's syndrome showing an ascending aortic diameter >25mm/m2 should be operated on (David et al., 2006).

3.3 Preoperative imaging

Transthoracic and transesophageal echocardiography are performed to define the anatomy of the valve and the phenotype of the ascending aorta (Roman et al., 1987). It remains critical in order to analyze the lesional mechanism of aortic insufficiency both pre- and postrepair in case of aortic valve repair procedures. It measures the 4 characteristics aortic diameters at end diastole, in the parasternal long-axis view, at 4 levels: aortic annular base, sinuses of Valsalva, sino-tubular junction and supra-coronary aorta. Measurements are made perpendicular to the long axis of the aorta using the leading edge technique in views showing the largest aortic diameters. (Fig. 2) (Roman et al., 1987). Analysis of the valve evaluates the number of cusps and direction of regurgitant jet. An eccentric jet towards the anterior mitral leaflet identifies a right coronary cusp prolapse whereas a jet directed towards the septum corresponds to a non or left coronary cusp prolapse (De Waroux et al., 2007).
Most patients are initially evaluated and followed with helical CT (computed tomography) scans, completed with a 3-dimensional reconstruction of the data to increase the accuracy of aneurysm measurements, determination of its proximal and distal extent, and differentiation between dissection, penetrating ulcera or intramural hematoma. Moreover, it allows preoperative coronary arteries assessment.
As a routine, it is recommended to perform both an echocardiography and a helical computed tomography in order to evaluate and confirm the size of the aneurysm.

3.4 Surgical techniques for dystrophic aortic roots

Treatment for dystrophic aortic root aneurysms can be either replacement of the aortic valve and root, or repair of the aortic valve, while replacing the dilated aortic root in case of aneurysms.

3.4.1 Aortic valve and root replacement procedure

Depending on root phenotype, it consists either of isolated valve replacement (isolated aortic insufficiency), composite valve and graft replacement (Bentall procedure, for aortic root aneurysms (Bentall & De Bono, 1968)) or supracoronary graft and/or valve replacement (supra-coronary aneurysm).

3.4.2 Aortic valve-sparing procedures

Owing to the improved understanding of aortic valve dynamics, reconstructive methods have been developed to treat aortic insufficiency, based on sparing or repairing the native aortic valve, while replacing or stabilizing the other components of the aortic root, in order to avoid complications of prosthetic valves.

4. Remodeling of the aortic root and reimplantation of the aortic valve

4.1 Description of the original valve sparing procedures

The two original valve sparing procedure - remodeling of the aortic root and reimplantation of the aortic valve - focused on root reconstruction to reduce the dilated root diameters in order to restore proper valve function (David & Feindel, 1992; Yacoub et al., 1983). The reimplantation technique offers aortic annulus support but withdraws the sinuses of Valsalva and includes the interleaflet triangles within a graft tube, thus impairing root dynamics (David et al., 1992, 2006, 2007). In contrast, the remodeling technique provides more physiologic movements of the cusps within three reconstructed neo-sinuses, thus preserving root expansibility through the interleaflet triangles, but without addressing annular base dilation (Yacoub et al., 1983, 1998).

These techniques spare the patient from anticoagulation and prosthetic valve morbidity with a 10-year survival rate ranging from 80.4 to 92% (mean 88.2%) (Aicher et al., 2010; Lansac & Di Centa, 2010c). In both techniques with proper patient selection, the results up to 10 years are equally excellent. However, in earlier series of the remodeling technique, the reoperation rate was higher after type A aortic dissection and in patients with Marfan syndrome (Lansac et al., 2006; Leyh et al., 2002; Luciani et al., 1999; Yacoub et al., 1998). In the unselected population of the original remodeling series, up to 30 % of patients presented recurrence of AI grade II or III (Erasmi et al., 2005; Furukawa et al., 1999; Lansac et al., 2006; Luciani et al., 1999). The only risk factor for failure was a dilated native aortic annulus (diameter ≥ 25 mm) (Hanke et al., 2009; Lansac et al., 2006; Leyh et al., 2002; Luciani et al., 1999; Yacoub et al., 1998).

4.2 Aortic root and valve dynamics after remodeling or reimplantation

4.2.1 In vitro studies

All studies show that the remodeling technique exhibits valve dynamics closest to those of the native aortic root. The recreation of the sinuses of Valsalva preserves vortex formation, as well as cusp opening and closing dynamics, thus, reducing cusp stress which theoretically improves their durability. The valve shows asymmetric motion after reimplantation. The cusp bending deformation index is increased with the reimplantation techniques and sinus prosthesis compared with the control and remodeling groups (Erasmi et al., 2005; Furukawa et al., 1999; Grande-Allen et al., 2000).

4.2.2 In vivo studies

Leyh and colleagues clearly demonstrated that distensibility of the aortic root and a proper valve motion were better preserved after the remodeling than after the reimplantation technique (Leyh et al., 1999). They showed that reimplantation with a straight tube abolished root distensibility at all levels; the cusps took longer for closing, and systolic contact of at least one cusp against the tube graft was constantly found. Reconstruction of the sinuses may assure a sufficient gap to avoid any such contact between the open cusp and the Dacron wall, which is known to be responsible for cusp thickening and accelerated degeneration (Aybek et al., 2005; De Paulis et al., 2002). The presence of vortices inside the neosinuses of Valsalva preserves the slow closing displacement of the cusps and is associated with a valve motion similar to that of normal subjects (De Paulis et al., 2002; Maselli et al., 2005). Although not significant, valve velocities after the remodeling procedure using the Valsalva graft (Gelweave Valsalva™, Vascutek, Inc.) are closer to normal than after reimplantation using the same graft (De Paulis et al., 2002).

Therefore, all dynamic studies suggest that cusp motion and flow patterns across the reconstructed aortic root are more physiologic (1) after remodeling of the aortic root than after reimplantation of the aortic valve and (2) after procedures using a prosthetic conduit fashioned with neosinuses of Valsalva than without.

4.3 Modification of original remodeling and reimplantation techniques

Numerous technical variations aimed to associate preservation of aortic root dynamics with vortices (neosinuses of Valsalva) and expansibility (interleaflet triangles) with the treatment of dilated native annulus (± cusp lesion) (Hopkins, 2003; Lansac & Di Centa, 2010c).

David et al. added an external Teflon strip on the aortomitral junction to the remodeling technique (David III) or oversized (+4 mm) the tube graft for the reimplantation technique (David IV) (David, 1999, 2005). The David V technique used an even larger graft size (+ 6-8 mm), which is "necked down" at both the bottom and the top ends to create graft pseudosinuses (Miller, 2007). Many authors suggested different methods to customize the tube graft for the reimplantation or remodeling in order to provide better neosinuses of Valsalva. More recently De Paulis et al. designed the Valsalva graft (Gelweave Valsalva™, Vascutek, Inc.) with vertical pleats in the proximal section for reconstruction of the aortic root and with the standard horizontal pleats for ascending aorta replacement (Cochran & Kunzelman, 2000; Gleason, 2005; Hess et al., 2005; Hetzer et al., 2008; Kollar, 2007; Miller, 2007; Morishita et al., 2002; Ruvolo & Fattouch, 2009; Scensson, 2003; Takamoto et al., 2006; Urbanski et al., 2009; Zehr et al., 2000).

We suggest combining advantages of both original valve sparing techniques by associating the Remodeling reconstruction of the aortic root with an expansible sub-valvular annuloplasty (Figure 5).

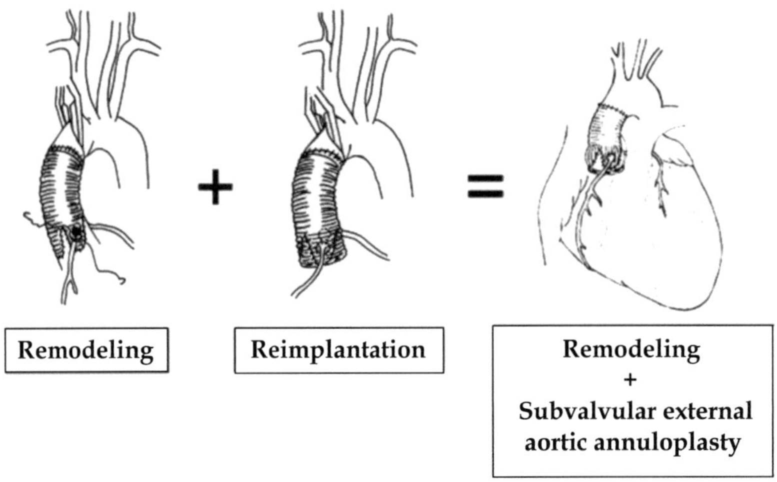

Fig. 5. Combination of Remodeling and Reimplantation procedures by placing an external subvalvular ring annuloplasty associated to the Remodeling procedure

5. From original valve sparing procedures to a physiological approach of aortic valve repair

Although restoration of root geometry is an important prerequisite for a successful valve sparing, preventing recurrence of aortic insufficiency remains a challenge. Most failures with valve sparing techniques are due to residual cusp prolapse, either as a primary unrecognized lesion or secondary to an induced prolapse after root reconstruction. Despite its more frequent detection intra operatively, cusp prolapse remains challenging to evaluate and treat. Schafers et al proposed to use a cusp caliper to obtain symmetrical cusp resuspension with an effective height ≥8 to 10 mm in order to restore cusp coaptation (Bierbach et al., 2010; Schäfers et al., 2006). In their report, an effective height ≥9 mm is an excellent predictor for a good haemodynamic outcome after valve repair. This technique allows correction of any residual or induced symmetrical prolapse after reduction of the STJ provided by the remodeling procedure. Indeed, Soncini et al., using finite element analysis showed that noduli of Arantius were lowered towards the valve orifice during valve closure after reimplantation (3.8 mm) and remodeling (3.3 mm) (Soncini et al., 2009). Subvalvular annuloplasty through an aortic ring or proximal suture of a reimplantation tube graft partially compensates the induced symmetric prolapse by increasing the coaptation height. However, in the absence of cusp resuspension, coaptation level may remain too low (at the level of the aortic annular plane or below). This can induce a billowing aspect of the cusps with progressive drop of the coaptation level and height (<4mm) which have been described as a risk factor for reoperation (De Waroux et al., 2007). Normalisation of effective height leads to a high probability of normal or near-normal aortic valve function (Bierbach et al., 2010; Schäfers et al., 2006).

As restorations of both root geometry and cusp coaptation are the prerequisite for a successful valve sparing procedure, we designed a standardized surgical management of dystrophic aortic roots towards a more systematic and physiological repair approach (Fig. 6). This approach is proposed based on the principles of reduction of dilated root diameters

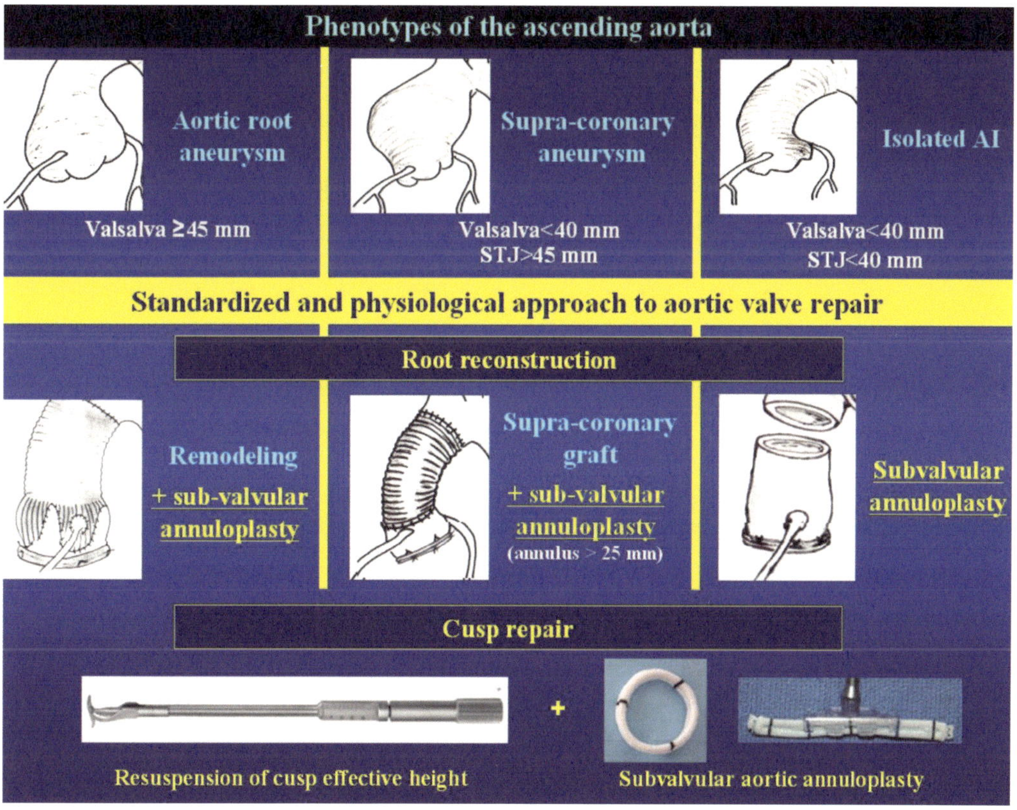

Fig. 6. Standardized and physiological approach to aortic valve repair according each phenotype of the ascending aorta

(aortic annular base and STJ); respect of root dynamics (expansibility through the interleaflet triangles and restoration of sinuses of Valsalva) and retoration of cusp coaptation height (measurement of the effective height). Depending on the phenotype of the ascending aorta, reduction of the sinotubular junction diameter will be achieved through a physiological reconstruction of the root according to the Remodeling technique (root aneurysm, sinuses of Valsalva≥45 mm), a supracoronary graft (supracoronary aneurysm, sinuses of Valsalva<40 mm). Valve repair is achieved in two steps: 1) before root reconstruction by aligning adjacent cusp free edges, excess of length is corrected using plicating central stitches or limited resection; 2) after root reconstruction, resuspending residual or induced cusp prolapse in order to obtain an effective height of 8 mm (distance between the free edge of the cusp to the aortic annular base). Expansible subvalvular annuloplasty is systematically added using an external expansible aortic ring in order to increase cusp coaptation height, while maintaining systolic expansibility. Ring is "open" in case of isolated aortic insufficiency or supra-coronary aneurysm, in order that it may be positioned below the coronary arteries without detaching them from the aortic root (Lansac et al., 2005a, 2006, 2009, 2010a, 2010b, 2010c, 2011a, 2011b).

6. An expansible aortic ring for a calibrated subvalvular aortic annuloplasty

To standardize this physiologically based approach to conservative aortic valve surgery, we designed a calibrated expansible aortic ring that reduces dilated diameters in diastole in order to increase cusp coaptation height, while maintaining root systolic expansibility (Figure 7) (Lansac et al., 2009).

The aortic rings (Extra-Aortic, CORONEO Inc., Montreal, Canada) are composed of two silicone elastomer cores covered by a polyester textile. Black indicator marks on the ring and suture windows in the ring-holder are incorporated to facilitate optimal suture placement between the two cores. Design prerequisites for the ring were: 1) target *in vivo* device expansion between 5% and 15% over the cardiac cycle, 2) minimized radial thickness of the ring while preserving the desired dynamic behaviour, 3) ring durability, 4) stable and predictable bioreaction with surrounding tissues.

Characteristics of this new device were established *in vitro* on the bench-top. Biocompatibility of the ring and the impact of its implantation on root dynamics were studied *in vivo* in the ovine model.

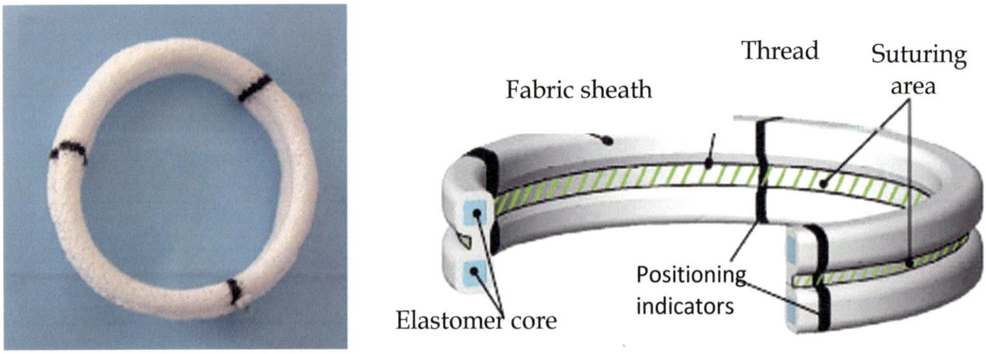

Fig. 7. Expansible aortic ring (left hand side) and its detailed constitution (right hand side)

Root dynamics were assessed using intracardiac echography before surgery, and at 6 months. Histological, scanning electron microscopy and mechanical studies were then performed on explanted samples. Prosthetic rings created a significant reduction of the aortic annular base diameter without significant transvalvular gradient (mean 3.4 ± 2.1 mmHg). Coaptation height was increased from 2.5 ± 0.7 mm to 6.2 ± 1.1 mm ($p<0.001$). Dynamics of the root were well preserved. The device was clearly visible in explanted sheep hearts at 6 months. There was no erosion of the external ring into the aorta or adjacent structures, neither at the level of the aortic annular base nor at the STJ level. Coronary arteries were patent in all cases. Mechanical testing on 6 month explanted samples revealed no significant differences in elastic modulus. Histomorphological studies showed incorporation of the material without degradation. Aortic cusps remained thin and pliable. Macroscopic examination of the hearts did not show calcification as confirmed by Alizarin red staining. Polyester fabric was fully integrated in the tissue and colonized by a dense extracellular matrix. Low and high magnifications of the samples showed the encapsulation of the elastomer core in a fibrous zone. No inflammatory reaction was noted around the device and no apparent degradation of the elastomer core was observed by SEM observation (Lansac et al., 2009).

7. Remodeling of the aortic root with cusp resuspension and subvalvular external aortic ring annuloplasty for aortic aneurysms

We describe a standardized procedure for aortic aneurysms with tricuspid valves (Lansac et al., 2011b). In all cases, intra-operative transesophageal echocardiography (TEE) remains critical in order to analyze the lesional mechanism of AI both pre- and post-repair (Lansac et al., 2011a).

7.1 Dissection of the subvalvular plane

After aortic cross-clamping, the aneurysm is opened and the aortic root and valve are carefully inspected (particularly the geometry of the aortic valve and leaflet morphology). Pliable non retracted cusps are suitable for valve repair. The presence of an intact fenestration, a bicuspid valve or limited calcification is not a contraindication. External dissection of the aortic root is performed down to the base of the aortic annulus which is liberated from the pulmonary artery and infundibulum and from the roof of the left atrium, in order to reach the subvalvular plane. The wall of the aortic sinus is totally removed leaving a fringe of aortic wall of approximately 2 mm. The internal aortic annular base diameter is measured with Hegar dilators. Measurement of the native aortic annular base diameter with Hegar dilators is the sole criterion to determine size of the expansible aortic ring which is undersized from one size in order to increase coaptation height while protecting cusp repair (Table 1).

	Aortic annular base Ø (Hegar dilators, mm)			
	25-27	**28-30**	**31-33**	**≥34**
Tube graft Ø (mm)	28	30	32	34
Subvalvular aortic ring Ø (mm)	25	27	29	31

Table 1. Criteria for choice of the aortic ring and tube graft diameters

7.2 Placement of 5 subvalvular anchoring stitches (fig. 8)

Five threads of 2.0 coated polyester fiber pledgeted (3/8 needle 25, Ethibond, Ethicon Inc., Somerville NJ, USA), are placed from the inside out as "U" stitches (width of 3 mm) circumferentially in the subvalvular plane, clock-wise beginning from the non-coronary sinus. Three stitches are placed 2 mm below the nadir of insertion of each cusp, and two stitches are placed below two of the three commissures at the base of the interleaflet triangles (no suture is placed at the base of the interleaflet triangle situated between the right and noncoronary sinuses to avoid potential injury to the bundle of His and membranous septum*)

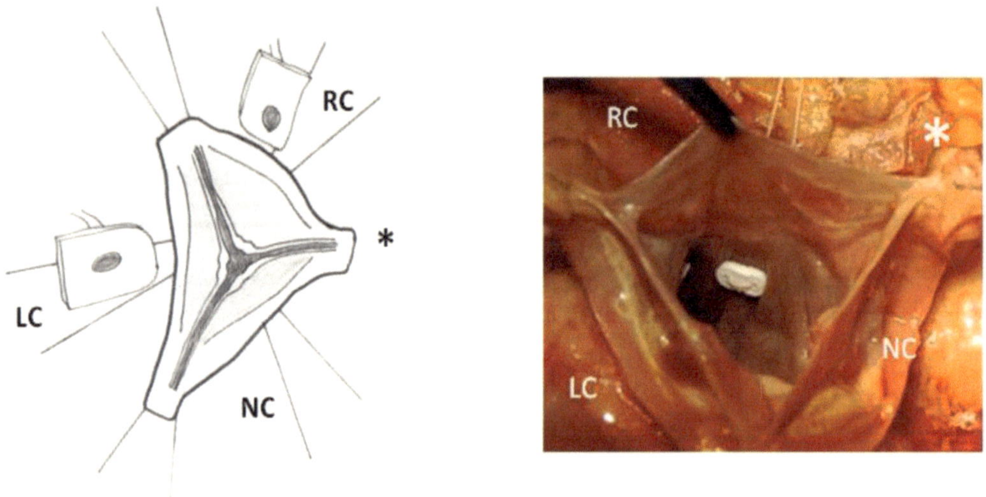

Fig. 8. Positioning of the stitches. RC: right coronary, LC: left coronary, NC: non-coronary, *: membranous septum

7.3 First step of valve repair: Alignment of adjacent cusp free edges (fig. 9)

A polypropylene 6/0 stay suture is passed through each noduli of Arantius. A grasper pulls outwards on the corresponding commissure while the two stitches at the level of the noduli of Arantia are retracted in the opposite direction. The excess length of free edge is then determined. Same step is performed for each hemi-cusp. Distance between the two stitches determines the area for the central plicating stitches to equalize each hemi-cusp (polypropylene 5 or 6/0-13).

7.4 Remodeling of the aortic root (fig. 10)

The Remodeling technique is performed using a Gelweave Valsalva™ graft. Remodeling of the aortic root is standardized by scalloping the Valsalva graft into three symmetrical neosinuses using the linear demarcations on the bulging part of the graft. The heights of the scallops to suture the commissures are cut up to the transition point between circumferential and axial folds in the graft. Suturing of the graft starts on the left coronary sinus at the nadir of the sinus (1) towards half sinus (2). Another running suture is begun at the tip of the commissure (3) towards corresponding hemi-sinus (4). (polypropylene 5.0). Right and non coronary sinuses are then sutured.

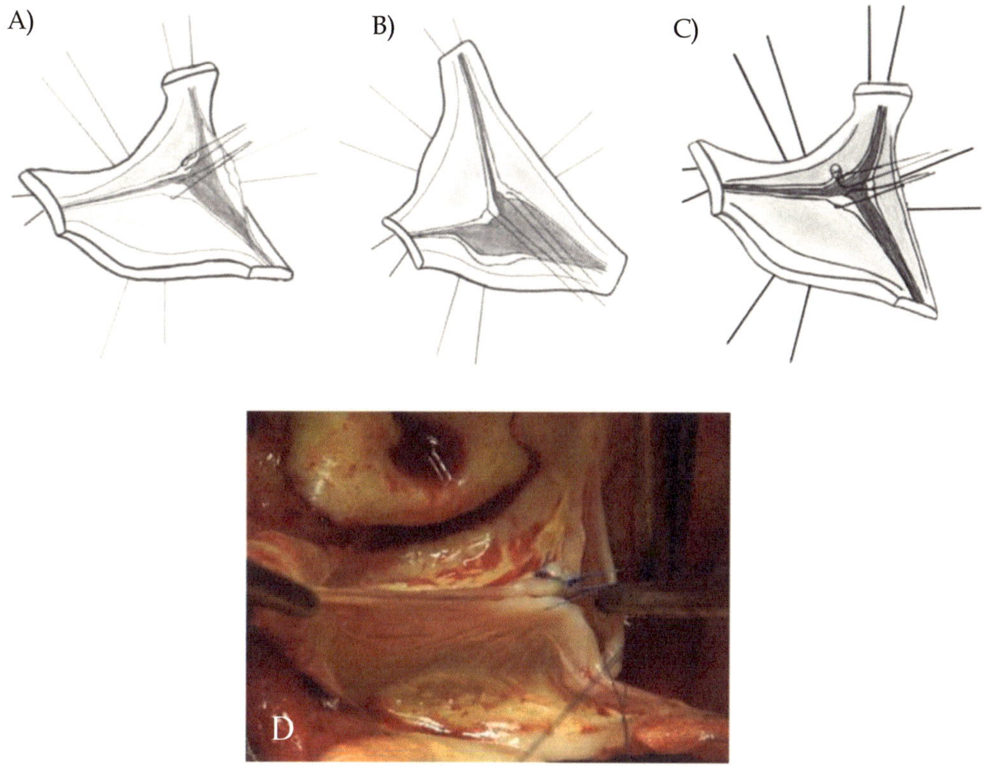

Fig. 9. First step of cusp repair. Alignment of cusp free edges to determine excess of length (A-B) and plicating of stitches to equalize each hemi-cusp (C-D)

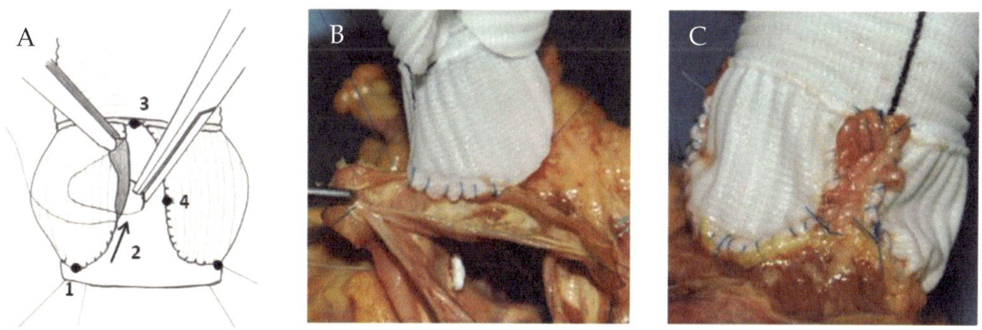

Fig. 10. Step by step suturing of the tube graft for Remodeling (A), from beginning (B) to the end (C)

7.5 Second step for cusp repair: Resuspension of cusp effective height (fig. 11)

Once suturing of the tube graft performed,, commissural traction sutures are placed to mimic a pressurized aortic root in order to measure the effective height of each cusp. A dedicated cusp caliper is used to evaluate any residual or induced cusp prolapse (Fehling

Instruments, Karlstein, Germany) (Schäfers et al., 2006). Plicating stitches are added on the free edge of the culprit leaflet until an effective height of 8 to 10 mm is obtained.

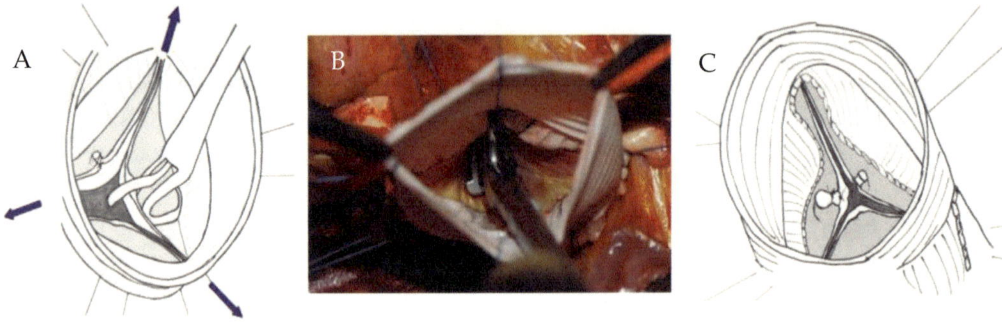

Fig. 11. Commissural traction and cusps measurement using a calliper (A-B) and cusps height correction (C)

7.6 Placement of the prosthetic aortic ring in the subvalvular position (fig. 12)

The five anchoring "U" stitches are passed through the inner aspect of the prosthetic expansible aortic ring (Extra aortic, CORONEO Inc., Montreal, QC, Canada). The attachment point between the handle and the ring-holder is aligned with the commissure between the non- and right coronary sinuses (atrioventricular node) where there is no anchoring stitch. The ring is then descended around the remodelled aortic root (a). The holder is released and knots are tied to secure the ring in subvalvular position (b).

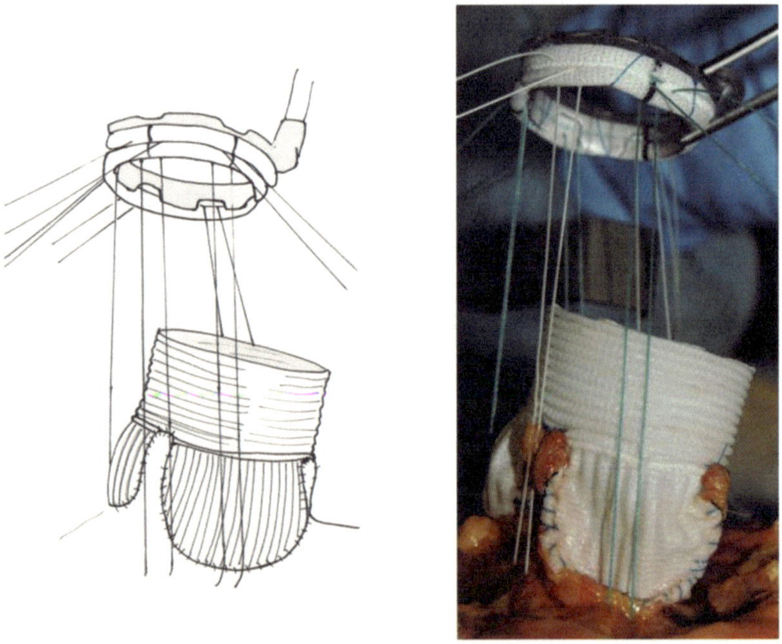

Fig. 12. Suture and descent of the prosthetic aortic ring

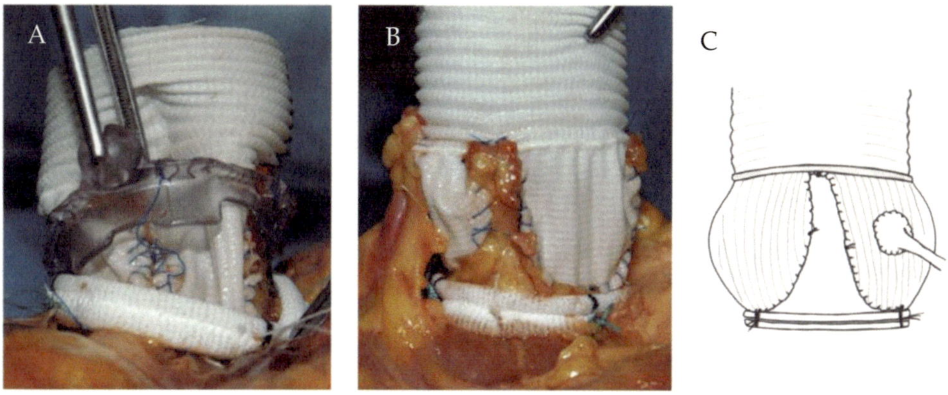

Fig. 13. Final steps of the procedure: the holder is removed (A) and final aspect of the neoaortic root after anastomosis of the coronary ostia (B-C)

Reimplantation of the coronary ostia buttons into the corresponding 'neo-sinuses' of Valsalva is obtained using 5.0 Prolene (fig. 13). The thicker part of the Gelweave graft can be cut to suture the coronaries ostia if they are ascensionned which is often the case for the right coronary button. Distal anastomosis is performed using a 4-5/0 Prolene running suture in a standard fashion.

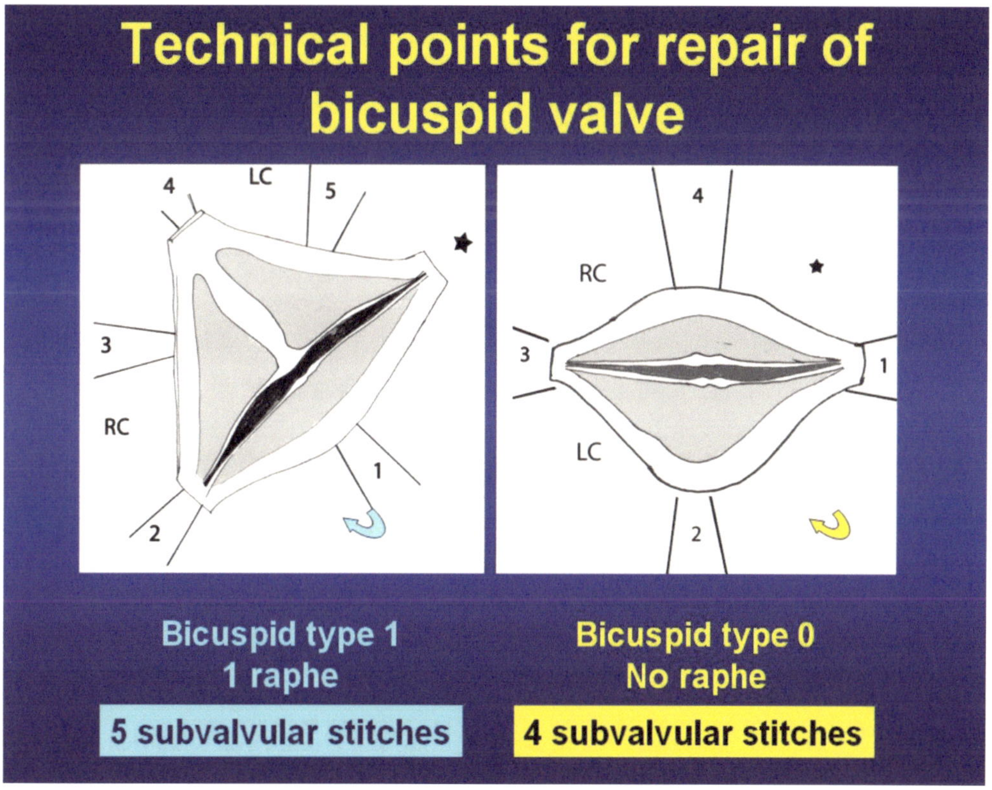

Fig. 14. Bicuspid valves: Placement of the 5 subvalvular "U" stitches

7.7 Specific aspect of repair for aortic root aneurysms with bicuspid aortic valves
Dissection of the subvalvular plane as well as sizing of the ring and graft are similar to tricuspid valves (Lansac et al., 2011b). Principle for repair, applicable to all types of bicuspid valves, consists of aligning the free edges of the two cusps, and placing the commissures in the neo-aortic root at 180° according to Schafers et al. Therefore, the Remodeling technique is performed by tailoring the Gelweave Valsalva™ graft into two symmetrical sinuses of Valsalva (Schäfers et al., 2010) (fig. 14-15).

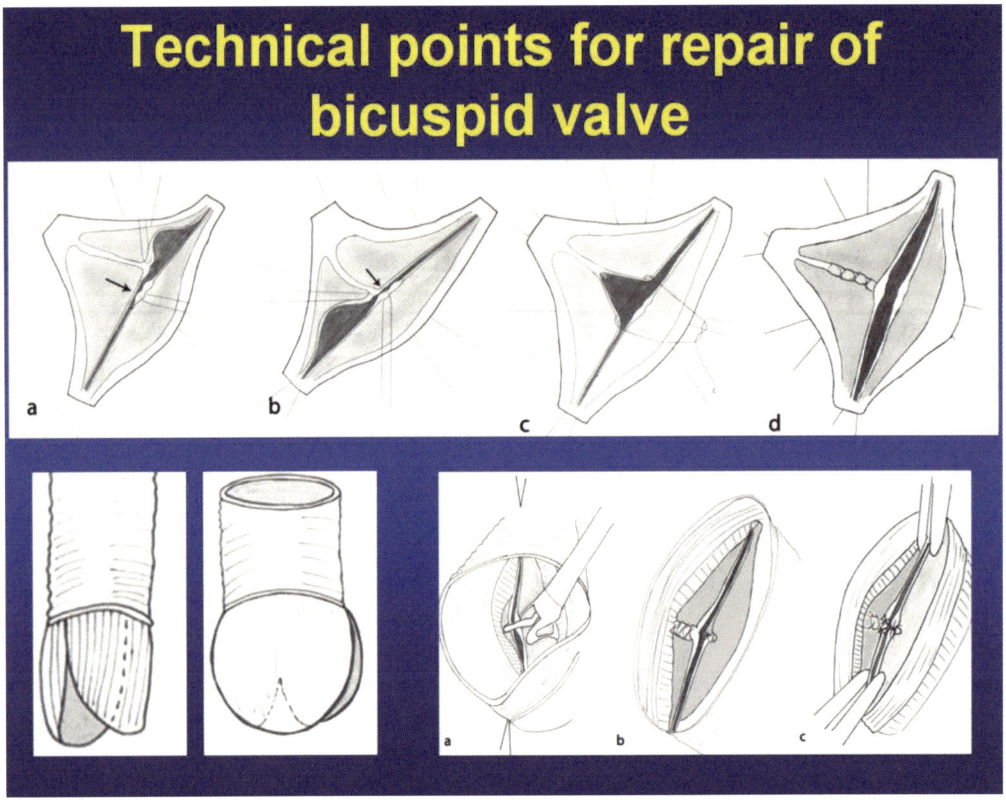

Fig. 15. Bicuspid valves: Valve repair and suture of the remodeling

8. Subvalvular aortic annuloplasty for isolated aortic insufficiencies

Principle of isolated aortic valve repair associates cusp repair (alignment of cusp free edge + effective height resuspension) with subvalvular aortic annuloplasty. The expansible aortic ring is of an open configuration in order to allow placement below the coronary arteries without detaching them from the aortic wall (Lansac et al., 2011a, 2011b).

8.1 Transection of the aorta and dissection of the aortic root down to the subvalvular plane

The aorta is completely transsected 1 cm above the sino-tubular junction. External dissection of the aortic root down to the aortic annular base is performed, passing under the coronary arteries, without detaching them from the aortic wall. The external aspect of the aortic wall is dissected free from the pulmonary artery and infundibulum and from the roof of the left atrium, in order to reach the subvalvular plane. The internal aortic annular base diameter is measured with Hegar dilators. It is the sole criterion to determine the size of the expansible external subvalvular aortic ring, which is downsized by one size (CORONEO, Inc.).

8.2 Placement of the five anchoring subvalvular "U" stitches

Five "U" stitches (2.0 coated polyester fiber, 3/8 needle 25) are circumferentially placed from inside out in the subvalvular plane, below the nadirs of each cusp and at the base of each interleaflet triangles except the one situated between the right and noncoronary sinuses to avoid potential injury to the bundle of His and membranous septum.

8.3 Valve repair: Alignment of adjacent cusp free edges followed by resuspension of the cusp effective height

Commissural traction stitches are placed. Alignment of adjacent cusp free edges is performed. Excess cusp length is corrected by plicating central stitches if <5mm and limited cusp resection if >5 mm. Effective height cusp resuspension is then re-evaluated on the un-fused cusp using a cusp caliper (Fehling Instruments, Karlstein, Germany). Plicating central stitches are added on the free edge of this cusp until an effective height of 10 mm is obtained. Re-alignment of the two cusps free edges is then performed by adding plicating stitches on the fused cusp (fig. 16).

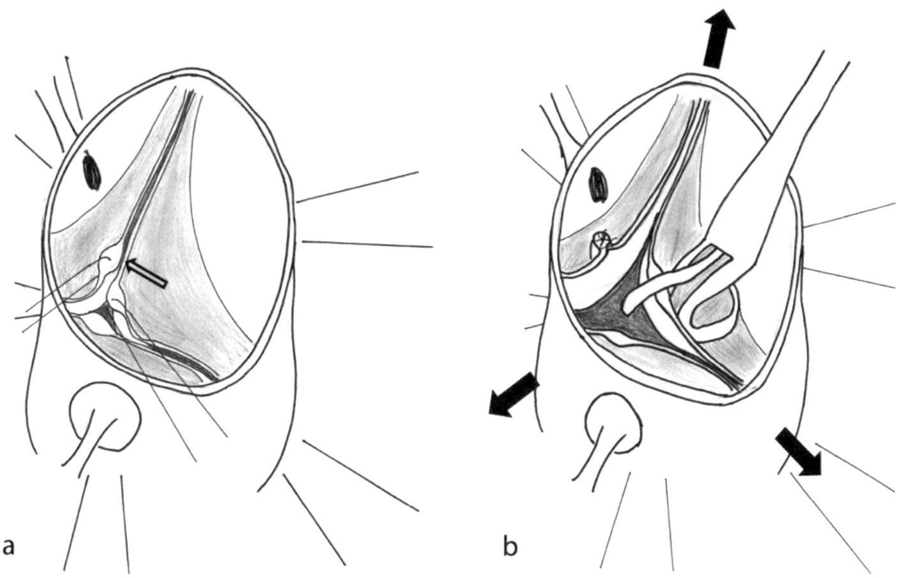

Fig. 16. Aortic valve resuspension for repair of isolated aortic insufficiency

8.4 Placement of the aortic prosthetic ring in subvalvular position and TEE control

The subvalvular stitches are passed through the inner aspect of the 'open' subvalvular prosthetic ring, in order that it may be positioned below the coronary arteries. The ring is closed with a series of "U" stitches. Transsection of the aorta is closed in standard fashion with running suture (fig. 17).

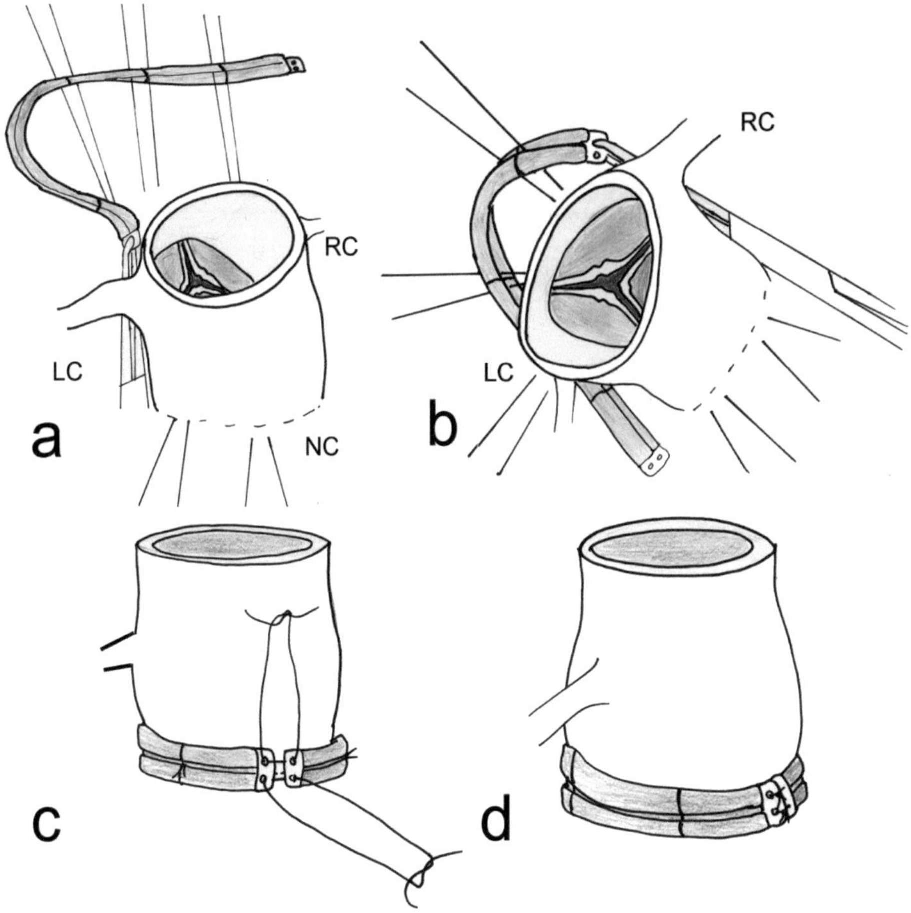

Fig. 17. Placement of the aortic prosthetic ring in subvalvular position

9. Preliminary results

From 2003 to 2009, 187 patients underwent Remodeling with subvalvular ring annuloplasty in 14 centers (24 surgeons). Preoperative AI≥grade 2 was present in 67.9% (127), and bicuspid valve in 20.8% (39). Need for cusp repair was assessed according to 3 strategies: Group 1: gross visual estimation (74 patients), Group 2: alignment of cusp free edges (62 patients), Group 3: two-steps approach associating alignment of cusp free edges with effective height resuspension (51 patients). A composite outcome was defined as recurrence of aortic insufficiency ≥ grade 2 and/or reoperation.
Valve sparing was successful in all but 2 cases. Operative mortality was 3.2% (6). Ring produced a significant annular base reduction from 27.3±0.6 to 20.5±1.7 mm ($p<0.01$) without significant mean transvalvular gradient (7.2±2.9 mmHg). Treatment of cusp lesion was most frequently performed in Group 3 (70.6%, versus 20.3% Group 1 and 30.6% Group 2, $p<0.001$). Nine patients required reoperation during follow-up (31.4±4.5 months (1-80)). At one year, no patients in Group 3 presented with composite outcome events (versus 28.1% Group 1, 15% Group 2, $p<0.001$). Residual aortic insufficiency and tricuspid anatomy were

independent risk factors for composite outcome in Group 1 and 2. Annulus diameter, Marfan syndrome and cusp repair had no effect on aortic insufficiency recurrence or reoperation. Repair of bicuspid valves showed better results than tricuspid valves anatomy. This might be partly explained by higher rate of cusp repair in bicuspid patients (72% of patients versus 28% of patients for tricuspid valves). Apart from high rate of cusp repair, better results in Group 3 also could reflect a learning curve or other confounding factors, since these patients were operated later (Lansac et al., 2010a, 2010b).

10. Evaluation of the standardized approach to aortic valve repair: CAVIAAR trial and registry (Conservative Aortic Valve surgery for aortic Insufficiency and Aneurysm of the Aortic Root)

Few series have compared valve repair with composite valve and graft replacement (Bassano et al., 2001; De Oliveira et al., 2003; Karck et al., 2004; Patel et al., 2008; Volguina et al., 2009; Zehr et al., 2004). Conclusions remain controversial since they were often retrospective, based on selected patients (Marfan), and compare different operating time periods, techniques and learning curve periods. Overall, rates of thromboembolism, bleeding, and endocarditis after valve repair seem lower than those reported for prosthetic valves. A current prospective international registry just provided 30-day morbidity and mortality data and shows equivalent results after a composite valve replacement or a valve-sparing procedure (despite various type of reimplantation) in a selected population of Marfan patients (National Marfans Foundation prospective aortic root replacement registry) (Volguina et al., 2009).

In order to evaluate the standardized approach of valve repair using the expansible aortic ring versus mechanical valve replacement, unselected population of patients with aortic root aneurysms (bicuspid and tricuspid valves) are currently enrolled in France in the ongoing prospective multicenter CAVIAAR trial (Conservative Aortic Valve surgery for aortic Insufficiency and Aneurysm of the Aortic Root), over the next 5 years. Aside from the trial, all patients operated according to the CAVIAAR technique outside France are enrolled in the prospective CAVIAAR registry.

11. Conclusion

Avoidance of anticoagulation and prosthetic related complications makes aortic valve repair an appealing procedure. Considering the increasing rate of cusp repair reported in the literature, conservative aortic valve surgery seems to be evolving from aortic valve sparing to aortic valve repair. However, the need remains for reliable long-term data comparing valve replacement and valve-repair procedures. A standardized management of dystrophic aortic roots towards a physiological approach to valve repair might improve long term durability of the results, and encourage more widespread adoption of these procedures.

12. Acknowledgements

We wish to thank the surgeons who operated the patients in the CAVIAAR trial: Pr C. Acar, Pr B. Albat, Dr E. Arnaud Crozat, Dr F. Baud, Pr D. Blin, Dr N. Bonnet, Dr O. Bouchot, Dr D. Chatel, Dr F. Doguet, Dr G. Fernandez, Dr JP Fleury, Dr T. Folliguet, Pr I. Gandjbakhch, Dr R. Hacini, Pr P. Leprince, Dr S. Lopez, Pr P. Menu, Pr P. Nataf, Pr A. Pavie, Dr A. Rama.

Authors thank the Ecole de Chirurgie de l'Assistance Publique Hôpitaux de Paris (Paris, France) for the use of its anatomical laboratory and organization of the yearly workshops on aortic valve repair.

13. References

Aicher D, Fries R, Rodionycheva S, Schmidt K, Langer F, Schäfers HJ. (2010). Aortic valve repair leads to a low incidence of valve-related complications. *Eur J Cardiothorac Surg*, Vol. 37, No. 1, pp. (127-132).

Anderson RH, Devine WA, Ho SY, Smith A, Mc Kay R. (1991). The myth of the aortic annulus: the anatomy of the subaortic outflow tract. *Ann Thorac Surg*, Vol. 52, No. 3, pp. (640–646).

Aybek T, Sotiriou M, Wohleke T, Miskovic A, Simon A, Doss M, Dogan S, Wimmer-Greinecker G, Moritz A. (2005). Valve opening and closing dynamics after different aortic valve-sparing operations. *J Heart Valve Dis*, Vol. 14, No. 1, pp. (114-120).

Bassano C, De Matteis GM, Nardi P, Buratta MM, Zeitani J, De Paulis R, Chiariello L. (2001). Mid-term follow-up of aortic root remodelling compared to Bentall operation. *Eur J Cardiothorac Surg*, Vol. 19, No. 5, pp. (601-605).

Bentall HH, De Bono A. (1968). A technique for complete replacement of the ascending aorta. *Thorax*, Vol. 23, No. 4, pp. (338–339).

Bierbach BO, Aicher D, Issa OA, Bomberg H, Gräber S, Glombitza P, Schäfers HJ. (2010). Aortic root and cusp configuration determine aortic valve function. *Eur J Cardiothorac Surg*, Vol. 38, No. 4, pp. (400-406).

Brewer RJ, Deck JD, Capati B, Nolan SP. (1976). The dynamic aortic root: its role in aortic valve function. *J Thorac Cardiovasc Surg*, Vol. 72, No. 3, pp. (413–417).

Cabanes L, Chalas C, Christin-Maitre S, Donadille B, Felten ML, Gaxotte V, Jondeau G, Lansac E, Lansac J, Letur H, N'Diaye T, Ohl J, Pariente-Khayat A, Roulot D, Thepot F, Zénaty D. (2010). Turner syndrome and pregnancy: clinical practice. Recommendations for the management of patients with Turner syndrome before and during pregnancy. *Eur J Obstet Gynecol Reprod Biol*, Vol. 152, No. 1, pp. (18-24).

Cochran RP, Kunzelman KS. (2000). Methods of pseudosinus creation in an aortic valve-sparing operation for aneurysmal disease. *J Card Surg*, Vol. 15, No. 6, pp. (428–433).

Dagum P, Green GR, Nistal FJ, Daughters GT, Timek TA, Foppiano LE, Bolger AF, Ingels NB Jr, Miller DC. (1999). Deformational dynamics of the aortic root: modes and physiologic determinants. *Circulation*, Vol. 100, No. 19 Suppl, pp. (II54–II62).

David T, Feindel CM, Webb GD, Colman JM, Armstrong S, Maganti M. (2006). Long term results of aortic valve sparing operations for aortic root aneurysm. *J Thorac Cardiovasc Surg*, Vol. 132, No. 2, pp. (347–354).

David TE, Feindel CM, Webb GD, Colman JM, Armstrong S, Maganti M. (2007). Aortic valve preservation in patients with aortic root aneurysm: results of the reimplantation technique. *Ann Thorac Surg*, Vol. 83, No. 2, pp. (S732–S735), discussion S785–S790.

David TE, Feindel CM. (1992). An Aortic Valve-sparing operation for patients with aortic incompetence and aneurysm of the ascending aorta. *J Thorac Cardiovasc Surg*, Vol. 103, No. 4, pp. (617–622).

David TE. (1999). Aortic valve repair for management of aortic insufficiency. *Adv Card Surg*, Vol. 11, pp. (129-159).

David TE. (2005). Sizing and tailoring the Dacron graft for reimplantation of the aortic valve. *J Thorac Cardiovasc Surg*, Vol. 130, No. 2, pp. (243–244).

De Oliveira NC, David TE, Ivanov J, Armstrong S, Eriksson MJ, Rakowski H, Webb G. (2003). Results of surgery for aortic root aneurysm in patients with Marfan syndrome. *J Thorac Cardiovasc Surg*, Vol. 125, No. 4, pp. (789-796).

De Paulis R, De Matteis GM, Nardi P, Scaffa R, Bassano C, Chiariello L. (2002). Analysis of valve motion after the reimplantation type of valve-sparing procedure (David I) with a new aortic root conduit. *Ann Thorac Surg*, Vol. 74, No. 1, pp. (53-57).

De Waroux JB, Pouleur AC, Goffinet C, Vancraeynest D, Van Dyck M, Robert A, Gerber BL, Pasquet A, El Khoury G, Vanoverschelde JL. (2007). Functional anatomy of aortic regurgitation: accuracy, prediction of surgical repairability, and outcome implications of transesophageal echocardiography. *Circulation*, Vol. 116, No. 11 Suppl, pp. (I264-I269).

Erasmi A, Sievers HH, Scharfschwerdt M, Eckel T, Misfeld M. (2005). In vitro hydrodynamics, cusp-bending deformation, and root distensibility for different types of aortic valve-sparing operations: remodeling, sinus prosthesis, and reimplantation. *J Thorac Cardiovasc Surg*, Vol. 130, No. 4, pp. (1044-1049).

Furukawa K, Ohteki H, Cao Z, Doi K, Narita Y, Minato N, Itoh T. (1999). Does dilatation of the sinotubular junction cause aortic regurgitation? *Ann Thorac Surg*, Vol. 68, No. 3, pp. (949-954).

Gallo R, Kumar N, Al Halees Z, Duran C. (1995). Early failure of aortic valve conservation in aortic root aneurysm. *J Thorac Cardiovasc Surg*, Vol. 109, No. 5, pp. (1011-1012).

Gleason TG. (2005). New graft formulation and modification of the David reimplantation technique. *J Thorac Cardiovasc Surg*, Vol. 130, No. 2, pp. (601–603).

Gorman JH 3rd, Gupta KB, Streicher JT, Gorman RC, Jackson BM, Ratcliffe MB, Bogen DK, Edmunds LH Jr. (1996). Dynamic three-dimensional imaging of the mitral valve and the left ventricle by rapid sonomicrometry array localization. *J Thorac Cardiovasc Surg*, Vol. 112, No. 3, pp. (712-726).

Grande-Allen KJ, Cohran RP, Reinhall PG, Kunzelman KS. (2000). Re-creation of sinuses is important for sparing the aortic valve: a finite element model. *J Thorac Cardiovasc Surg*, Vol. 119, No. 4 Pt 1, pp. (753-763).

Hanke T, Charitos EI, Stierle U, Robinson D, Gorski A, Sievers HH, Misfeld M. (2009). Factors associated with the development of aortic valve regurgitation over time after two different techniques of valve-sparing aortic root surgery. *J Thorac Cardiovasc Surg.*, Vol. 137, No. 2, pp. (314-319).

Hansen B, Menkis AH, Vesely I. (1995). Longitudinal and radial distensibility of the porcine aortic root. *Ann Thorac Surg*, Vol. 60, No. 2 Suppl, pp. (S384-S390).

Hess PJ Jr, Klodell CT, Beaver TM, Martin TD. (2005). The Florida sleeve: a new technique for aortic root remodeling with preservation of the aortic valve and sinuses. *Ann Thorac Surg*, Vol. 80, No. 2, pp. (748–750).

Hetzer R, Komoda S, Komoda T. (2008). Remodeling of aortic root by annular reconstruction and plication of sinuses of valsaleft ventricular a. *J Card Surg*, Vol. 23, No. 1, pp. (49–51).

Higashidate M, Tamiya K, Toshiyuki B, Yasaharu I. (1995). Regulation of the aortic valve opening: in vivo dynamic of aortic valve orifice area. *J Thorac Cardiovasc Surg*, Vol. 110, No. 2, pp. (496-503).

Hiratzka LF, Bakris GL, Beckman JA, Bersin RM, Carr VF, Casey DE Jr, et al. (2010). ACCF/AHA/AATS/ACR/ASA/SCA/SCAI/SIR/STS/SVM guidelines for the diagnosis and management of patients with Thoracic Aortic Disease: a report of the American College of Cardiology Foundation/American Heart Association Task Force on Practice Guidelines, American Association for Thoracic Surgery, American College of Radiology, American Stroke Association, Society of Cardiovascular Anesthesiologists, Society for Cardiovascular Angiography and Interventions, Society of Interventional Radiology, Society of Thoracic Surgeons, and Society for Vascular Medicine. *Circulation*, Vol. 121, No. 13, pp. (e266-369).

Hopkins RA. (2003). Aortic valve leaflet sparing and saleft ventricular age surgery: evolution of techniques for aortic root reconstruction. *Eur J Cardiothorac Surg*, Vol. 24, No. 6, pp. (886–897).

Houel R, Soustelle C, Kirsch M, Hillion ML, Renaut C, Loisance DY. (2002). Long-term results of the bentall operation versus separate replacement of the ascending aorta and aortic valve. *J Heart Valve Dis.*, Vol. 11, No. 4, pp. (485-491).

Iung B, Baron G, Butchart EG, Delahaye F, Gohlke-Barwolf C, Levang OW, Tornos P, Vanoverschelde JL, Vermeer F, Boersma E, Ravaud P, Vahanian A. (2003). A prospective survey of patients with valvular heart disease in Europe: The Euro Heart Survey on Valvular Heart Disease. *Eur Heart J*, Vol. 24, No. 13, pp. (1231–1243).

Karck M, Kallenbach K, Hagl C, Rhein C, Leyh R, Haverich A. (2004). Aortic root surgery in Marfan syndrome: Comparison of aortic valve-sparing reimplantation versus composite grafting. *J Thorac Cardiovasc Surg*, Vol. 127, No. 2, pp. (391-398).

Kollar A. (2007). Valve-sparing reconstruction within the native aortic root: integrating the Yacoub and the David methods. *Ann Thorac Surg*, Vol. 83, No. 6, pp. (2241–2243).

Kunzelman KS, Grande KJ, David TE, Cochran RP, Verrier ED. (1994). Aortic root and valve relationships: impact on surgical repair. *J Thorac Cardiovasc Surg*, Vol. 107, No. 1, pp. (162–170).

La Canna G, Maisano F, De Michele L, Grimaldi A, Grassi F, Capritti E, De Bonis M, Alfieri O. (2009). Determinants of the Degree of Functional Aortic Regurgitation in Patients With Anatomically Normal Aortic Valve and Ascending Thoracic Aorta Aneurysm Transesophageal Doppler Echocardiography Study. *Heart*, Vol. 95, No. 2, pp. (130-136).

Lansac E, Di Centa I, Arnaud Crozat E, Bouchot O, Doguet F, Daroca T, Nijs J. An external open ring for isolated aortic valve repair. (2011a). *MMCTS* (February 14, 2011). doi:10.1510/mmcts.2009.004119 (http://mmcts.ctsnetjournals.org/cgi/content/abstract/2011/0214/mmcts.2009.004119).

Lansac E, Di Centa I, Arnaud Crozat E, Bouchot O, Doguet F, Hacini R, Demaria R, Chatel D, Sleilaty G, Debauchez M. (2011b). Remodeling of the aortic root combined to an expansible aortic ring annuloplasty. *MMCTS* (April 1, 2011). doi: 10.1510/mmcts.2006.001958 http://mmcts.ctsnetjournals.org/cgi/content/full/2011/0401/mmcts.2006.001958.

Lansac E, Di Centa I, Bonnet N, Leprince P, Jault F, Rama A, Acar C, Pavie P, Gandjbakhch I. (2006). Aortic prosthetic ring annuloplasty: a useful adjunct to a standardized aortic valve-sparing procedure? *Eur J Cardiothorac Surg*, Vol. 29, No. 4, pp. (537-544).

Lansac E, Di Centa I, Raoux F, Al Attar N, Acar C, Joudinaud T, Raffoul R. (2008). A lesional classification to standardize surgical management of aortic insufficiency towards valve repair. *Eur J Cardio Thorac Surg*, Vol. 33, No. 5, pp. (872–880).

Lansac E, Di Centa I, Raoux F, Bulman-Fleming N, Ranga A, Abed A, Ba M, Paolitto A, Letourneur D, Meddahi-Pelle A. (2009). An expansible aortic ring for a physiological approach to conservative aortic valve surgery. *J Thorac Cardiovasc Surg*, Vol. 138, No. 3, pp. (718-724).

Lansac E, Di Centa I, Sleilaty G, Arnaud Crozat E, Bouchot O; Hacini R; Blin D, Doguet F; Bessou JP, Albat B, De Maria R, Villemot JP, Portocarrero E, Acar C, Chatel D, Lopez S, Folliguet T, Debauchez M. (2010a). An aortic ring: from a physiological reconstruction of the root to a standardized approach of aortic valve repair. *J Thorac Cardiovasc Surg*, Vol. 140, No. 6 Suppl, pp. (S28-S35).

Lansac E, Di Centa I, Sleilaty G, Bouchot O, Arnaud Crozat E, Blin D, Acar C, Debauchez M. (2010b). An aortic ring to standardize aortic valve repair: a preliminary results of a prospective multicentric cohort of 144 patients. *Eur J CardioThorac Surg*, Vol. 38, No. 2, pp. (147-154).

Lansac E, Di Centa I, Varnous S, Rama A, Jault F, Duran CMG, Acar C, Pavie A, Gandjbakhch I. (2005a). External aortic annuloplasty ring for valve-sparing procedures. Ann Thorac Surg, Vol. 79, No. 1, pp. (356-358).

Lansac E, Lim HS, Shomura Y, Lim KH, Rice Nt, Goetz W, Duran C. (2002). A four-dimensional study of the aortic root dynamics. *Eur J Cardiothorac Surg*, Vol. 22, No. 4, pp. (497–503).

Lansac E, Lim HS, Shomura Y, Lim KH, Rice NT, Goetz WA, Duran CM. (2005b). Aortic root dynamics are asymmetric. *J Heart Valve Dis*, Vol. 14, No. 3, pp. (400–407).

Lansac, E. Di Centa, I. (2010c). From dynamic anatomy to conservative aortic valve surgery: the tale of the ring, In: *Aortic root surgery*, Yankah, CA. Weng, Y., Hetzer, R., pp. (102-132), Springer, ISBN 978-3-7985-1868-1, Germany.

Leyh RG, Fischer S, Kallenbach K, Kofidis T, Pethig K, Harringer W, Haverich A. (2002). High failure rate after valve-sparing aortic root replacement using the "remodelling technique" in acute type A aortic dissection. *Circulation*, Vol. 106, No. 12 Suppl 1, pp. (I229-I233).

Leyh RG, Schmidtke C, Sievers HH, Yacoub MH. (1999). Opening and closing characteristics of the aortic valve after different types of valve-preserving surgery. *Circulation*, Vol. 100, No. 21, pp. (2153-2160).

Luciani GB, Casali G, Tomezzoli A, Mazzucco A. (1999). Recurrence of aortic insufficiency after aortic root remodeling with valve preservation. *Ann Thorac Surg*, Vol 67, No. 6, pp. (1849-1852).

Maselli D, Montalto A, Santise G, Minardi G, Manzara C, Musumeci F. (2005). A normogram to anticipate dimension of neo-sinuses of valsalva in valve-sparing aortic operations. *Eur J Cardiothorac Surg*, Vol. 27, No. 5, pp. (831-835).

Miller DC. (2007). Valve-sparing aortic root replacement: current state of the art and where are we headed? *Ann Thorac Surg*, Vol. 83, No. 2, pp. (S736–S739).

Morishita K, Murakami G, Koshino T, Fukada J, Fujisawa Y, Mawatari T, Abe T. (2002). Aortic root remodeling operation: how do we tailor a tube graft? *Ann Thorac Surg*, Vol. 73, No. 4, pp. (1117–1721).

Muriago M, Sheppard MN, Ho SY, Anderson RH. (1997). Location of the coronary arterial orifices in the normal heart. *Clin Anat*, Vol. 10, No. 5, pp. (297–302).

Nataf P, Lansac E. (2006). Dilation of the Thoracic aorta: medical or surgical management. *Heart*, Vol. 92, No. 9, pp. (1345-1352).

Pang DC, Choo SJ, Luo HH, Shomura Y, Daniel S, Nikolic SJ, Cheung DT, Oury JH, Duran CMG. (2000). Significant increase of aortic root volume and commissural area occurs prior to aortic valve opening. *J Heart Valve Dis*, Vol. 9, No. 1, pp. (9-15).

Patel ND, Weiss ES, Alejo DE, Nwakanma LU, Williams JA, Dietz HC, Spevak PJ, Gott VL, Vricella LA, Cameron DE. (2008). Aortic root operations for Marfan syndrome: a comparison of the Bentall and valve-sparing procedures. *Ann Thorac Surg*, Vol. 85, No 6, pp. (2003-2010).

Reid K. (1970). The anatomy of the sinus of Valsalva. *Thorax*, Vol. 25, No. 1, pp. (79–85).

Roberts WC, Ko JM, Moore TR, Jones WH 3rd. (2006). Causes of pure aortic regurgitation in patients having isolated aortic valve replacement at a single US tertiary hospital (1993 to 2005). *Circulation*, Vol. 114, No. 5, pp. (422–429).

Roberts WC. (1970). The structure of the aortic valve in clinically isolated aortic stenosis: an autopsy study of 162 patients over 15 years of age. *Circulation*, Vol. 42, No. 1, pp. (91–97).

Robicksek F. (1991). Leonardo da Vinci and the sinuses of Valsalva. *Ann Thorac Surg*, Vol. 52, No 2, pp. (328-335).

Roman MJ, Devereux RB, Niles NW, Hochreiter C, Kligfield P, Sato N, Spitzer MC, Borer JS. (1987). Aortic root dilatation as a cause of isolated, severe aortic regurgitation. Prevalence, clinical and echocardiographic patterns, and relation to left ventricular hypertrophy and function. *Ann Intern Med*, Vol. 106, No. 6, pp. (800–807).

Ruvolo G, Fattouch K. (2009). Aortic valve-sparing root replacement from inside the aorta using three Dacron skirts preserving the native Valsalvasinuses geometry and stabilizing the annulus. *Interact Cardiovasc Thorac Surg*, Vol. 8, No. 2, pp. (179–181).

Schäfers HJ, Bierbach B, Aicher D. (2006). A new approach to the assessment of aortic cusp geometry. *J Thorac Cardiovasc Surg*, Vol. 132, No. 2, pp. (436-438).

Schäfers HJ, Kunihara T, Fries P, Brittner B, Aicher D. (2010). Valve-preserving root replacement in bicuspid aortic valves. *J Thorac Cardiovasc Surg*, Vol. 140, No. 6 Suppl, pp. (S36-S40).

Silver MA, Roberts WC. (1985). Detailed anatomy of the normally functioning aortic valve in hearts of normal and increased weight. *Am J Cardiol*, Vol. 55, No. 4, pp. (454–461).

Soncini M, Votta E, Zinicchino S, Burrone V, Mangini A, Lemma M, Antona C, Redaelli A. (2009). Aortic root performance after valve sparing procedure: a comparative finite element analysis. *Med Eng Phys*, Vol. 31, No. 2, pp. (234-243).

Sutton JP III, Ho SY, Anderson RH. (1995). The forgotten interleaflet triangles: a review of the surgical anatomy of the aortic valve. *Ann Thorac Surg*, Vol. 59, No. 2, pp. (419–427).

Svensson LG. (2003). Sizing for modified David's reimplantation procedure. *Ann Thorac Surg*, Vol. 76, No. 5, pp. (1751–1753).

Takamoto S, Nawata K, Morota T. (2006). A simple modification of "David-V" aortic root reimplantation. *Eur J Cardiothorac Surg*, Vol. 30, No. 3, pp. (560–562).

Tamás E, Nylander E. (2007). Echocardiographic description of the anatomic relations within the normal aortic root. *J Heart Valve Dis*, Vol. 16, No. 3, pp. (240-246).

Thubrikar M, Bosher LP, Nolan SP. (1979). The mechanism of opening of the aortic valve. *J Thorac Cardiovasc Surg*, Vol. 77, No. 6, pp. (863-870).

Thubrikar M, Harry L, Nolan SP. (1977). Normal aortic valve function in dogs. *Am J Cardiol*, Vol. 40, No. 4, pp. (563–568).

Thubrikar M, Heckman JL, Nolan SP. (1993). High speed cine-radiographic study of the aortic valve leaflet motion. *J Heart Valve Dis*, Vol. 2, No. 6, pp. (653-661).

Tops LF, Wood DA, Delgado V, Schuijf JD, Mayo JR, Pasupati S, Lamers FPL, van der Wall EE, Schalij MJ, Webb JG, Bax JJ. (2008). Noninvasive evaluation of the aortic root with multi-slice computed tomography: implications for transcatheter aortic valve replacement. *J Am Coll Cardiol Img*, Vol. 1, No. 3, pp. (321–330).

Turner K, Navartnam V. (1996). The positions of coronary arterial ostia. *Clin Anat*, Vol. 9, No. 6, pp. (376 -380).

Urbanski PP, Zhan X, Frank S, Diegeler A. (2009) Aortic root reconstruction using new vascular graft. *Interact Cardiovasc Thorac Surg*, Vol. 8, No. 2, pp.(187–190).

Vahanian A, Baumgartner H, Bax J, Butchart E, Dion R, Filippatos G, Flachskampf F, Hall R, Iung B, Kasprzak J, Nataf P, et al. (2007). Guidelines on the management of valvular heart disease: The Task Force on the Management of Valvular Heart Disease of the European Society of Cardiology. *Eur Heart J*, Vol. 28, No. 2, pp. (230-268).

Volguina IV, Miller DC, LeMaire SA, Palmero LC, Wang XL, Connolly HM, Sundt TM 3rd, Bavaria JE, Dietz HC, Milewicz DM, et al. (2009) Valve-sparing and valve-replacing techniques for aortic root replacement in patients with Marfan syndrome: Analysis of early outcome. *J Thorac Cardiovasc Surg*, Vol. 137, No. 5, pp. (1124-1132).

Vollebergh FE, Becker AE. (1977). Minor congenital variations of cusp size in tricuspid aortic valves: possible link with isolated aortic stenosis. *Br Heart J*, Vol. 39, No. 9, pp. (1006–1011).

Yacoub M, Fagan A, Stassano P, Radley-Smith R. (1983). Result of valve conserving operations for aortic regurgitation [abstract]. *Circulation*, Vol. 68(suppl):III321.

Yacoub MH, Gehle P, Chandrasekaran V, Birks EJ, Child A, Radley-Smith R. (1998). Late results of a valve sparing operation in patients with aneuryms of the ascending aorta and root. *J Thorac Cardiovasc Surg*, Vol. 115, No. 5, pp. (1080–1090).

Zehr KJ, Orszulak TA, Mullany CJ, Matloobi A, Daly RC, Dearani JA, Sundt TM 3rd, Puga FJ, Danielson GK, Schaff HV. (2004). Surgery for aneurysms of the aortic root: a 30-year experience. *Circulation,* Vol. 110, No 11, pp. (1364-1371).

Zehr KJ, Thubrikar MJ, Gong GG, Headrick JR, Robicsek F. (2000). Clinical introduction of a novel prosthesis for valve-preserving aortic root reconstruction for annuloaortic ectasia. *J Thorac Cardiovasc Surg,* Vol. 120, No. 6, pp. (692–698).